To Rosemarie,
With love and
find inspiration and strength in
your life, as did the unmackable
Sister of Mercy who founded
The Mater Misericordia hospitals
in
Brisbane.

Grace.

EXPRESSIONS OF MERCY
Brisbane's Mater Hospitals 1906–2006

ABOUT THE AUTHOR

Helen Gregory is a professional historian and practises as a consultant in Queensland history and cultural heritage conservation. She has written many commissioned histories including a history of the Queensland Law Society, a history of Maroochy Shire, and a bestselling history of the Brisbane River. Helen has also lectured and tutored in Queensland and Australian history, and has written many articles for various historical journals.

EXPRESSIONS OF MERCY
Brisbane's Mater Hospitals 1906–2006

Helen Gregory

UQP

First published 2006 by University of Queensland Press
PO Box 6042, St Lucia, Queensland 4067 Australia

www.uqp.uq.edu.au

Typeset in 11/15pt Berkeley by Post Pre-press Group, Brisbane
Printed in Australia by McPherson's Printing Group

Distributed in the USA and Canada by
International Specialized Books Services, Inc.,
5824 N.E. Hassalo Street, Portland, Oregon 97213-3640

Cataloguing-in-Publication Data
National Library of Australia

Gregory, Helen.
Expressions of mercy: Brisbane's Mater Hospitals 1906–2006

Includes index.
ISBN 0 7022 3539 3.
ISBN 0 7022 3552 0 (pbk.).

1. Mater Health Services (Qld.) – History. 2. Sisters of
Mercy (Qld.) – History. 3. Hospitals – Queensland –
Brisbane – History. 4. Medical care – Queensland – History.
I. Mater Health Services (Qld.). II. Sisters of Mercy
(Qld.). III. Title.

362.11099431

CONTENTS

INTRODUCING
THE FAMILY

'He was rushed off to the Mater after his heart attack!'
'Our baby was born at the Mater.'
'Asthma in a three year old is terrifying; she's in the Mater now.'
'Mum's having her hip replacement in the Mater Private.'
'I'll go to the Mater Redlands, it's closer.'

Such statements regularly trip off the tongues of Brisbane people. 'The Mater', as it is always known, has become so familiar that the nickname is much preferred in ordinary conversation to the original name, Mater Misericordiae, Mother of Mercy, or the twenty-first century name, Mater Health Services. Perhaps it is more than the habit of abbreviation; perhaps 'running to mother' is actually an entirely appropriate way to think of instinctive behaviour when people are hurt, or worried, or ill, or full of joys, hopes, and plans for the future.

'The Mater' is a simple term to cover an enterprise of great complexity. The Mater is not one hospital, but seven. Six members of the hospital family still live in the family home on Mater Hill at Woolloongabba in South Brisbane. The newest member of the Mater family has left home for Redland Bay, at the southern end of picturesque Moreton Bay.

This history is the life story of the Mater Misericordiae hospitals, from their gestation in the minds of a remarkable group of women, the Irish Sisters of Mercy, to their eminence in health care in Queensland.

In every era, the people who made the Mater – the Sisters, the doctors, the nurses, the researchers, the technologists, the administrators, the volunteers, the fundraisers – had a single aim: the best possible health care for Mater patients. This, then, is also a story of a building and growing, mending and maintaining, planning and managing, challenges and changes, faltering and succeeding.

The Mater lives in several realms – the world of the Roman Catholic church and the Sisters of Mercy, the medical world, and Queensland's social and political world, where it has often been the bane of governments. Social, economic and political forces, changes in the church and innovations in the wider world of health care are all reflected in the Mater story. The Mater has changed and grown in response to these influences, but its central mission – to care for the poor, the sick and the needy, irrespective of religious belief – has remained constant. The Mater has always been very much part of the society which envelops it and the city which surrounds it. In this, it reflects the foundation of the Sisters of Mercy, who began their work as 'walking nuns', very much engaged in society's preoccupation and needs.

The Mater story begins in the nineteenth century in two very different cities: Dublin, a large, ancient city in the northern hemisphere, and Brisbane, a tiny, new city in the southern hemisphere. Some distinctively unappealing features link the nineteenth-century experiences of these two cities – poverty, dirt, disease, and governments unwilling, or unable, to provide adequate health care or education for the disadvantaged. Catherine McAuley established her Sisters of Mercy in Dublin in 1831, when Brisbane was still the headquarters of a remote penal settlement. Thirty years later, the first Sisters arrived in Brisbane. The Sisters' experiences in the forty years before they established the Mater set the tone for the future. They developed their work, despite their small numbers, to encompass several dimensions of society's needs in a climate of government indifference, disputes with the diocese, and financial stringency.

Growth was the keynote from the time the first Mater Private Hospital was established in rented premises in 1906. The first expansion occurred in both the physical and philosophical dimensions. A move to a large new site on a hill on the southern side of the Brisbane River was accompanied by the development of a second hospital which achieved the Sisters' dream of providing health care to all who needed it, irrespective of material circumstances, creed or condition. This, too, was pioneering. A public and a private hospital sharing a single site was a new departure in the development of Queensland's hospitals in the early twentieth century.

This major change in the Mater's circumstances, and further expansion in the decades that followed, was supported by many in the community and the city's leading doctors, but it was not accomplished without difficulty. Fundraising, economising, dealing with pressures on available ward space, training nurses and doctors, accommodating technical advances in medical care, wrestling with governments, planning additional hospitals, and dealing appropriately with staff, the church and advisors, accompanied the Mater through the twentieth century.

It was always a struggle to feed and clothe the growing Mater family and to provide a growing range of extracurricular, but necessary, activities – research, health promotion, education support and community outreach programs. Stellar individuals have come to the fore and exercised leadership in meeting the demands of various times and circumstances, often in a climate of vigorous debate.

Social pressures didn't make the task any easier. The difficulties of economic depression, staff absences during the world wars, changes in the church and declining vocations for the Sisters of Mercy in the turbulent 1960s and 1970s, not to mention medical discoveries producing ethical challenges as well as exciting opportunities in the Mater's first century, have all been powerful influences on the Mater's personality and stance in the world.

The complex and fascinating modern Mater Health Services is a dynamic system, still growing and developing, and still dedicated to the original aim of the Sisters of Mercy – to provide the best possible health care to all who need it.

PART ONE

GETTING ESTABLISHED

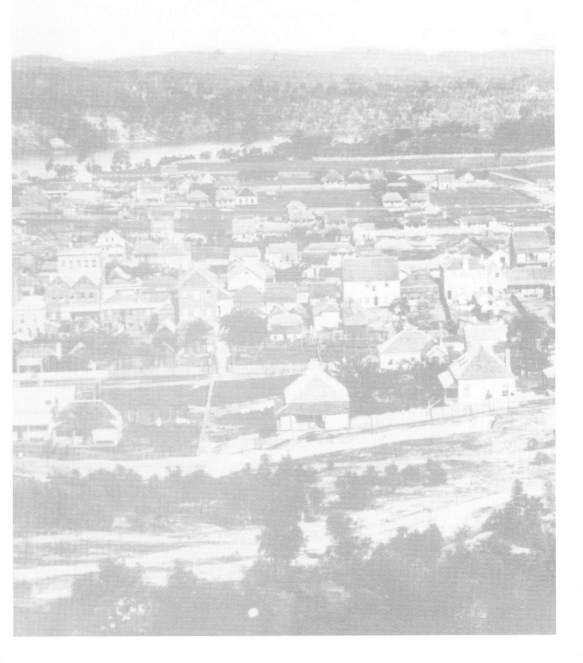

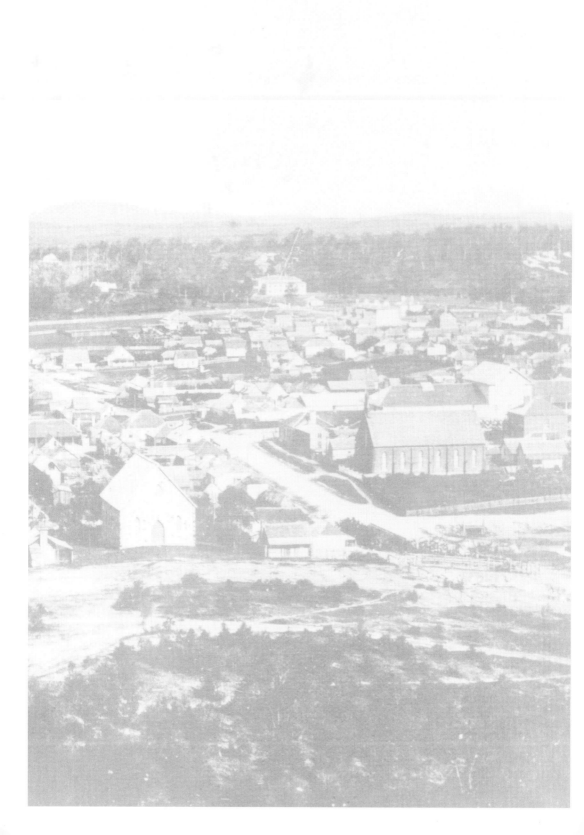

CHAPTER ONE

BEGINNING A 'BIG WORK'

This, I hope is the beginning of a big work that will do much good . . .

Mother Patrick Potter, 27 February 1906

Brisbane was a tiny, shabby, struggling town in 1861 when the Sisters of Mercy arrived.

A mere handful of some 7,000 people formed a tiny outpost of Britishness in the southern seas, positioned about halfway between the extreme south-east of the Australian continent and its far north-east. It was only twenty years since the first free settlers had been allowed within the borders of the original Moreton Bay convict settlement. The new settlers of the 1840s and 1850s were generally an enterprising lot – entrepreneurial storekeepers and publicans, pastoralists passing through on their way to take up rich lands on the Darling Downs to the west and in the fertile river valleys to the north and south, and workers in search of opportunity in a labour-starved domain.

In the 1840s, Brisbane had few of the finer touches of civilised life, and very little religion. It was a fertile field for missionaries. Bishop John Bede Polding, first Catholic Bishop of Sydney, celebrated the first Mass ever held in Brisbane, on 14 May 1843, in an old barn, a disused government store in the centre of town. Polding's mission to

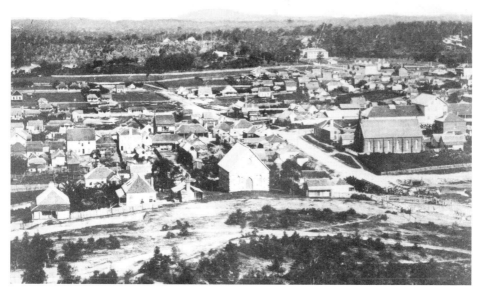

A view of Brisbane from Wickham Terrace looking towards South Brisbane in 1862, not long after the first Sisters of Mercy arrived. JOHN OXLEY LIBRARY

the Aboriginal people on nearby Stradbroke Island was unsuccessful, and he was upbraided by his flock for bringing missionaries for the unconverted rather than priests for the faithful. Polding appointed Father John Hanly to Brisbane. As well as ministering to a few dozen loyal Catholics who subscribed to his salary, Hanly established the first school in Brisbane's free settlement era, St Stephen's School, which became the Sisters of Mercy's first charge on their arrival some fifteen years later.[1]

The population grew slowly in the 1840s and 1850s, much to the chagrin of the promoters of the Moreton Bay district. Immigrant ships went first to Sydney, where new settlers were immediately enticed to stay; very few moved north. There were many dark mutterings that the government was unfairly favouring the Sydney region over Moreton Bay, not only in the matter of immigration but also in provision of basic public services. Very little government money was spent in Brisbane on water supply, drainage, roads, schools and hospitals.[2]

The struggle to find sufficient labour to develop the Moreton Bay district eased a little when the *Artemisia* arrived in Brisbane, carrying some 240 artisans, labourers and domestic servants, including one Catholic family. There were also those who had very definite ideas about the appropriate composition of the colonial population. Dr John Dunmore Lang, who visited Brisbane in 1846, was a feisty Presbyterian clergyman with definite ideas about ensuring that the proportions of Irish Catholics, roistering materialists and pretentious squatters in the former convict colonies were leavened by sober, thrifty, hard-working Protestants. He was immediately impressed by the colony's potential for a prosperous future based on awesome timber reserves and tropical crops, which he envisioned in the rich river soils of the areas around Brisbane.[3] Much to the surprise of the town of Brisbane and the New South Wales government, three shiploads of immigrants organised by Dr Lang arrived in 1849. They were an interesting group of mainly urban people, fundamentalist in religion and radical in their political leanings.

The combination of Langite urban radicals, opportunist traders, publicans and English squattocracy was a heady, disputatious mix. The urgent need for a separate government for the northern districts was one major issue on which they did agree. Brisbane, still very much a frontier town, gradually acquired some of the infrastructure of a modern administrative centre. The north side of the river remained the headquarters of the New South Wales administration but, paradoxically, most of the commercial life of the city was generated from the wharves on the south side of the river. There was no bridge, merely an inefficient ferry. On the north side, there was a customs house, managed by William Duncan, a leading Catholic layman, and a few substantial houses such as Duncan's Dara in Ann Street, Dr William Hobbs' Adelaide House, and Dr George Fullerton's Adderton on a bluff overlooking the Brisbane River, directly opposite Dara. A new Catholic church, St Stephen's, was built on the northside in 1854. It was a small but very handsome Gothic stone building, following the style brought to the colonies by Pugin, the renowned English architect.

The British government finally acceded to increasingly strident petitions for self-government and Queen Victoria signed the Letters Patent creating Queensland on 6 June 1859. Despite recent improvements, Brisbane was by no means ready to assume the responsibilities of a capital city with all the accoutrements of representative government. There was no Government House for Sir George Bowen, the first Governor; he made do in Adelaide House for some years. There was no Parliament House; the first legislators, led by Robert Herbert, the first premier, met in the old convict barracks. The Brisbane City Council, also created in 1859, had no Town Hall.

Most of the people lived in cramped, inadequate houses lining badly drained streets. They had no reliable water supply and were forced to share a muddy waterhole with livestock. As the local newspaper the *Daily Guardian* pointed out acerbically: 'Brisbane is no doubt a most pretentious city. It pretends to be famous without gas, without water, without sewerage, without any of the requisites in fact of a tenth rate English town.'[4]

Nevertheless, the first Queensland Parliament, dominated by pastoralists and landowners, dreamt big dreams. They had a definite social vision. This was to be a democratic, secular society in which no Christian denomination was to enjoy the privileges and government aid accorded the Church of England in Britain. This was bad news for the Anglican Church in Queensland, which had appointed its first Bishop in 1860. It wasn't promising for the Catholic Church either. The decision presaged an end to the New South Wales system, which had provided land, and some financial subsidy, to religious bodies to establish churches and schools.

Legislators during the 1860s shared one dominant priority – a determination to develop the huge land area under their charge, an area as large as France, Italy and Spain combined. They wasted little time on education of any kind, or on such matters as the proper organisation of health and medical services. Early governments focused their effort on legislation organising the profitable disposal of Crown lands, and on an ambitious immigration scheme. New settlers who could afford to pay their own passage were rewarded with grants of land; less affluent settlers were granted free passage, but no land. Within a very short time, thousands of immigrants leapt at the chance to come to Queensland.

Health care was quickly dismissed, with legislation in 1861 proclaiming that the chronically ill would be cared for in acute care hospitals and, in 1862, confirmation that voluntary committees would govern the hospitals of the colony.[5] Brisbane's one and only hospital, the original convict settlement hospital, was revived by the establishment of a 'committee of gentlemen' after the government peremptorily closed it in 1848. It struggled on as a voluntary hospital, supported by subscribers, people of some financial means who believed in providing charity to the sick poor. Subscribers much preferred to pay for the attention of their own doctors in their own homes. Nevertheless, the hospital committee continued to call for subscriptions with the reminder that 'in every community at all distinguished for Christian charity and general philanthropy such institutions for the relief of human suffering exercise a claim upon individuals which may almost be called sacred'.[6] It was sacred to Protestants and Catholics alike.

On 10 May 1861, six women who had dedicated their lives to works of charity and mercy arrived in this unpromising, unruly, materialistic environment, only a few of the hundreds of immigrants who arrived in Brisbane that year. Like the first Sisters to come to Australia, Sister Ursula Frayne who arrived in Western Australia in 1845, and Mother Mary Xavier Maguire who started work in Melbourne in 1859,[7] these six Sisters of Mercy had not chosen to leave their homeland in search of a better life or to enhance a family fortune. Instead, they had responded to a challenge to bring education and religion to a rough colonial population. The leader of this little group, Mother Mary Vincent Whitty, was already a woman of considerable achievement, quite accustomed to dealing with daunting situations. Born in 1819 in Country Wexford, Ireland, she was a trained teacher when she joined the Sisters of Mercy in 1839, only eight years after their official foundation by Catherine McAuley.

Catherine McAuley was an unusual woman. Her father, an architect and dealer in real estate, was a rare Catholic of means in eighteenth-century Dublin. He practised charity in his everyday life, bringing the poor to his home for sustenance. Catherine was very young when her parents died, and she went to live with her distant relatives, William Callaghan and his Quaker wife. In her formative years, she was also influenced by the wealthy Protestant apothecary William Armstrong, whom she regarded as a person of high moral principle. Catherine was drawn to the notion of a lay Catholic social service, a society of ladies to 'devote themselves to the poor without making vows', an idea which she later said derived from her Protestant relatives.[8]

In this aspiration, Catherine reflected a movement stirring among comfortably affluent, serious-minded women in Britain and Europe. During the late eighteenth century, the industrial revolution had created a new 'middle class', successful people who had prospered as factory and mine owners, merchants, traders and expansionist farmers who benefited from greater access to land. They were not part of the old landed aristocracy, nor were they part of the burgeoning new class of industrial workers. The wives and daughters of the entrepreneurial middle class, moved either by Christian duty to the poor or simply by human compassion for the disadvantaged, embarked on ambitious social work. Dispossessed rural workers flocked to cities and towns searching for opportunities in factories and businesses, but many fell between the cracks into a world of poverty, dirt and disadvantage. Throughout the nineteenth century, in the old world and the new, committees of women, often led by charismatic leaders, reformed prisons, cared for 'fallen' women and single girls, established hospitals, and promoted education.

Even apart from such urban pressures, the first decade of the nineteenth century was a dangerous time in Dublin. A brief period of Irish political independence ended in 1800 when an Act of Union merged the Irish Parliament with the British Parliament. Wolf Tone's movement to create a united Ireland formed of Catholics, Protestants and Dissenters, free of English rule, had failed. Catholic emancipation seemed a long way off when the Church rejected the offer of emancipation on condition that the British government could veto the appointment of Bishops. Yet another Irish nationalist insurrection failed in 1803. Poor economic times added to the atmosphere of political and religious dispute. The Callaghans, taking Catherine McAuley with them, joined a middle-class move to sanctuary away from the city.[9] Catherine lived with the Callaghans at Coolock, their estate outside Dublin, and cared for them until their deaths. Both converted to Catholicism, but Catherine was also influenced by Mrs Callaghan's Society of Friends' philosophy with its emphasis on human relationships. Combining ministry to the better off with work for the poor was a powerful, enduring amalgam, once described as the 'Mercy secret'.[10]

William Callaghan left his fortune to Catherine to use for her good works. With the help of a priest who had befriended her, Catherine selected a property at the corner of Baggot and Herbert Streets in Dublin to be her organisational centre. This was not a poverty-stricken part of Dublin – it was considered to be no bad thing for the wealthy to see the poor in their midst. The foundation stone of Catherine's new building was laid in July 1824. Education, always a keynote of Mercy work, was one of Catherine's first preoccupations. She studied teaching methods in Dublin schools and in France in preparation for opening a school for the poor at Baggot Street. A loyal supporter, Anna Maria Doyle, arrived at Baggot Street on 24 September, the Feast of Our Lady of Mercy, prompting the decision to name the building the House of Mercy. Archbishop Murray, who became Catherine's friend and advisor, consented to the title 'Institute of Our Lady of Mercy' for the new social service organisation. For some years, Murray had wanted to establish a religious order to work among the poor; they would be 'walking nuns', working in the world rather than cloistered in the contemplative life.

Adopting the multiple concerns of the world led to diversity, always a powerful theme in Mercy work. In the first year, a residence for working women and an employment agency were established. An orphanage, made even more necessary by an outbreak of fever among Dublin's poor, was added shortly afterwards. Attracting the interest and support of powerful people has also been a consistently important tool in advancing Mercy work. Daniel O'Connell, the lawyer whose non-violent campaign against political and religious injustice was generally supported by the Catholic Church, carved the meat at the Mercy House Christmas dinner in 1828, some nine years after his election to the English parliament. His two daughters had joined Catherine's growing group of helpers. By the end of 1828, the Mercy women had added visits to the sick in their homes and in two Dublin hospitals to their responsibilities. But it wasn't easy. Pressures close to home severely strained the quality of mercy. Some influential priests resented a charity backed by private money; others regarded lay charity as the trivia of the church; many felt that charity, business and finance should remain the province of men,[11] a cross also borne by many other able women throughout the nineteenth century and most of the twentieth.

Eventually, Catherine was persuaded that her Institute had taken on the appearance of an irregular convent. In 1830, still with many reservations about the conventual life, Catherine served her novitiate with the Presentation Sisters. She was professed in December 1831 and, with some simplifications, adopted the Presentation Sisters' Augustinian Rule for her Institute. From the very beginning the Sisters of Mercy adopted the 'walking nuns' concept pioneered by Mary Aikenhead's Sisters of Charity, rather than the concept of enclosure favoured by the Presentation Sisters. Practical religion among the people was to be the key. Four principles, distilled from Catherine's religious life, upbringing and experience of early nineteenth-century Irish life, underpinned the Sisters of Mercy – mercy to the afflicted, union and charity among the Sisters, obedience, and the discipline of common life. Catherine was also determined to maintain a 'charity-imbued simplicity in every Convent of Mercy, believing that a single-minded kindliness should characterise every member of the congregation'.[12]

The 1830s and 1840s were very difficult years in Ireland, even more overlaid with tragedy than the turbulent early decades of the century. Cholera struck Dublin in 1832, with appalling death rates in homes all over the city and in the hospitals. The Dublin Board of Health appealed to the Sisters for help. Theirs was an effective response to a prevailing fear among the poor that hospitals were places where death was certain. This was no irrational fear. In the English-speaking world, 'voluntary' hospitals supported by charitably minded people were generally ignored by governments. Private doctors gave what time they could spare to attend the sick poor on an honorary basis. The patients were cared for by untrained women, often no cleaner or more sober than the patients. The more affluent would not dream of entering such places, no matter how ill they were. Things were considerably better in Europe. Religious orders, particularly the Order of the Visitation of Mary and the Daughters of Charity of St Vincent de Paul, had been working since the seventeenth century to establish hospitals and to improve health care for the poor. The Irish Sisters of Charity followed the French model when they established St Vincent's Hospital in Dublin in 1834.[13]

The Sisters of Mercy's work improved conditions to the extent that the death rate in the Townsend Street hospital was slashed. Nevertheless, cholera left a nasty aftermath of parentless children and homes without breadwinners. There was much for the Sisters to do – but they needed the wherewithal to do it. Voluntary donations from supporters continued, but much more was needed. Archbishop Murray was initially most reluctant to sanction a bazaar as a money-raising venture. Catherine prevailed, however, and the first bazaar was a great success, doubtless helped by the donation of some of Princess Victoria's handiwork.

Expansion outside Dublin came next. The Sisters founded convents and schools throughout Ireland and in London, Birmingham and Liverpool in England. The Mercy Rule, with its constitutional adherence to Rome rather than government by the 'mother house' in Dublin, meant that all the convents and their attached schools formed a loose federation of independent institutions rather than a hierarchical structure of branches administered by a central convent.[14]

Much had been achieved when Catherine died in 1841, attended by the newly professed Sister Mary Vincent Whitty for whom she had developed a high regard. Sister Mary Vincent served a period as Novice Mistress before being elected Reverend Mother in 1849, when she was only 30. She shared Catherine's view that the education of women was the key to the improvement of the whole society. Neither believed that the National School system, established in 1831 with a rigid separation between

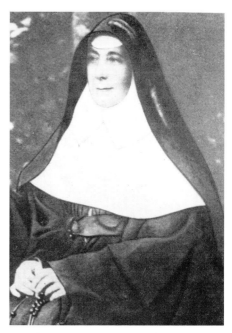

Mother Mary Vincent Whitty, first Superior of the Sisters of Mercy in Brisbane. SOMCA

secular and religious instruction in schools, was the way to improve society or to educate women adequately.

The pleas of visiting Bishops during the 1840s persuaded Mother Vincent to send Sisters overseas, even though human and financial resources were very stretched by continuing expansion at home. The aftermath of famine in Ireland in the 1840s escalated the need for the works of Mercy. Poverty, illness and death in the Irish countryside and congestion in the cities, where ever-increasing numbers of desperate people sought food and work, was one towering challenge; the strain on struggling church and educational infrastructure in new societies in North America and the southern hemisphere, to where Irish refugees had fled seeking respite from starvation and poverty, was another.

Mother Vincent stretched Mercy work to include a home for unmarried mothers and an industrial school, and yet managed to keep her eye firmly on the McAuley vision of providing health care to the poor. In 1851, she purchased land in Eccles Street, Dublin, for a hospital. The Sisters had already been invited to manage the nursing at the Jervis Street charitable infirmary in Dublin when another, much more surprising, opportunity came their way in 1854: a plea for help from the British government.

In the early stages of the Crimean War, the British government was thoroughly shamed by the shoddy standard of care its wounded and sick soldiers received at the hands of untrained male orderlies, the 'worn out pensioners' made infamous by the London *Times*.[15] Higher nursing standards in French military hospitals run by nuns were rewarded by much lower death rates. Mother Vincent believed that her Sisters could improve the British system and sent Sisters to care for some 10,000 Irish soldiers fighting in the British army. This was their chance to demonstrate that the Mercy mission to the sick extended to people of all religious faiths, no small consideration in the climate of anti-Popery still strong in Britain in the mid-century. Catherine McAuley had known what it was to fight for her faith, but she also knew how to love those who didn't share it. Mother Vincent was also aware, as she told the other Sisters, that this war work would 'be of service to the Catholic cause in Ireland hereafter'.[16] Sisters from several convents in Ireland and England served in the Crimea, but the religious and political climate of the day ensured that Florence Nightingale, the English advocate of trained nursing, who had studied the nursing methods of religious orders at Kaiserwerth in Germany, came home with most of the credit for cleaning up the military hospitals.

Although Mother Vincent was not part of the Crimean excursion, she was not devoid of adventurous missionary spirit. After her term as Superior at Baggot Street, she regularly sought permission to join a Mercy venture overseas. It was, she said, 'the real desire of my heart' which she had held for twenty years.[17] Unsurprisingly, her abilities and her close connection to Catherine McAuley were too highly regarded by her Sisters for them willingly to let her go, particularly with their vision of a new hospital well within sight. Archbishop Cullen of Dublin assisted the newly appointed Bishop of Brisbane, James Quinn, in overcoming the Sisters' opposition.[18] Quinn's association with the Sisters of Mercy when he accompanied them to the Crimea doubtless made him well aware of their ability to achieve much with little. As a previous headmaster of St Laurence's College in Dublin, his focus was on education, not health.

The call to the new mission in Brisbane came at a pivotal time in Mother Vincent's life. She left behind her the new Dublin Mater Hospital nearing completion, as much tangible evidence of her organisational and administrative skills as of her faith and the support of the Mercy community. She certainly had the right attitude for the conditions she faced during her thirty years in Brisbane, telling her Superior that: 'nuns might as well stay at home as go on Missions without holding themselves ready for any work required, according to the circumstances of the place they go to'.[19]

In Mother Vincent's case, the circumstances were more than a little alarming. After a long voyage to Sydney and thence to Brisbane, the Bishop, Mother Vincent, Sister Catherine Morgan from Liverpool, Novices Mary Benedict McDermot and Cecilia McAuliffe, and two postulants, Jane Townsend and Emily Conlan, disembarked in Brisbane from the coastal steamer *Wonga Wonga* on 10 May 1861, only two hours before midnight in the darkness of an autumnal night. After some conviviality at the priest's house at St Stephen's, the nuns set off on foot for the cottage on Spring Hill which had been rented for them.

It was spartan accommodation, furnished only with bedsteads and bedding. Fortunately, Mother Vincent had already said that she was willing to 'take day by day and live only for the day'.[20]

Daylight revealed that, as new arrivals among hordes of immigrants, Mother Vincent's party was well off, as 'the crowds of people are now coming in such flocks that we see many tents up for the newcomers'. Some of the existing housing was evidently not much better. The Sisters made their first sick calls within days of their arrival and found 'wretched dirty places'.[21] It was also a religious desert – Brisbane people had become accustomed to being left for more than a month without Mass when their priest travelled hundreds of miles to stations in the bush.

Bishop Quinn's ideas, and the challenges he faced, influenced the work of the Sisters in Queensland. Their challenge was ensuring that the Sisters of Mercy ideal could adapt, flourish and grow in a new landscape richly studded with discouragements, disappointments and disagreements and poorly decorated with willing hands and financial support. Flexibility in adapting both the Sisters of Mercy structure and the work they did to new environments set the tone for their work in the next century and a half. Within a month of their arrival, the Sisters were supervising and teaching in St Stephen's school, hoping to start work in Ipswich, and visiting the acutely ill and the benevolent asylum patients in the Brisbane Hospital.

The Brisbane Hospital was still struggling in the old convict hospital building, helped by government grants for capital expenditure and some of the running costs. The small Brisbane community was, however, generally unheeding of pleas for financial assistance.[22] Wrenching such assistance from the government and winning the charity of the public remained potent forces challenging the Sisters of Mercy and their hospitals during their whole history in Queensland. Mother Vincent also remarked on more than one occasion that 'people never think of giving money – everyone in Australia must work for that'.[23]

Queensland was a secular society, unlike the United States, where the first colonies had been founded by people escaping religious persecution and possessing strong Christian principles emphasising thanksgiving and philanthropy. In the Australian colonies, getting and spending in this world were far higher priorities than laying up treasure for the next. Queensland was also full of independent souls. Twenty years of neglect by the New South Wales government had bred an independence not easily curbed by either government or church. Both struggled to establish authority.

By 1863, the Sisters' work had extended to the nearby town of Ipswich. They managed a flourishing school and were so well received on their visits to the local hospital that Mother Vincent held high hopes that the Ipswich hospital 'will be yet under nuns'. She had worked hard to reduce Protestant apprehensions and was able to report that:

> without changing their Religion, we make improvement in the Protestant patients, [who] welcome us as warmly as if they were Catholics. I never in my life had so much to do with Protestants as I had since I came on this Mission, and I find them so very good.[24]

She had much less time for official government policy, which she thought was bigoted against Irish immigration: 'Chinese, and people from other nations are admitted, but the poor dear Irish, well, no matter, they will come and plant their own Faith in this distant land – let the Government plan and say what they please'.[25]

And the Irish were coming. In a scheme reminiscent of John Dunmore Lang's determination to plant Protestant seed in the colony, Bishop Quinn and his able ally, Father Robert Dunne, a former member of the staff of St Laurence's who followed him to the colony, brought almost 4,000 Irish settlers to Queensland. The Sisters of Mercy worked frantically during the 1860s and 1870s to keep educational and social service supply up to the demand. Then, without Mother Vincent's knowledge, the Bishop bought Dr Fullerton's house, Adderton, to become the Sisters' convent. Quinn's high hopes for Catholic prominence in Queensland gave the Sisters the terrifying problem of debt at a time when need proliferated. The convent was named All Hallows', rather than the names Mother Vincent appeared to favour, Mater Misericordiae or Auxilium Christorianorum.[26]

This surprising step was characteristic of the Bishop. In the mould of all the Irish bishops in colonial Australia, Quinn regarded himself as the source of all authority in the diocese.[27] He removed Mother Vincent from her position as Superior, largely because he thought that she would not be amenable to his view that in matters of management and direction he should be, in effect, the superior.[28] Many of the Sisters resented this distortion of the Mercy constitution, which required obedience to Rome, not the local diocesan, and left the diocese. Mother Vincent understood the Bishop's reasons for compromising with the National School system, which he saw as a meeting ground for all faiths, but continued to repine against the ending of state aid to religion, believing that her schools could be successful in promoting harmony and unity in the whole community. The All Hallows' property proved her point. The large four-storeyed house allowed the Sisters to establish the only girls' secondary school in Brisbane, supported by Protestants and Catholics alike.[29]

All Hallows' enabled the Sisters to expand their practice of charging fees to those who could afford it, but Mother Vincent worried constantly about repaying the debt – £6,000 at 6 per cent interest 'in this poor Mission without government aid for anything'.[30] There was much to do among those who could not afford to pay fees. The influx of Quinn's immigrants and those brought to Queensland under the government's scheme increased the need for schools, strained accommodation at the Sisters' St Vincent's Orphanage and revealed an urgent need for a House of Mercy to care for single or destitute women. Nevertheless, the Sisters managed to follow the settlers in the 1870s and established schools on the Darling Downs, in the Wide Bay district and in central Queensland.

When she was overseas recruiting new Sisters in 1871, Mother Vincent received a letter that was a wonderful bolt from the blue. Miss Florence Honoria O'Reilly wrote from London:

> I have heard a good deal of your struggles in Brisbane to promote the charitable works which there as well as anywhere else, engage the whole attention of the Sisters of Mercy. I feel a great interest in your charities and I hope to see you and all of your good institutions in less than a year from this . . . I have no present intention of becoming a nun, but I wish to serve God in my own humble way.[31]

Her first 'humble' gesture was to lend the Sisters £4,000 at 3 per cent interest, greatly reducing their debts, but this paled into insignificance with Miss O'Reilly's announcement in 1872 that the loan was now a gift because she had inherited even more money.[32]

Miss O'Reilly brought her accountant, George Wilkie Gray, into the Sisters' lives. He became a valued mentor, their trustee and one of their greatest supporters. Gray arrived in Brisbane in 1863. He married a member of the Quinlan family, converted to Catholicism and joined the family firm, Quinlan Gray & Co., which amalgamated with the Victorian Fitzgerald family business. Castlemaine Brewery and Quinlan Gray & Co. established a brewery at Milton in Brisbane. Gray was a clever entrepreneur with investments in enterprises such as schooners in the 1860s Brisbane–Ipswich river trade, the Bendigo pottery, land in Melbourne and the Queensland sugar industry. He became a director of leading Queensland companies, including the Queensland National Bank and the *Daily Mail* newspaper.[33]

Miss O'Reilly's beneficence was well-timed. The Bishop's accommodation with the state over the education question lasted only until 1875. Legislation in that year proclaimed that government education in Queensland would be free, compulsory and secular. Catholic schools were on their own. Replacing lay teachers with nuns wherever possible was important in reducing costs, but balancing the books was always a battle. In 1880, a year before Bishop Quinn's death, Mother Vincent was forced to dampen diocesan expectations that the All Hallows' convent could supply endless numbers of sisters, or bottomless purses of educational support. She told the Bishop:

> All Hallows' Convent has to bear the expense of training, educating and supporting all the young untrained Sisters . . . All Hallows' School which is supposed to support all the Brisbane Schools is giving this year gratuitous instruction to Catholic children to the amount of £468.[34]

The need to raise funds overcame the Bishop's opposition to bazaars and other public appeals for funds. Several bazaars in the last decades of the nineteenth century had the added benefit of further planting in the Queensland mind the idea that the Sisters of Mercy intended to integrate their work into the affairs of the wider community. The bazaars were attended by governors' wives and a wide range of people of all denominations, from the wealthiest and most prominent to working people on a day out. Donations of substantial prizes for art unions demonstrated that the Sisters were attracting significant support. The first prize at the 1883 art union bazaar, conducted under the patronage of the premier, Sir Arthur Palmer, was a wagonette complete with horse and harness valued at £100.[35]

More than the finances were changing. Bishop Quinn died in 1881, and was succeeded by Robert Dunne. Although Dunne did not develop a particularly good relationship with Mother Vincent, he nevertheless protested Quinn's usurpation of authority over the Sisters and was instrumental in helping them to establish St Vincent's Orphanage.[36]

Life was hectic for the new Bishop and the Sisters in the 1880s. It was a period of prosperity and rapid growth in Queensland. Gold mining and burgeoning sugar fields in the north, a boom in the wool-growing areas in the west, and the development of intensive agricultural cultivation inflated community and government coffers and produced a strong demand for labour. Immigration was steady. Governments were hard pressed to provide the necessary infrastructure – railway lines, ports and communications. Social infrastructure – schools, hospitals and welfare services – were lower priorities. Prosperity transformed Brisbane. Entrepreneurs, among them successful Irish immigrants including the retailer T C Beirne, built large houses in the growing suburbs and erected substantial business premises, striking in their Victorian grandiosity, in the city, more than matched by banks and government agencies.

Medical services improved, despite government neglect and the struggle of voluntary committees to maintain the city's three major hospitals, the Brisbane Hospital, the Children's Hospital and the Lady Bowen maternity hospital. Diseases such as typhoid fever and diphtheria were rampant in the city in the 1880s, but the happy coincidence of the arrival of several very talented young doctors began to rescue the medical situation. One of them, Dr Ernest Sandford Jackson, established a training school for nurses at the Brisbane Hospital in 1886.[37]

Although they did not yet have their own hospital, the Sisters of Mercy had largely replicated the pattern of works established in Dublin. By the time Mother Vincent died in 1892, 222 Sisters of Mercy in Brisbane and regional Queensland managed twenty-six schools with 7,000 pupils, a training college for teachers, a secondary girls' school, an orphanage, an industrial school, and a Magdalen asylum for unmarried mothers. Although a hospital was an ambition which Mother Vincent enunciated soon after her arrival, first things had had to come first. Ironically, within a year of her death, the purchase of a large area of land at South Brisbane laid the basis for the achievement of her health care dream.

The year following Mother Vincent's death, 1893, was a horrible year in Brisbane. Enormous floods in February washed away bridges, devastated suburbs, and laid waste to much of the city. The economy of all Australian colonies was in deep depression; floods added to the misery in Brisbane and much of south-eastern Queensland. Homelessness, ruined businesses and high unemployment made life almost impossible for the poor, and severely dented the prosperity of the better off. Banks failed, once-thriving businesses looked in vain for customers, and the building and immigration booms of the 1880s seemed like phenomena from another planet.[38] Success in managing a major enterprise in such a climate, and then developing it further, required a remarkable leader. That outstanding person was Mother Mary Patrick Potter.

Like Mother Vincent, Sister Mary Patrick had been professed for only ten years when she was elected Superior of the All Hallows' Congregation. She held that office, or that of assistant Superior, for forty-eight years. In addition to her profound spirituality, she demonstrated an intellectual grasp of business, an astute understanding of the ways of politics and politicians, a flair for public relations, a lively interest in people and the skills required to manage them. She became well known and highly respected in Brisbane, and forged a much more productive relationship with Archbishop Dunne than had Mother Vincent with either Dunne or Bishop Quinn. She was a 'people person'. One of her pupils at All Hallows' remembered Mother Patrick as a good teacher, but remarked 'it was more as a

NORAH MARY POTTER was born near Longford, Ireland, in 1849. After education in the Irish National School system and at the Mercy convent in Longford, Norah entered the Mercy convent at Athy, the springboard for many who found their vocations in Queensland in the 1860s.[39] The young Novice arrived in Brisbane in 1868 when she was only nineteen. She was professed in 1869 and spent the next period of her life as a teacher in Ipswich and then at All Hallows'. She was an ardent advocate of education for women, expanding both the academic and cultural program at All Hallows', and encouraging as many of her pupils as possible to enter Sydney University. Mother Patrick became a determined advocate for the establishment of a university in Queensland, a passion she shared with Archbishop Dunne.

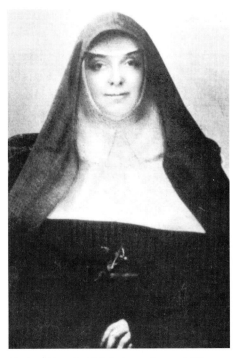

Mother Mary Patrick Potter, whose ability in business was responsible for raising and managing the funding to build the first three Mater hospitals. SOMCA

moulder of character that she stood prominent, for she was very firm, and ruled us not by fear, but through love of her and her wonderful example'.[40] Relationships were important to her. She kept in close contact with newer Mercy foundations in regional Queensland, as well as with the Sisters in her own congregation. Her correspondence is peppered with letters to her former pupils many years after they left school, and gentle chidings of those who neglected to reply.[41]

The Potter era was a period of great expansion – the Mercy congregation in Brisbane grew from thirty to 500 between 1879 and 1927. As well as opening more schools, Mother Patrick eagerly adopted Mother Vincent's vision for a Mater hospital in Brisbane. The first step was the purchase of ten acres of land at a cost of £7,000 adjacent to St Killian's College, a Catholic secondary school which also educated trainee teachers and seminarians.[42] The land was in a beautiful position. It was high on a hill overlooking South Brisbane and Woolloongabba, clearly visible from the city side of the Brisbane River. This lovely spot came to be known as Mater Hill.

For thousands of years, this was a treasured part of the traditional homelands of the Coorpooroo-jaggin group of the Jagara people, speakers of the Yuggera dialect of the Turrubul language. The lands of the Coorpooroo people stretched along the south bank of the river between Oxley and Bulimba creeks and inland to Mt Gravatt. The South Brisbane area was glorious, clothed in dense bush, and fed by several small creeks flowing from nearby swamps. Food was plentiful – there were ducks and swans in their hundreds, and plenty of running game on the wedge of flat land bounded on three sides by the river. Coorpooroo men fished in bark canoes made from broad sheets of stringy bark or by casting heart-shaped tow-row nets to encircle mullet shoals. Women and children dived for lily roots in the swamps, dug yams, collected edible fern roots, and wove baskets from swamp grasses.[43]

The richness of this environment endured because only those animals needed for food were killed, and only those plants necessary for food or shelter were culled. The Coorpooroo people were active and healthy. They were excellent swimmers, adept tree climbers and skilled at manoeuvring their canoes. Several early white observers noted that the Aboriginal people of the Brisbane area were far superior physically to their European counterparts. In the 1840s, some twenty years after Europeans first came to the Brisbane area, Aboriginal people still occupied the watercourse campsites. Ceremonial grounds dotted the South Brisbane–Woolloongabba area. People from Ipswich and the Moreton Bay coast periodically visited the area, camping at Woolloongabba, the main gathering place.[44] On special occasions, 500 people would spread along the Vulture Street ridges and Mater Hill. Close by, Musgrave Park, with its bora ground near the Russell Street and Cordelia Street corner, was another important meeting place.

More and more new settlers moved into South Brisbane in the nineteenth century. Aboriginal and European children often played

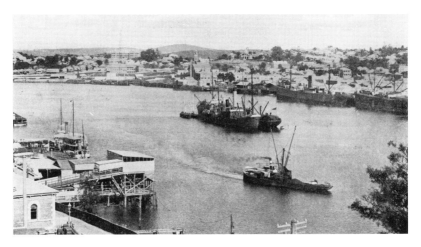

A view of South Brisbane in about 1911, showing the newly completed Mater Private Hospital high on its hill in the background at centre left. JOHN OXLEY LIBRARY

together. They enjoyed swimming in the popular 'corella', or water-hole, where the Gabba cricket ground was eventually developed; their diving competitions were invariably won by Aboriginal boys. In the 1850s and 1860s, the Coorpooroo people regularly visited homes and businesses, carting water from swamps in buckets placed on their heads and trading fish, game and honey. Although the Aboriginal population in the South Brisbane area declined in the mid nineteenth century with the growth of European settlement, many remained and, as late as the 1880s, hundreds of people still gathered near the site of the Boggo Road gaol.[45]

Although the Sisters bought the land in 1893, it was years before a new building appeared. In the troubled circumstances of the 1890s, spending £7,000 on land was enough – building a hospital had to wait. The Sisters continued to visit sick people in their homes and at the Brisbane Hospital, where standards of care had improved after the introduction of nurse training in 1888. Trained nursing greatly improved public perceptions of hospital care. The nurse came to be accepted by the community as a professional person of intellectual accomplishment, ethical standing and high moral character.[46] Nursing, like teaching, was one of the few career opportunities for women accepted by families in all social strata. Nevertheless, sick people all over the world who could pay for medical attention continued to eschew the large public hospitals where nurses were trained, preferring to be nursed in their own homes. The Dublin Mater, for instance, earned valuable income by hiring out many of its nurses to private patients.[47] Some Brisbane Hospital-trained nurses cared for private patients in their own homes, or found employment in the growing number of private hospitals. The new private hospitals, among them St Helen's at South Brisbane, were a compromise between hospital care, as the public continued to misunderstand it, and nursing in their own homes. As the *Queenslander* explained:

> These private hospitals are necessary and deserving institutions, they cater exclusively for the benefit of those who are willing and able to pay for the requisite attendance and accommodation and upon whom the prospect of being laid up in a public institution would have an irritating and possibly disastrous effect.[48]

By the early years of the twentieth century, Queensland had recovered from the flood and the depression, and by 1903 the economy was reviving after a nasty series of droughts. In many ways, the time was right for a Mercy hospital. William Naughton, a grazier from Gin Gin

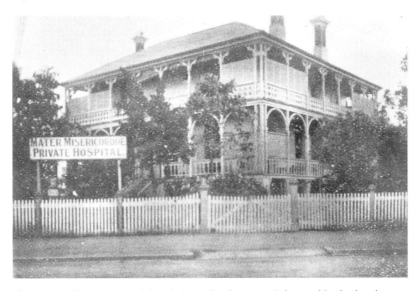

The Mater Private Hospital, North Quay, in about 1906, housed in the lovely Aubigny building. JOHN OXLEY LIBRARY

in the Burnett district, was so impressed by the Sisters' care of his wife during her illness that he donated £500 to the Sisters to establish their own hospital.[49] Premises had to be found. Fortunately, Aubigny, a house overlooking the river at North Quay, became available.

Aubigny was designed by the distinguished nineteenth-century Queensland architect Benjamin Backhouse for the merchant Samuel Davis, a founder of Brisbane's Hebrew congregation. The house, built in 1865, with a small synagogue in its grounds, was a handsome three-storeyed building surrounded on all sides by verandahs. The basement level, where the servants lived, extended five feet above ground level. The first floor was reached by a small flight of external stairs and the second floor by an internal staircase. The brewer Patrick Perkins bought the house in 1882 and the Perkins family lived there until 1899, before leasing it to the government as office accommodation for, among others, the Police Criminal Investigation Department.[50] In 1905, only one year after the Dublin Mater created its private hospital by linking five adjoining houses in Eccles Street, the Brisbane Sisters leased the house from Mrs Perkins for £5 per week, a rental which worried Mother Patrick; the many other works of Mercy had to be supported and she was still coping with pressing requests for new schools.[51]

Mother Patrick's religious outlook did not prevent her from having her feet firmly planted in the material world. Her way to heaven was not paved only with good intentions – good strategic planning and meticulous financial management formed a resilient tarmac. She consistently demonstrated sound business sense, winning the admiration of leading Brisbane business people and Archbishop Dunne, who had been trained in the family drapery business before entering the priesthood and regarded keeping a close eye on the books as the key to successful management.[52] Financial management, including a keen appreciation of value for money, remained one of Mother Patrick's preoccupations.

Worrying rentals notwithstanding, the lease for Aubigny was signed in December 1905. The Mater Misericordiae Private Hospital opened its doors on 4 January 1906 with accommodation for twenty patients. There were six single rooms on the first floor, all well ventilated and painted a cool pale green with pale blue linoleum on the floors, the same shade as the bedsteads. The operating theatre, at the rear of the first floor, had two glass walls and a glass roof, in accordance with the fashion of the day but not with Brisbane's subtropical climate. Three two-bed rooms and two single rooms were fitted out on the second floor, which also sported a bath carved from a solid block of marble and decorated with sculptured heads representing the god Pan, a strangely pagan symbol in a Catholic hospital. River views from the verandah on the upper floor enhanced the relaxing environment for convalescent patients. Three plainer two-bed wards shared the basement with the kitchen and a storeroom. Lay staff were accommodated in the rear wing. The Sisters lived in an adjoining cottage; their chapel was the little building in the grounds, originally constructed as a synagogue for Samuel Davis and used by the Perkins family as a billiard room.[53]

The inauguration of the new hospital on 4 January 1906 was celebrated at an afternoon tea attended by leading members of the Brisbane community, including a dozen prominent doctors. The Mater was welcomed by the *Brisbane Courier* as 'an important addition to the hospitals of the city' which would be a 'boon to those in need of medical or surgical treatment, and of good nursing'.[54] The Mater staff were led by the Superior, Sister Mary Felix McInerney, and the Matron, Sister Mary Antonia Brosnan. An emigrant from Killarney, County Kerry, Minnie Brosnan trained at the Brisbane General Hospital in 1897, receiving her certificate in 1899.[55] She entered the All Hallows' Convent and was professed in April 1904. There were, as well, two lay trained staff on the opening day, also former trainees of the Brisbane Hospital, Nurses Molly Malone and Norma McLeod. Three newly professed Sisters, Francis Mary Fitzgerald,

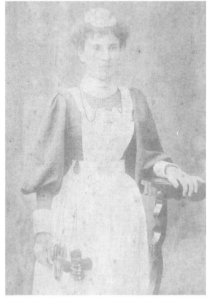

Sister Mary Antonia Brosnan, first Matron of the Mater Private Hospital.
ILLUSTRATION COURTESY OF MRS MARY (O'SHEA) DARMODY

Mary Edmund Stritch and Mary Assissium Dunne completed the staff.[56] They were joined a few months later by Sister Mary Chanel England.

The concept of a fee-paying private hospital was both a means of addressing the new hospital's immediate financial needs and a stepping-stone to the ideal of providing a public hospital for people who could not afford fees. This mimicked arrangements at All Hallows' school, where fees were charged to help support schools where fees were either not charged or were set at a very low rate.

To succeed at all, the new hospital had to attract patients; the key to this was winning the trust of private doctors. Dr Fred Page was the first doctor to make the required leap of faith and referred the Mater's very first patient, a young man with pneumonia. The next patient, a young priest, suffered from a fatal combination of two diseases plaguing Brisbane – typhoid fever and dengue fever.[57] Another early patient, Sister Mary Consilio's mother, led her doctor, Dr Lilian Cooper, and insisted on the new Mater.[58] Although Dr Cooper was initially very reluctant, as she feared that the Mater staff were not adequately trained, she overcame her concerns and became one of the early Mater's strongest supporters. Dr Cooper shared with the Sisters the experience of being a woman determined to succeed in a man's world.

By the end of 1906, with more doctors trusting the Mater, the new hospital had treated 141 patients. Competition from the other private hospitals was brisk, but by 1907 all beds at the Mater were usually full – indeed, the hospital treated 275 patients in its second year, an almost 100 per cent increase. Prospective patients soon had to be turned away, despite the fee of £3.3.0 per week. By March 1908, the *Telegraph* reported that the original Mater was too small, 'bed after bed having been added, till not a sitting room or verandah has been left unused'.[59]

The private hospital sector remained competitive, but business was growing for all hospitals, including public hospitals where patients were still expected to pay for their care unless they were subsidised by subscribers. The new enthusiasm for hospital care was largely due to the increasing success of modern surgery. Abdominal surgery advanced with the development of anaesthesia and asepsis. By 1905, surgeons in Brisbane had discarded their frockcoats for washable white garments and caps, instruments were sterilised, and rubber gloves were more accepted.[60] The Brisbane surgeon Dr David Hardie made the revolutionary suggestion that public hospital care should be free of charge, supported by a tax on all 'amusements', including race meetings and concerts. But the time was not yet ripe. The voluntary hospitals struggled on, charging fees when they could.

The climate was, however, right for Mother Patrick to press on with the next stage of development – building two brand new Mater hospitals at South Brisbane.

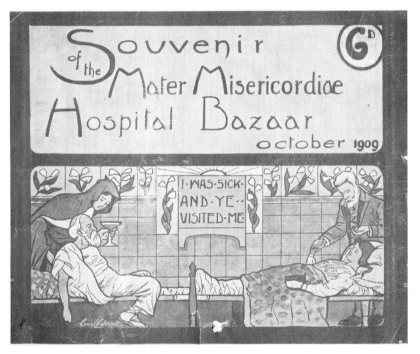

This booklet produced to aid in fundraising to build the first Mater Hospitals at South Brisbane reflects Mother Patrick's flair for public relations. MHHC

CHAPTER TWO

ADVANCING TO 'GREATER TRIUMPHS'

. . . from the 'day of small things', the good Sisters are
advancing to the glories of greater triumphs.

Brisbane Telegraph, 7 March 1909

In approaching the task of building the new hospitals, Mother Patrick
demonstrated both her determination and her business acumen. Her
flair for public relations was scarcely less important than her strategic
outlook, capacity for financial management and skill in dealing with
people of all kinds. In 1907, Mother Patrick revealed her plans to
finance the venture. She intended to hold a 'Grand Drawing' art union,
if the Sisters' remaining sugar investments at Innisfail did not sell,
and if an appeal to the public did not bring in the necessary funds.
Mother Patrick watched her timing, waiting until after Christmas 1907
because 'Brisbane has been overdone with hospital collections of late'.[1]
Her appeal was a direct open letter to the 'Charitable and Generous
Residents of Queensland on behalf of their Sick and Suffering Fellow Countrymen', making it clear that there would be both a private,
fee-paying hospital and a public hospital for the less affluent. Mother
Patrick explained that recent increases in vocations had relieved pressure on the Sisters who, when 'their duties were many and their hands
were few', had not found it possible to establish their own hospital

to fulfil all dimensions of the Mercy mission to the sick, poor and ignorant.[2]

The Brisbane press responded. The *Telegraph* reported in March 1908 that 'rumours' had been circulating for weeks that a new hospital was to be built on a hill 'facing the cool summer breezes, and protected by the rising hill behind from the westerly winds'. The reference to the perfect Brisbane aspect is likely to have been no chance remark, but carefully placed to help reduce the reluctance of doctors and patients to venture to the southern side of the river which, despite the beautiful homes built along the river at West End and on the slopes of Highgate Hill, was generally regarded as the less salubrious side of town. Very similar reports in the *Brisbane Courier* and in newspapers on the Darling Downs indicated that a press release had been carefully distributed. The newspapers cooperated, publishing lists of donors to the appeal. By May 1908 donations had reached £4,088.14.3, and, following the bazaar and art union held in October that year at the skating rink near the Central railway station in the city, the funds stood at £8,875.8.6.[3]

It was an impressive sum, but this was an ambitious project. The plans were in the experienced hands of the Brisbane architectural firm Hall and Dods, architects of the Lady Lamington Nurses' Home at the Brisbane General Hospital. The Mater Private Hospital was to be a three-storeyed brick building with verandahs on all sides. Quality was the keynote. Many elements in the design, including the detailing of the verandah railings, were similar to those at the Lady Lamington Nurses' Home, and were characteristic of Robin Dods, one of the most distinguished Australian architects of his generation.[4] The Mater Private Hospital plans, reproduced in the newspapers as part of the fundraising effort in 1908, were little different from the completed building.

The foundation stone was laid with great celebration on 24 May 1908, the Feast of Our Lady Help of Christians, by Cardinal Moran of Sydney, nephew of Archbishop Cullen of Dublin who had laid the foundation stone of the Dublin Mater just over fifty years earlier. The ceremony attracted enormous public interest – about 12,000 people clustered around the site.[5] The crowd readily responded to the call to place donations on the stone and contributed £4,000, supplemented

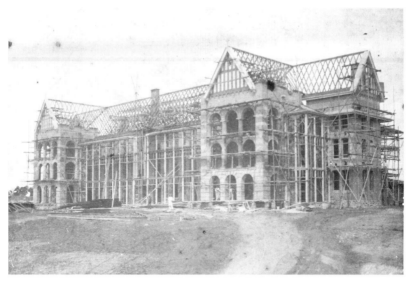

The Mater Private Hospital under construction in 1909–1910. MHHC

by a bequest of £3,000 from Father Connolly, parish priest of Sandgate, and a further £1,000 donated by William Naughton. Donations were approaching the £25,000 target set by Mother Patrick, and covered the initial building contract of just over £20,000 for the Private Hospital. Sixteen months later, on 24 September 1909, the Feast of Our Lady of Mercy, Archbishop Dunne laid the foundation stone of the public hospital, also designed by Robin Dods, to be built further down the hill. It was to be Brisbane's second adult public hospital.

On 14 August 1910, a lovely sunny day in late winter, the new Mater Private Hospital was blessed by Cardinal Moran and officially opened by the Governor, Sir William MacGregor. The hospital grounds were brightly decorated with flags and bunting and crammed with a crowd of 8,000 people overflowing to the hillside overlooking the hospital. One newspaper noticed particularly the 'beautiful house flag' – a blue background with the intertwined letters 'MM' worked by hand. The band of the Queensland Rifles Regiment provided the music, and cadets from Nudgee College formed a guard of honour for arriving dignitaries.

The press remained firmly supportive. The widely circulated weekly journal, the *Queenslander*, published a lengthy pictorial report on Cardinal Moran's visit to Brisbane to open the hospital. Another paper reported:

Already the good work of the Mater Misericoridiae Hospital has established a reputation that is widely and honourably known, and one that doubtless, under more improved conditions, will become more indissolubly bound up with the welfare of a great State.[6]

The *Brisbane Courier* praised the new hospital's elegant silky oak staircase, wide balconies, and bathrooms at the end of each corridor, noting approvingly that their 'walls are tiled and floors impermeable'. There were single rooms for fourteen patients on the ground floor, and, on the first floor, nineteen private rooms and many more beds in shared wards. Patients' rooms were furnished by the hospital's well-wishers, supplemented by tray cloths and table covers made by Sisters in various convents throughout the Archdiocese. Two operating theatres were separated from the eastern end of the ground floor by a gangway. The larger theatre had five plate-glass windows facing south, with separate rooms for anaesthesia and sterilising.[7]

In his speech opening the hospital, the Governor praised the Sisters of Mercy. This was much more than mere tact. In his earlier career as a doctor in Britain's colonial service, he had supervised hospitals

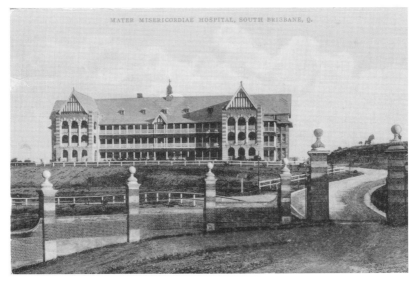

MATER MISERICORDIAE HOSPITAL, SOUTH BRISBANE, Q.

The Mater Private Hospital, completed in 1910. The imposing gates and fence marked the entry from Raymond Terrace. The driveway visible at the left of the main drive inside the gates led to the site of the Mater Public Hospital. MHHC

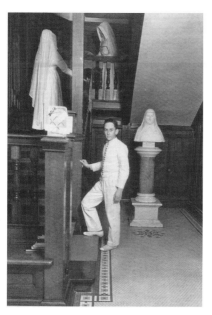

The entrance hall at the Mater Private Hospital, showing the beautiful tiled floor and silky oak staircase which later made way for a modern lift. The page in the foreground was always known as 'Buttons', presumably in reference to his uniform. MHHC

in Port Louis, Mauritius, where religious sisters formed the nursing staff.[8] In his work in Mauritius, Fiji and New Guinea, MacGregor had consistently demonstrated his concern for the health of disadvantaged people. He had been appointed Governor of Queensland in 1909, towards the end of his career, with his passion for medicine and science intact. His dispatches to England revealed that, like Archbishop Dunne and Mother Patrick, he was appalled that Queensland had no university.[9]

On 8 September 1910, the hospital's first patient, Mrs Bolger from Fortitude Valley, was transferred from Aubigny. Five months later, on 2 February 1911, the new Mater Public Hospital was opened without fanfare or special celebrations. This V-shaped building was light and airy. French doors in each of the four ten-bed wards allowed beds to be pushed out on to the balconies. The walls were painted cream with chocolate-coloured dados. Each patient had a gunmetal locker, topped with marble. A pleasant terrace for recuperating patients occupied the space between the arms of the V on the Stanley Street side. The generous public again came to the aid of the Mater. The women's wards were furnished by an anonymous donor; Brisbane's jockeys and horse trainers furnished the men's surgical ward.[10] A great deal had been accomplished in little more than five years. The idea of a Mater Private Hospital was an undoubted success, and the Sisters' years of hoping to care for the sick poor had become reality. But there was no time for resting on laurels.

Buildings, no matter how new and up to date, form only the skeletons of hospitals. Many vital elements must be added and coordinated to enable them to do their work. Human and financial resources must be pumped in and circulated or hospitals will not function, workers must provide the muscle or nothing will be done, the administration must provide goals and brain power or there will be no direction, the vision that the sick must be cared for must be central or hospitals will have no life. All must be coordinated to deal with the outside world, or a health service will not grow. The two new Mater hospitals were conceived for a specific purpose – as vehicles for Mercy values in action. These values – compassion and service to the poor and the afflicted – were to be the guiding spirit of the hospitals' developing personalities.

The new Mater Public Hospital was born in a turbulent period for Queensland's public hospitals. Secular public hospitals were still voluntary, community-based organisations, funded by subscribers and supplemented, more in theory than reality, by fees paid by patients who could afford to do so. In 1911, when the first patients were admitted to the Mater Public, the day when patients could expect hospital care free of charge was still decades away. To grow and develop, or even to keep going, the Mater hospitals have always had to deal with the tough realities of the secular world. Somehow ends had to be made to meet in the present, in order to provide for future development. A few months after the Mater Public opened in 1911, Archbishop Dunne seemed well pleased with the Sisters' progress:

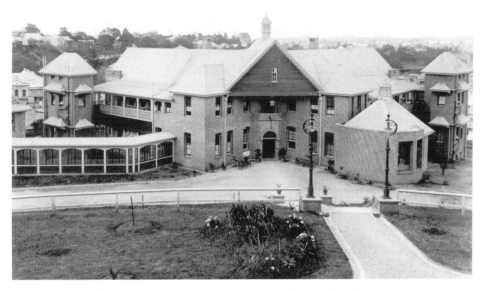

The Mater Public Hospital photographed from the Mater Private Hospital showing the main entrance and the roof-line of the two wings comprising the original 'V' shape. A terrace for recuperating patients stretched between the wings of the V on the Stanley Street side. MHHC

> Looking back one is simply astounded at seeing what has been done by a handful of ladies . . . in an absolutely new country. The community now numbers over 300 . . . Altogether it is a campaign for God Almighty that has few, if any, parallels.[11]

However, the Archbishop had been reluctant to provide anything more tangible than moral support to the Mater. Mother Patrick found in 1908 that 'the Archbishop wishes to have his name out of the deed of land where the hospital is to be built, as in the case of a mortgage, he wishes to be quite out of it'.[12]

Many of the opportunities, pressures and challenges the Mater hospitals faced in their first century were revealed in the twenty years after the first two hospitals were built on Mater Hill. In inveigling support from reluctant governments and in keeping up to date with health facilities in both the public and the private hospital sectors, much depended on good public relations, retaining public support in fundraising campaigns, enrolling the assistance of powerful and effective advocates – and making judicious compromises. The Sisters' funds did not extend to building a convent at South Brisbane. The top floor of the Private Hospital became the Sisters' convent, instead of accommodating fee-paying patients. Two rooms on the first floor served as the chapel, furnished with the altar Mother Vincent had brought from Dublin fifty years earlier. Nevertheless, in the Mater Public's first year, the Private Hospital managed to contribute £300 – just over one-quarter of the Public Hospital's income.[13]

Financial strain was, to some extent, lessened by the advantage of composing staff in both hospitals entirely of religious Sisters who did not need to be paid. Sister Mary Felix McInerney continued as Superior until 1913 when Mother Damian Dunne took over the reins. Sister Mary Antonia Brosnan was Matron of both hospitals until her death in 1912. She was succeeded by Sister Francis Mary Fitzgerald, another veteran of the North Quay days. For some years, the same Sisters' names appeared on staff lists at both the Private Hospital and the Public Hospital: a great deal of work was covered by very few people.

Fortunately, the Sisters were able to draw on public support.

Fundraising by voluntary committees was essential to success from the very beginning. The volunteers worked extremely hard; in the first three years alone, their hospital balls, linen club and Hospital Saturday collections raised almost £1,000.[14] Much depended on good public relations. Subscribers' names were regularly published in the press and in annual reports; donations of everything from pumpkins to pillow slips were faithfully acknowledged in published material.

Wringing assistance from government was far more difficult than enthusing volunteers. The Queensland government, still holding at arm's length any obligation to provide a health service for its citizens, provided paltry subsidies.[15] The State's biggest hospital, the Brisbane Hospital, had reached such a low financial ebb in 1904 that it had to plead with the government for increased subsidies; patients' fees and voluntary subscriptions came nowhere near covering costs. In 1905, a government attempt to compel the Brisbane City Council to share the deficit failed, and the Brisbane Hospital continued to flounder. Part of the problem was undoubtedly the debt incurred by patients who could afford to pay fees but did not. Then, as now, public hospitals faced the pressures of a continually growing population producing ever-increasing numbers of patients, and steadily developing scientific and technological innovations that were always costly to implement.

Far from assisting the development of Brisbane's second public hospital, the government actually made it harder. In December 1911, only nine months after the new hospital opened, the government closed its South Brisbane 'outdoor relief' depot where needy people found medical aid as well as daily sustenance. Leaving people without help was not the Mercy way, and the Sisters opened their outpatient department in July 1912. This department, housed in its own specially built brick building, treated 1,440 people in its first six months.[16] Despite the fact that more than 3,000 inpatients – presumably people who would otherwise have added to the pressures at the Brisbane Hospital – were treated in the Mater Public in its first three years, the government did not provide any bed subsidy for public patients until the 1913–14 year.[17] The lack of government subsidy was not for want of the Sisters' trying.

Mother Patrick began her campaign for government assistance in November 1912. Her correspondence with government authorities reveals her skill in developing winning arguments. The ground was well prepared. The illustrated booklet *The history of the movement for the establishment of the Mater Misericordiae Hospital Brisbane from 1 January 1906 to 31 October 1911*, published to support appeals to the public as well as to government, was enclosed with her letter. The booklet included impressive statistics, demonstrating that the Sisters had already done much to help themselves: initially, the donation of £7,500 from Sisters of Mercy funds, then the Brisbane and Warwick bazaars which had raised £7,725.6.0 and £1,125.16.0 respectively, donations from the public amounting to £10,880.13.0, 'entertainments' which had raised £1,303.2.11, art unions at Sandgate and Toowoomba which between them raised £508.18.0, and bequests totalling £3,560.1.5 – a grand total of almost £30,000. The bank loan of £12,000 was also included. This ammunition supported Mother Patrick's main salvo:

> I, of myself, and under considerable pressure from the Citizens in general, request you to consider whether this Public Hospital is not entitled to the generous recognition of the State, taking the form of an endowment, as in the other Public Hospitals, of forty shillings to the pound subscribed by the Public.[18]

The argument that the Mater Public deserved the same support as secular public hospitals was logical. However, if it chose to reject the submission, the government had legislative authority on its side. The Mater Public did not fit the definition of a public hospital in the *Hospitals Act 1862*, still the only hospital legislation on the statute books. It was owned by the Sisters of Mercy, its land and buildings were not vested in trustees for hospital purposes, and it was managed by the Sisters rather than by a committee elected by hospital subscribers to which a government representative was appointed.[19] Despite the strictly legal position, the government did not close the door, and held the matter over for further consideration.

The press did what it could to hasten government cogitation. In

March 1913, the *Darling Downs Gazette*, under a headline proclaiming 'Needs not creeds' jabbed tender government electoral sensitivities:

> It is almost needless to remark that the Premier of Queensland will meet with universal approval if he is able to include the Mater Misericordiae hospital in Brisbane within the list of the institutions that receive an annual subsidy.[20]

The paper forestalled any possible suggestion that sectarianism was practised at the Mater. Pointing out that 'charity knows no creed', the paper reported that Protestant patients had outnumbered Catholics, and quoted a Protestant member of the Mater's honorary medical staff as saying that his creed mattered 'not at all' to the Sisters or to the other doctors. At this stage in Queensland's political history, the premier, D F Denham, was all too aware that the rising Labor Party, led by the Catholic politicians T J Ryan and Edward Theodore, was rapidly closing the electoral gap. Archbishop Dunne had overcome his fear that the Labor Party was godless socialism in action, coming to regard the new political force as the only party beyond religious prejudice and concerned for all citizens.[21]

The government had much to lose in not appeasing the Mater, but it was besieged by impecunious hospitals. The Brisbane General Hospital again pleaded for help, and was rewarded by a government loan in February 1911, just as the Mater Public was opening its doors. Mother Patrick kept up the pressure. In June 1913, she produced a crunching argument, using the premier's praise of the Mater Public at its first annual meeting as a sign that he recognised that it deserved government endowment.[22] The Mater's battle was won. Mother Patrick's gracious, cleverly expressed gratitude left no room for government retreat:

> I really cannot find words to express our deep gratitude for your kindness in placing £1000 on the Estimates for the Mater Misericordiae Hospital. The manner in which you have given this grant to the Hospital enhances its value, as it shows your confidence in us, and you may be assured that this confidence is much appreciated.[23]

Influential support from another quarter helped to ensure that the government amended its local government legislation to compel the South Brisbane City Council to waive the rates on the Mater property. The Governor, Sir William MacGregor, departed from the usual vice-regal protocol of never commenting on government policy matters when, as guest of honour at the Mater Public's first annual meeting, he said he 'begrudged' the £125 paid in municipal rates.[24]

Jostling for funding equity was not the only arena of competition between the Mater and secular public hospitals. When the Mater Public opened its doors in February 1911, it was modern in every respect. On the other hand, the Brisbane General Hospital, with its main building dating from the 1860s, was hopelessly old-fashioned. In the first decades of the twentieth century, when surgery was rapidly developing, operating theatres were key facilities. Within a few years of the first operations performed at the Mater Public, the Brisbane General had enrolled the Mater's architects to design a similar large modern operating theatre, made possible by an allocation of £3,000 from the Walter and Eliza Hall Trust. In contrast, the Mater's allocation from the Trust was only £200.[25]

The Mater Public's popularity showed no signs of waning. Pressure on beds – originally for forty patients in four ten-bed wards – was so great that, in 1913–14, the hospital was extended to double the accommodation for surgical patients and to provide space for an X-ray department, a pathology room and two small wards for 'extreme cases', the first intensive care facility.[26] Patient care in the Public Hospital was supervised by honorary physicians and surgeons, with a resident medical officer on the spot at all times. Mother Patrick had developed good relationships with leading Brisbane doctors and had consulted many of them on the design of the new hospitals to ensure that they would meet modern standards. The doctors continued to refer patients to the Private Hospital, and many volunteered to serve at the Public Hospital. No voluntary hospital of this era could operate without the honorary medical officer system. Paying a full medical staff would be completely impossible when patient fees and small government subsidies did not cover costs.

The doctors did reap some reward – honorary medical service

helped young specialists to become known, increasing their chances of developing successful private practices. Material advantages for senior, successful doctors were less clear, but all regarded service to the needy as a key professional obligation. In its first ten years, the Mater attracted many of Brisbane's distinguished doctors to the honorary staff. They included the pioneers from the North Quay days – Doctors Fred Page, W F Taylor and Lilian Cooper – and additions such as the ear, nose and throat specialist W N Robertson, the surgeon L P Winterbotham, and the radiologist Andrew Doyle.[27]

Appointment to the Mater staff was clearly desirable to young specialists. In 1913, a surgeon newly arrived in Brisbane applied to Mother Patrick for an honorary position after hearing that one of the senior honorary surgeons was ill and unlikely to resume a full workload. He suggested that older surgeons become consultants, as was the practice overseas, 'thus giving a chance to younger men for doing the strenuous part of the business and leaving the older man liberty to do as he likes'. Many of the doctors who held honorary appointments to the Public Hospital were also permitted to admit patients to the Private Hospital. The same young doctor saw a dual appointment as important to career advancement in the competitive private hospital world:

> . . . there is a good deal of jealousy displayed towards the Mater and it is becoming known that I have been sending a lot of my patients to the Mater. Some of these [private] hospitals . . . were very friendly to me . . . but they are beginning to growl and tax me with sending my cases to you and if I continue to do so they will campaign against me. I would like to support the Mater exclusively but if I do I would like to have some standing on your public staff so that I would at least get the same advantage as your other patrons.[28]

Appointment of medical staff was yet another administrative challenge facing the Sisters. The Congregation retained all decision-making power for many decades but, in the Mater's earliest days, appointed an advisory Medical Board to recommend doctors for appointment to the visiting staff. Most doctors in this era were members of the Queensland

Branch of the British Medical Association (BMA), the doctors' professional association. The BMA was a powerful influence in medical circles and, on occasion, took stances reminiscent of the powerful trade unions in protecting the interests of its members. Around the time of the First World War, Dr H J Windsor, who eventually became a longstanding Mater identity, was initially rebuffed by the Mater's medical board because he was not a member of the BMA.[29]

In penetrating the complexity of Brisbane's medical and hospital world, the Sisters chose wisely in appointing Dr William Frederick Taylor to be first president of their Medical Advisory Board. Dr Taylor was influential in the three main arenas – medicine, government and Protestantism – in which the Sisters' intentions needed to be accepted and endorsed. W F Taylor had studied at La Charité in Paris where he became familiar with the work of religious Sisters before starting his Brisbane practice in 1882. As well as being honorary ophthalmologist and in charge of the ear, nose and throat department at the Brisbane General Hospital, Taylor had broader professional interests. He was a member of the Central Board of Health, the Medical Board of Queensland and the Queensland Medical Defence Society, and President of the Queensland branch of the BMA in 1894, 1899 and 1901. As a Member of the Legislative Council, the upper house of the Queensland parliament, Dr Taylor fought to maintain the independence of the health care professions.

Medical staffing was only one area of connection between Queensland's public and private hospitals. The confused issue of who should be entitled to free treatment in the public hospitals was a complicating factor. There was a worrying implication for private hospitals if people with means were admitted to public hospitals free of charge. The *Telegraph* newspaper ventilated the issue in 1908 by stating the obvious problem – the Brisbane Hospital was supported by subscribers who never used it, and used by people who never subscribed. The Mater solution, two hospitals – one for patients who must pay and one for those who could not – was a solution that could forestall an alarming future prospect:

> Put this proposition to the test. Suppose a paying patient is occupying a room or bed, and, when not another [bed] remains unoccupied . . . a

non-paying patient is carried to the door . . . and admission refused. It might lead to the downfall of a government possessing fewer lives than our present Ministry.[30]

This dilemma has never been solved in the government system, and the political nerve it touches remains sensitive.

The development of hospital care in the early decades of the twentieth century also put the spotlight on the nurses who cared for the patients. Nursing at the Mater Private Hospital was exclusively in the hands of religious Sisters, but the rapid growth of both hospitals was likely to outstrip the Sisters' capacity to supply nurses from their own ranks. Pressure on nursing at the Mater also came from an entirely different source. Although it did not fit the legislative definition of a public hospital, the Mater was in the anomalous position of coming under legislation governing other aspects of health care. Queensland governments were very slow in enacting modern legislation to run the state's hospitals, but they had introduced legislation to regularise the health professions. In the first two decades of the twentieth century, pharmacists, dentists, optometrists and nurses felt the effect of government determination to insist on adequate qualifications.[31]

The Australasian Trained Nurses Association (ATNA) had maintained a register of qualified nurses for years. It persuaded the government to create a separate nurses' registration board – the first of its kind in the nation – instead of registering nurses under the Medical Board established by the *Health Act 1911*. The nurses' own board established a three-year training course and set examinations. Unlike his counterpart in Sydney, Archbishop Dunne did not resist the imposition of state regulation on nurses in Catholic hospitals. During his entire episcopate, he maintained his determination that the Church would be part of the community and in no way retreat into separateness or sectarianism.[32] The Mater was able to claim in its first annual report that it had implemented all the new regulations. Six Sisters, some of whom qualified for registration through their experience at the first Mater, were registered in 1913. However, only the Matron, Sister Mary Antonia Brosnan, and Sisters Mary Lucien Salmond and Mary Vincentia Roe had completed formal courses of nurse training.[33]

The Mater Public training school for lay trainees was formally established in 1912. Sisters of Mercy were trained separately at the Mater Private. By 1914, seventeen Sisters of Mercy had secured their registration. Some Sisters did not wish to be nurses but, like dozens more in succeeding decades, were subject to the Mother Superior's direction. Mother Patrick did not shirk this task, telling one reluctant Sister that 'you are going to be in the hospital while the grass is green on the ground'.[34] Whether religious or lay, life for the nurse trainee was far from easy. Long shifts in the wards were the trainee's lot in hospitals everywhere, but at the Mater some Sisters worked two shifts each day, sewed the hospital linen at night and, in what scarce free time remained after fulfilling their religious obligations, attended lectures and studied for examinations.

Provision for the training schools added to the Mater's financial burdens, even though the hospital had followed the custom of the day in all training schools and charged lay trainees for their education.[35] All training hospitals required their trainees to live on the premises. The strict regime in nurses' homes in secular and religious hospitals under the rule of 'Home Sisters' was akin to conditions in military barracks, and, like life in the military, rules and ranks in the nurses' homes reinforced hierarchical structures in the workplace; uniforms and insistence on polite, chaste behaviour reproduced the convent model. The first fourteen lay probationers entered the training school in 1914, the year the St Mary's Nurses' Home was built close to the Mater Public.

The extensions to the surgical wards at the Mater Public were also completed in 1914 – just in time to meet the challenge of the First World War. The war demonstrated beyond any doubt that the Mater Public was an essential part of the life of the whole community. Archbishop Dunne's policy of inclusion, rather than separateness, saved Brisbane from most of the bitter sectarianism raging in Sydney and Melbourne, where all Catholics tended to be suspected of disloyalty after the 1916 Easter rebellion against British rule in Dublin, shortly followed by Archbishop Mannix's vociferous opposition to conscription for war service.[36] The Sisters immediately made twenty beds available at the Mater Public to treat injured soldiers. Over the next few years, a steady stream of soldiers flowed through the wards. Like other public hospitals, the Mater worked under duress with many of its honorary medical staff and resident medical officers on war service. There was also a financial cost. Appeals to the public for donations to support the hospital were suspended during the war so that community patriotic appeals could claim the public's attention.[37]

Before long, Mother Patrick was forced to report that 'the stress of war reacts with terrible force on our slender resources', even though the medical and nursing staff limited themselves to using the bare minimum of equipment. By 1916, 34 per cent of the hospital's funds came from patient fees, 34 per cent from large donations, 25 per cent from the government and 7 per cent from community contributions.[38] Mother Patrick looked to government to lift its game. The annual subsidy was £1,000 – £25 per bed for the Mater Public's forty beds. However, even when the daily average of patients treated in the recently expanded hospital rose to 83.9 in 1915, the £1,000 grant did not increase, despite several promptings from the Sisters.[39]

After the 1915 election, Mother Patrick's target was the new Labor government. Its policy of bringing all the old voluntary hospitals under state control was likely to have given her some cause for disquiet, because, strictly interpreted, the nationalisation policy would mean the end of any hope of funding for the Mater Public while it remained in private ownership. Nevertheless, Mother Patrick kept up the pressure. In August 1919, supported by her usual array of carefully compiled statistics and costings, she wrote:

> We fully realise the great strain that war conditions and their effects have brought upon the Government's financial resources, but we believe that whatever the claims may be for help to other objects, the Government will recognise that none are more urgent than that of the sick poor which the Hospital is designed to assist.

Her case proved irresistible. The Home Secretary, John Huxham, Member of Parliament for the Mater's electorate, took her plea to Cabinet and noted 'Provided £2,000 instead of £1,000 on estimates'.[40]

This softening of the government heart may well have been

prompted by the Mater's role in a major public health emergency. The Spanish influenza pandemic swept the world in 1918 and 1919, taking millions of lives. Returning soldiers brought the disease to Australia, rapidly overcrowding the hospitals. Matron Bourne at the Brisbane General Hospital was hastily appointed to make arrangements for flu victims. The Mater readily agreed to her request that 25 per cent of the nursing staff, the same proportion as at Brisbane's secular hospitals, be made available for flu victims. The Archdiocese went further than this, and arranged to turn the adjacent St Laurence's school into a special flu hospital. The Mater's place as an essential community facility was further confirmed when it treated Brisbane General Hospital outpatients and elective surgical cases. The General was so besieged that influenza patients were nursed in tents in the hospital grounds and in horse stalls in the exhibition grounds. Some teaching Sisters from All Hallows' were pressed into service to help with the nursing at St Laurence's – a critical measure because only three of the Mater's trainee nurses avoided the illness.[41]

Even without the influenza emergency, the war years had taken a toll on the Mater Public staff and increased the financial strain, only partly relieved by donations, bequests, allocations from the Mater Private and gifts of food. The overdraft in the building fund had grown, but the Public Hospital was faced with the need to expand, having treated as many as 110 patients at peak periods in accommodation designed for only seventy. Patient demand fuelled a series of pressures: more nurses were needed, but the Nurses' Home was full; more drugs were essential, but the war had restricted supplies and raised prices.

A modicum of relief was on the way. In 1920, Mother Patrick received the welcome news that the Mater Public would receive some of the proceeds of the government's Golden Casket Art Union on the same basis as other public hospitals. The Golden Casket lottery, begun as a means of raising money for the Queensland War Council during the war, remained popular with the public and very profitable for the government. Although governments always had some qualms about financing hospitals through the proceeds of gambling, the Golden Casket remained a valuable source of hospital funding. However, the Mater was the last in a long list of beneficiaries and received only £235.15.9 in the first distribution, less than half of its entitlement of £620.8.4, calculated at the rate of 5 shillings in the pound based on its maintenance expenditure.[42] Nevertheless, it was better than nothing, and Mother Patrick could remark at the end of 1920 that she could 'place the flower of satisfaction rather than the marble of disappointment over the grave of the old year'.[43]

A series of innovations made the decade after the First World War even more satisfying. The first extensions to the Public Hospital had provided space under the new Ward 1 for basic diagnostic X-rays and a 'pathology experiment room'. By the mid-1920s,

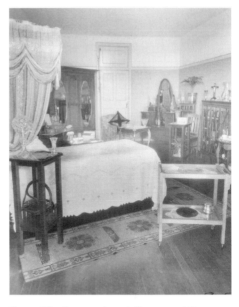

One of the famous 'crystal' rooms at the Mater Private Hospital, furnished like a domestic bedroom. MHHC

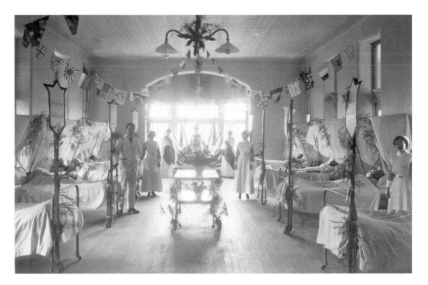

Ward 1, Mater Public Hospital, during the First World War, decorated with patriotic flags. The beds are placed at regular intervals, as typical of 'Nightingale' wards in all public hospitals. The French doors that led onto the verandah, visible at right, and the pressed metal ceiling indicate the quality of construction. MHHC

the diathermy machine treated conditions such as rodent ulcers and early cancers of the tongue and tonsils. The Sisters also planned to install a 'deep X-ray' machine to treat other cancers, described at the 1924 annual meeting as being the consequence of 'too much high living'. At this time, the radiologist, Dr A T Nisbet, was treating cancer patients from the public hospital in his private rooms at a cost of £30 per treatment from his own pocket. The Brisbane General Hospital was not convinced of the efficacy of deep X-ray therapy, so the Queensland Cancer Campaign installed Queensland's first deep therapy machine at the Mater Public in 1928. In 1930, the new unit treated ninety-four cancer patients by radiation therapy and a further 122 by deep X-ray.[44] The X-ray department developed rapidly in the 1920s. In 1926, new equipment diagnosed gallstones by means of 'iodine and bromide salts', the major means of diagnostic testing in the era before ultrasound scanning. In 1927, 946 diagnostic X-rays were taken and sixty-eight patients were treated for various conditions. A new 'Victor' X-ray machine was installed in 1928 and there were soon calls for a portable machine to take to patients in the wards.[45]

The development of the laboratory was another remarkable innovation. The Mater was very fortunate to have its first honorary pathologist, Dr James Vincent Duhig, who returned to Brisbane after war service and a course of study in pathology at King's College Hospital in London.[46] He found a willing partner at the Mater in a family friend, Sister Mary Chanel, first supervisor of the nurse training scheme. Sister Mary Chanel began her study of pathology at the state laboratories as soon as the one-room Mater laboratory was built in 1914. She saved for her first microscope by doing the laundry for patients at the Mater Private, a time-consuming task in the days of pin-tucked, lacy nightdresses.[47] Her fascination with scientific developments in bacteriology, biochemistry and microbiology was fuelled by a gift subscription to the American *Journal of Hospital Progress*.

In the first few months of 1919, when the hospital was still dealing with the flu epidemic, Dr Duhig and Sister Mary Chanel established Queensland's first hospital laboratory at the Mater. Histology was initially Sister Mary Chanel's major interest, but when biochemistry developed in the Mater laboratory she revelled in the chemistry of

proteins, carbohydrates and fats.[48] Biochemistry became more prominent in diagnosis, and during the 1920s the Mater laboratory churned
out ever-increasing numbers of test results for conditions such as goi-
tre and kidney disease, both of which were becoming more common
in Queensland. Dr Duhig and Sister Mary Chanel did not hold back in
pressing for more resources:

> Scientific work of this kind is costly and shows no immediate cash return.
> But medical science can only progress with the progress on the laboratory
> side. And this side is worthy of generous endowment.[49]

Dr Duhig resigned from the Mater in 1929 to fight bigger battles in
developing pathology at the Brisbane General Hospital. His nephew,
Dr George Taylor, succeeded him at the Mater. Work continued apace
with improved equipment and more staff, after Sister Mercia Mary
Higgins, a trained pharmacist, joined the laboratory staff in 1930.

Sister Mary Chanel was a doughty soul. In developing the laboratory at the Mater, as in developing nurse education, she was recognised
as a 'mighty warrior', but, in one doctor's opinion, her forthright ways
had not made her the ideal person to be Matron of the Private Hospital, a position she held during the war.[50] Although science was her
consuming passion, sparking correspondence with doctors in the
United States whose articles she devoured, Sister Mary Chanel also
had gentler interests. With Sister Mary de Chantal James, she spent
hours converting the bare Mater hillside into pleasant gardens and
delighted in supplying flowers to the Private Hospital and some of the
honorary doctors.[51]

Developments in the 1920s were not only medical and scientific.
Once again, the builders were back on Mater Hill. This was an era of
major development throughout the Archdiocese. Archbishop James
Duhig, who succeeded Archbishop Dunne in 1917, was convinced
that the standing of the church in the community could be promoted
by the grandeur of its physical stature. The presence of the church
in the communities of the faithful was enhanced by Duhig's policy of
creating many more parishes, and parish churches, so that no Catholic was far from a church and its parish school. Placing churches

and schools in the centre of communities helped to develop a strong sense of Catholic identity which had been growing in Australia since the 1880s.[52]

The Mater Public underwent its second extension in only ten years, supported by an art union. Mother Patrick prepared the ground, securing prizes from Brisbane retailers: furniture from John Hicks and Co. and McDonnell and East, a violin worth £15.15.0 from Palings, and a sewing machine from Barry and Roberts. The pièce de résistance was the first prize – a Ford touring car made available by the Queensland Motor Agency at a considerable discount. One well-known donor did not wish to blow his own trumpet. The prominent retailer and Member of the Legislative Council Thomas Charles Beirne wrote to Mother Patrick: 'I still wish to have the Prize given as from T C Beirne, not the Honourable, not Mr, and not T C Beirne & Co – just T C Beirne'.[53]

The design of the 1920s extension reflected increasing specialisation

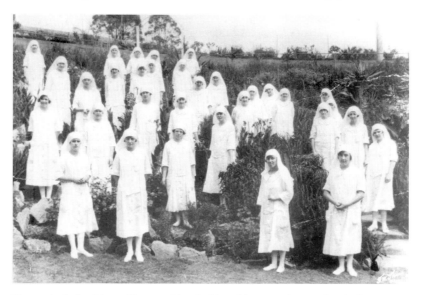

Nurses in their white uniforms with a fashionable 1920s lowered waistline, white stockings and white shoes, on the hill near the eventual site of the Mater Mothers' Hospital. The gardens on the hill matured in the 1920s and 1930s. Sister Mary Chanel England and Mother de Chantal James created most of the landscaping around the Mater through their own physical efforts. Construction of hospital buildings has, over the years, removed most of the hillside garden. MHHC

in medicine. Operating theatres suited to the particular needs of oph-
thalmological and ear, nose and throat surgery were provided, as well
as more surgical beds. The surgical load increased each year. In 1927,
for instance, honorary surgeons performed 466 abdominal operations, mainly appendectomies and hernia repairs, 230 gynaecological
procedures, thirty-eight operations on bones and joints, eighteen
amputations, forty-four excisions of tumours, nine chest operations,
500 ear, nose and throat procedures and 192 eye operations.[54]

The variety of medicine and surgery practised at the Mater provided plenty of experience and a daunting workload for trainee nurses.
The profession was gradually becoming more organised and more
determined to ensure that the value of nurses would be recognised.
Poor pay and excessive workloads persisting after the end of the war
boiled over at the Brisbane General Hospital. Nurses there formed the
Queensland Nurses Association to campaign for a proper industrial
award. The Award, handed down by the Industrial Court, contained
a nasty surprise for the Mater. Hospitals owned by churches were
included, despite the Mater nurses' application for exemption.[55] As
well as raising salaries, the Award imposed a limit of 112 hours a fort-
night on the nurses' duties and provided statutory off-duty time – one
whole day and one half-day each week. Lectures were still attended in
the nurses' own time. In addition to expense, the reduction in hours
meant that more trainees were needed. They rapidly filled an additional storey at St Mary's Nurses Home.

The growth of the hospitals brought many more Sisters of Mercy
to work on Mater Hill. The temporary convent on the second floor
of the Private Hospital could no longer accommodate them, and, in
any case, increasing demands meant that this space was needed for
patients. During 1925 and 1926, a new convent building was attached
to the western end of the Private Hospital. The convent echoed the
design of the hospital, with the same attention to quality in materials
and construction. As befitted its function, there was less attention to
decoration in the convent building, but beautiful silky oak timber and
leadlighting were used to good effect, particularly near the graceful
staircases linking the floors.

The slightly easier financial climate of the 1920s allowed the Sisters to build a permanent chapel to be the heart of the Mercy mission at the Mater. Planning for the chapel actually began in secret during the First World War. Robin Dods, the architect for the hospital buildings, was consulted even though he had moved to Sydney. The steep Mater hillside posed particular challenges in placing the chapel so that it could be conveniently reached from both the hospital buildings and the new convent. Dods was anxious that 'this job should be as good as human effort can make it'. He favoured a site between the Public Hospital and the Private Hospital, connected to both by cloisters or covered walkways, so that the chapel 'would appear to belong to the whole hospital and not . . . look as if it belonged solely to the private block'.[56] In this plan, Sister Mary Chanel's garden would be a feature, allowing the chapel to 'stand in the centre surrounded by beautiful flowers'.

Compromises had, however, to be made. The chapel design was finalised by the architect, T R Hall, and was built in front of the convent, closer to the Private Hospital than to the Public, using Dods' less favoured concept of connection to the Private Hospital by a continuation of the arcaded front verandah.

Archbishop Duhig also made his views known, and in 1917 Dods wrote to Mother Patrick:

> . . . to meet the express wish of the Archbishop, I have made the whole thing less severe in character, putting some tracery in the windows and suggesting a little ornament here and there, with the result that the Chapel as now designed will be lighter and more ornamental in appearance.[57]

In the end the chapel was, in the view of one of the Sisters, a 'gem of Romanesque architecture' with beautiful decoration. A large stained-glass window of Christ healing the sick child in its mother's arms, placed at the rear of the Altar, was imported from Munich, the statue of Our Lady of the Assumption was selected by Archbishop Duhig in Chicago, and the Carrarra marble statue of St Joseph was imported from Italy. There was also a close connection with the war: the crucifix on the Tabernacle was donated by a Colonel Joss, who had found it in a devastated region of northern France.[58]

By the mid-1920s, the Mater Public was a big hospital. With the addition of another wing containing two large wards and ancillary services, its original forty beds had trebled to 120, in which almost 2,000 patients were treated each year. The honorary medical staff had grown to seventeen and there were three Resident Medical Officers. Although there had been 'masseuses' on the staff for years, the formal 'Massage Department' was opened on 1 January 1923. By 1927 four physiotherapists worked flat out, using a range of equipment which included hot-air machines. The breadth of requests also expanded, with calls for a hospice for those who could not be cured.

The doctors' Clinical Society tackled the emerging medical problems of the day and held at least three meetings each year during the 1920s. Kidney disease was a major concern. In 1924 one-quarter of the 120 deaths in the Public Hospital was attributed to chronic nephritis. The hospital warned that a 'concerted effort must be made to try and stem the tide of a disease annually taking its toll throughout the State, not only of elderly people, but of children and young adults'.[59] However, medical science took another thirty years to unravel the link between kidney disease and phenacitin, a component of popular headache powders.

The extensions to the Mater Public immediately after the First World War had not been cheap. In 1921, the debt on the building account stood at £12,000 and there was also a small deficit in the hospital's operating account. Nevertheless, the Sisters had developed considerable assets at South Brisbane. In 1922, the value of the Mater site was estimated at £50,533.9.3, augmented by judicious investment in nearby property in Stanley Street and Raymond Terrace, valued at almost £14,000 in 1925. By 1929, the land and buildings on and around the Mater site were valued for insurance purposes at £82,785.[60]

Despite the scale of building activity in the 1920s, Mater Hill remained a very pleasant environment:

> The lawns are bright with flowers, the terraces are grassed and planted with flowering shrubs and palms, the cliffs are converted into rock gardens, and shady nooks are filled with ferns and orchids, all of which, combined with the chirping and whistling of birds, tend to

soothe the convalescing patient and carry his thoughts from the city to the bush.[61]

The chirping, whistling birds were, however, to be disturbed once more. Mother Patrick was determined to add a children's hospital to the expanding campus, saying that the pressing need for another children's hospital 'has been urged on the Sisters',[62] doubtless because Brisbane's only paediatric hospital, the Brisbane Children's Hospital, was groaning under the strain. It had treated 3,542 inpatients in 1923, and a further 6,000 children in its outpatients department.[63] There was little chance that the workload would decrease. Peace had revived the city. The population was growing in new suburbs spreading out from the old urban cores of North Brisbane and South Brisbane.

Once again, the Sisters' old friend George Wilkie Gray provided the solution. In 1916, Gray appointed the Sisters as beneficiaries of his life insurances. When Gray died in 1924, these were valued at £2,691.12.0. Gray had also transferred a property, Shalimar, at Sandgate to the Sisters and left them city land which sold for £1,000.[64] The Gray legacy and further success in public fundraising reduced the building debt considerably. Planning for the Mater Children's Hospital could begin in earnest. Even better, it appeared that at last the government was more strongly supportive of health services. The acting premier, W N Gillies, a Presbyterian, said in 1924:

> It has been said that the real test of good government in any country is the high percentage of happy, healthy men, women and children . . . The test of whether a people are highly civilised or have a right to call themselves Christian . . . depends on how they care for the sick and suffering, the aged, and the helpless little children. If higher forms of education do not develop a social conscience among the people, so as to ensure that this [the Mater] and kindred institutions caring for the sufferers shall never want for funds, then we are not advancing.[65]

Mrs E G Theodore, the premier's wife, put her shoulder to the wheel and raised £1,500 for the Children's Hospital in 1927, the year the excavators began work on the new hospital's site facing Annerley

Road. Hall and Prentice, the remaining partners in Robin Dods' practice, designed the building. Work was deferred in 1928 when the Sisters visited children's hospitals in southern Australia to ensure that the new hospital would be thoroughly up to the medical mark. Unfortunately, the prosperity of the 1920s was short-lived and by 1930, when the building was almost complete, the Great Depression was well and truly making its presence felt. The government reduced its annual grant, and most of the people who usually gave so generously were hard pressed to keep their own heads above water financially.

There was no hope of building the large hospital Mother Patrick had planned. However, when the Mater Children's Hospital was officially opened on 6 July 1931, its eighty beds were ready to make a substantial contribution to the health of the city's children. Every bed was occupied immediately. In its first eleven months, the hospital admitted 1,266 patients, drawn from a wide area of southern Queensland, and coped with 7,375 outpatient attendances. A common woe of childhood, respiratory illnesses, accounted for a large number of admissions, as did fashionable tonsillectomies, and the inevitable accidents. More worrying, as far as the long-term health of Queensland children was concerned, were forty-seven admissions for diseases of the kidney and urinary tract. Poliomyelitis topped the list of infectious diseases, with twelve admissions in the first year. Most polio patients stayed in hospital for months, so the Sisters made arrangements for their education to continue at intervals between painful treatments.[66]

Mother Patrick watched Archbishop Duhig lay the foundation stone of the Mater Children's Hospital in 1926, and saw the excavations begin in 1927. Sadly, she did not live to see the Mater Children's Hospital at work. She died on 13 November 1927, aged 78. The funerals of most Religious are quiet affairs; not so Mother Patrick's. She had become so well known in the life of the Church and the city that her funeral procession from St Stephen's Cathedral attracted a huge crowd. The careful selection and training of postulants was a less prominent side of her work, but in doing this, and steadily developing the Congregation to 600 Sisters, she had laid strong foundations for the future development of schools, social works and the hospital. Three new hospitals were a vital part of her legacy. In this, she had ensured that the work of the Sisters of Mercy would be widely appreciated in the Queensland community. In an era when sectarianism divided other communities, Mother Patrick had been a valuable ally to Archbishops Dunne and Duhig in their efforts to resist it in Brisbane. In this sense, Monsignor Byrne could pay her no higher compliment than in saying in his panegyric that she had become a household name.[67]

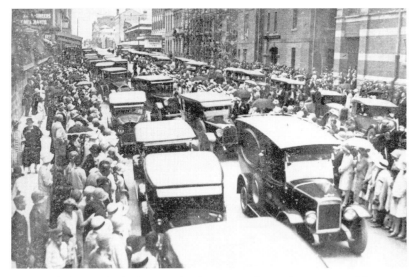

The crowds lining Elizabeth Street for the cortege for Mother Mary Patrick Potter's funeral in 1927. SOMCA

CHAPTER THREE

CHALLENGING MANAGEMENT

In regard to the administration of the Hospital, I wish
to state that owing to the mutual and involved interests
of the hospital in our charge, we intend to hold the
complete administration of the Hospital in our hands.
We shall, however, be glad to have the assistance and
advice of the Honorary Staff at all times.[1]

Sister Mary Ursula Lavery, 1931

In 1931, when the Children's Hospital opened, the Superior of the
Sisters of Mercy was, effectively, the sole point of authority over the
Mater hospitals and the Sisters' schools and social works. However,
the Sisters' ministries were growing larger and more complex. At the
Mater, for instance, services encompassed adult and child health,
public and private hospital care, a rapidly growing religious and lay
nursing service, a developing range of medical specialties, and ancillary services ranging from cancer treatment to physiotherapy. During
the 1930s and 1940s, managing the Mater tested a suite of management prerequisites – conserving and allocating resources, planning
for the future, dispute management and leadership. Even apart from
the effects of a severe economic depression and a world war, life at
the Mater was turbulent, difficult and very unsettling. The death of

MARGARET SALMON was born in County Kilkenny, Ireland, in 1880. She was trained as a teacher at Carysfoot, Dublin, and came to Queensland in November 1902 as one of thirty young Irish girls who responded to an appeal for Sisters for the Queensland mission. After teaching in various Sisters of Mercy schools, including All Hallows', Sister Mary Alban was Mistress of Novices until she became Superior for the first time in 1923. Mother Alban's tall stature, queenly bearing and strict control of the classroom marked her early as a person not to be trifled with. Even though she characteristically removed her spectacles and polished them while she talked, nothing escaped her notice. Many years later, she was recalled as 'one of the really memorable women of the Community'.[2]

Mother Patrick Potter brought to the fore Mother Alban Salmon, a shrewd, determined leader with a strong sense of direction.

Mother Alban had a profound insight into the workings of the human mind, an ability exercised regularly, as some antagonists at the Mater discovered to their cost. In the troublesome years of the 1930s and 1940s, Mother Alban showed herself willing to take substantial risks, yet able to hold her nerve and courageously face major onslaughts. In all that she did, Mother Alban was determined that the Mater would be the phoenix, not the ashes.

Mother Alban's charge was both large and complex. The Mater hospitals were only one part of a spreading Mercy Apostolate. Parish and secondary schools, orphanages and refuges for unmarried mothers, as well as medical services, were in the charge of some 600 Sisters. Taken as a whole, the Sisters of Mercy was a large business. Like any commercial corporation, it needed to turn a profit in order to expand, it had to be accountable to its clients,

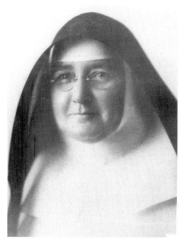

Mother Alban Salmon, who had the unenviable task of guiding the Mater hospitals through the Depression and the Second World War, and then took on the task of raising funds to build the Mater Mothers' Hospital. SOMCA

and it needed strategic plans in order to develop. The Mother Superior retained all decision-making power and control of administrative matters, including finance.[3] Local Superiors in each Mercy convent and the Matrons in each of the Mater hospitals were her branch managers.

In several vital respects the Sisters of Mercy as an entity differed from the commercial model. It had to obey two sets of laws – church law as well as secular law – and its 'stakeholders' were far less easy to identify. They included the Sisters themselves, the church, schoolchildren, patients in the hospitals, children in care, people in need of help and support, and professional staff always pressing for the development of their areas of expertise. The return the Sisters sought to deliver to all these stakeholders – better education, better care and better health – was far more difficult to quantify and to deliver than a merely monetary dividend.

Monetary dividends were very scarce in the 1930s in any business. Although the 1930s Depression was less severe in Queensland than in other parts of Australia, largely due to the strength of its agricultural industries, this Eden for the entrepreneur and Paradise for the worker was, nonetheless, envenomed by unemployment, business failures and

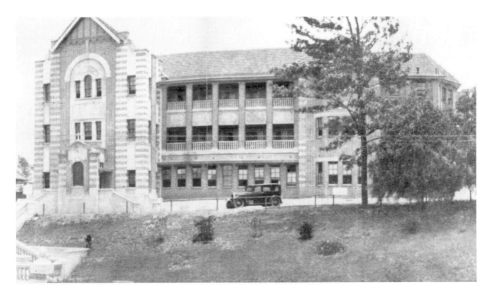

The brand new Mater Children's Hospital in 1931. The imposing entrance façade at left was intended to be balanced by an identical wing, to the right, but could not be built due to financial conditions during the Depression. MHHC

homelessness. By 1931, the effects were felt acutely. The new Children's Hospital was full to the rafters and the daily average number of patients treated in the Mater Public approached 138. Debts on big building projects – the Children's Hospital and extensions to the Public Hospital and the Nurses' Home – remained, and the deficit in the maintenance account had risen to more than £800. Clearly, the government's maintenance grants were insufficient to stem the downward financial slide. Worse was to come. In 1932, the government slashed the maintenance grant to £500.[4]

Careful conservation of the Mater's property assets was important in this situation. In 1927, Mother Alban had managed to resist Archbishop Duhig's request to place the Sisters' property in Archdiocesan ownership. The canon lawyer, the Reverend Dr John English, advised the Sisters that Canon 531 gave religious communities juridical capacity of ownership, and that only Rome could command the Sisters to cede their rights through the vow of obedience. This was fortunate for the Sisters. Land and buildings adjacent to the Mater property,

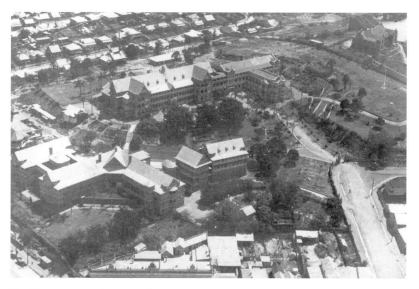

The Mater campus in the early 1930s, showing St Laurence's College at far right and, below it, the landscaped hillside with its paths and walkways. The new Mater Children's Hospital is shown at far left. The entrance gates at centre right led into the main driveway. The vacant space to the left of the gates became the site where Second World War army huts accommodated nurses when St Mary's Nurses Home (centre) became too small. MHHC

acquired over the years with a view to future expansion, had returned valuable rentals. During the Depression, however, the value of the Mater's properties declined and rental incomes fell.[5]

Donations from members of the public still arrived in creditable amounts, but fundraising through public appeals was much more difficult until the Depression began to wane in the mid-1930s. By the end of the decade, public street collections with associated stalls had again become a major means of raising extra revenue. Lay committees and the Sisters were dedicated fundraisers. Sister Mary St Rita Monahan, for instance, when not working in the laboratory, dragooned other Sisters into making goods for street stalls and fetes, growing plants by the thousands, weaving baskets, and collecting stamps which she often soaked in the laboratory sinks. Sister Mary St Rita did much of the work herself. She produced beautiful embossed leather work and ornamental boxes made from old X-ray film. These she sold to anyone who came within reach, including the staff of the old Frost's clothing factory across the road.[6] During the war, her charitable approach extended further. She and Sisters Mary Chanel and Mercia Mary were so moved when a patient was summarily dispatched to exile in the leprosarium on Peel Island in Moreton Bay that for many years they made the trip across the Bay with gifts of cigarettes, soap, and Christmas cakes and puddings made by one of their colleagues, Sister Anne.

There were also more formal events to raise funds during the 1930s. The Mater Ball was always the most celebrated. The 1936 ball, for instance, was extensively advertised on the radio, in the trams which rattled around the city and on the screen at suburban cinemas. Three of the thirteen debutantes in 1936 were trainee nurses – Sue O'Connor, Joan Williams and Jean Shannon.[7] The value of events such as balls, bridge parties and luncheons lay as much in public relations, inculcating and communicating the Mater spirit, as in the money they raised.

However hard the voluntary committees worked, more substantial contributions were urgently required. The corporate sector was an obvious target, as it had been in the past. The radio station 4BH distributed Christmas gifts donated by its audience to patients in the Children's Hospital for the first time in 1932, and maintained this

Christmas generosity for decades. Mother Alban approached Associated Breweries for a substantial donation, because 'the upkeep and expenses are always on the increase, and in reverse ratio, the income drops'. Sometimes, corporate help came unexpectedly. In 1937, a British firm, Morris Industries, sent a cheque for £2,250, one of several donations to Australian charities.[8]

Even though the government grant was reinstated in 1935, and public and corporate appeals were reasonably successful, a more reliable income stream was essential. Debt grew during the Depression, when even fewer patients could pay their fees. The government had taken over all the old secular public hospitals through the *Hospitals Act 1923*, but patients were still expected to pay to the extent of their means. The state covered deficits in its hospitals, but the Mater was on its own, apart from its small maintenance grants. The answer seemed to lie in health insurance.

Health insurance was not new. Various Friendly Societies associated with Masonic Lodges had run medical benefit plans in Brisbane for many years, as they had in other parts of Australia and the United Kingdom. Friendly societies paid medical and hospital expenses for members who contributed weekly subscriptions. Mother Alban saw the Queensland Public Service as an appropriate constituency for the Mater Public and Children's Hospitals Assistance Fund established in 1934. It was, in effect, a 'friendly society' for public servants. There were some similarities with the traditional idea of the voluntary hospital. Subscribers to the Mater scheme would nominate the people entitled to treatment through their subscriptions.[9]

The scheme was to operate on the basis of 'endowed' beds. Treatment in the two Mater public hospitals would be free of charge to subscribers and their nominees. Tetanus treatment, which could cost between £20 and £100 for serum for one patient, and expensive splints for polio patients were not covered. At an average inpatient stay, then seventeen days, Mother Alban calculated that each bed could accommodate twenty-two patients in one year. In the case of individual subscribers, this average might not be maintained, as a prolonged illness might exhaust the endowment for the year. It was equally possible that a series of patients suffering from short illnesses might enable the bed endowment to provide for a greater number. Therefore, each endowment was calculated in terms of 'bed weeks': one year's endowment entitled a nominee to a total of ten weeks' hospitalisation free of charge. Donors or subscribers were to be accorded the additional privilege of extended visiting hours, an incentive particularly attractive to parents, who were restricted to visiting their sick children only on Sunday afternoons, and then only for two hours.

These elements of the scheme might have been workable, but Mother Alban planned an incentive to encourage public servants to join which threw the whole concept into disarray. Subscribers' nominees were promised early admission to hospital, jumping the queue of public patients waiting for beds. This raised the ire of the Mater's honorary doctors who, in an era when patients often faced long waits between outpatient attendance and admission as an inpatient, objected strongly to preferential admission on any grounds other than medical urgency.[10] Doctors in Brisbane were particularly sensitive to any incursion into their areas of responsibility: this was a tense time for the medical profession.

Through the *Hospitals Act 1923* the government had, in effect, taken control of the Brisbane General and Children's Hospitals.[11] For all intents and purposes, state hospitals had become a section of a government department. While the Act's provision that state and local government would finance state hospitals was an undoubted relief, not one doctor was appointed to the board administering the state hospitals in Brisbane and, even worse, its chairman was Charles Edward Chuter, the public servant in charge of health. The General Medical Superintendent, Dr J B McLean, was highly respected by his peers, but he was responsible to the Board, not to the honorary medical staff. This new government arrangement enacted the long-established Labor policy that state hospitals should be controlled and managed by representatives of their owners – the taxpayers of Queensland. The doctors feared that this form of control would imperil their right to choose the most appropriate forms of treatment for their patients. The Mater's structure had clear parallels with the state system. Its administration was controlled entirely by its owners, the Sisters of Mercy, and three separate hospitals – the Mater Public, the Mater Private and the Mater Children's – came under a single administrative structure.

Alarm bells clanged throughout the medical profession. A Royal Commission, appointed by a conservative government in office between 1929 and 1932, appeased the doctors briefly by recommending that the government replace Chuter as chairman with a former Mater honorary, Dr W N Robertson, a distinguished ear, nose and throat surgeon. By 1935, when the doctors' concern about the Mater's contributory health scheme came to a head, the reinstated Labor government intended to replace the honorary system with full-time medical staff in state hospitals. The Brisbane General Hospital staff notified the Mater's Medical Board of their fear of the imminent removal of prestigious honorary appointments.[12] This was a particularly alarming prospect in Depression conditions when medical practice was not particularly remunerative. Honorary appointments continued to be the basis for the reputation upon which many a private practice was based.[13]

In this fraught atmosphere, the apparent challenge to medical authority raised by Mother Alban's plan for preferential treatment for subscribers to the public service health scheme was too much. The doctors enrolled the support of the British Medical Association,

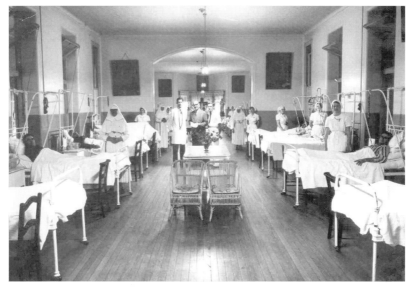

An honorary specialist and a staff doctor photographed in the centre of a ward at the Mater Public Hospital with the Sisters and nurses standing near their patients. Note the patients' marble-topped lockers and the large windows which let in breezes and sunlight. MHHC

an action Mother Alban regarded as an attack on the probity of the Sisters of Mercy. Nevertheless, she believed that 'the doctors' views are not groundless',[14] and agreed that the original scheme would be replaced by a new scheme modelled on those in operation in Victoria and New South Wales. The new scheme allowed ten weeks' treatment in the Public Hospital, valued at £2.17.8 per week, for each contributor, including dependants, but no preferential admission. The value of the rebate on private hospital treatment was less, at £2.9.0 per week. Mother Alban explained this difference as entirely consistent with Mercy objectives:

> Obviously private patients must be prepared to accept less benefit under the scheme than the indigent poor and this is an additional protection for the Public Hospital patient . . . Private patients are of no benefit to the scheme and are only encouraged to join to hold subscriptions for the Public Hospital.[15]

Nevertheless, the new scheme was risky. It would need 18,000 contributors, more than six times the number who had been members of the 1934 scheme. Mother Alban was also well aware that, if health insurance attracted members and therefore more patients for the Mater Public and the Mater Children's Hospitals, accommodation would be insufficient. The scheme was designed to pay benefits: no money would be diverted to buildings. And there was a further risk: neither the hospitals' accommodation nor the scheme's finances could possibly cope with even a mild epidemic, let alone a major catastrophe like the 1919 Spanish influenza.

The new plan was also designed to address another of the doctors' complaints. Many felt that, if an insurance scheme covered a patient's hospital fees, the doctors should be able to charge a fee, albeit at a lower rate than the fee charged to patients in private hospitals. This raised the question of a new class of hospital beds – the 'intermediate' category, which had been foreshadowed by the government in 1929 but not implemented until the Brisbane Women's Hospital opened in 1938.[16] In 1936, Mother Alban introduced intermediate beds for patients who would pay the doctor of their choice at the Mater Public.

In doing this, she was walking a fine line between accommodating the doctors' concerns, which she saw as reasonable, and maintaining the viability of the Mater Private Hospital. In order to maintain the distinction between the Mater Public and the Mater Private, intermediate fees were set at half the level of Mater Private fees.[17]

Discussed for more than a year, these concessions appeared to appease the Mater honoraries' concerns. Dr Ellis Murphy, secretary of the Medical Board for eleven years, felt able to relinquish the position, assuring the honoraries that 'they would always have a sympathetic hearing from the administration', admitting that 'any unpleasantness in the past was in great part due to his own remissness in not keeping more in touch with the management'.[18] Murphy's gracious statement perhaps masked the real problem. The Mater's operations had become large and complex with consequent expansion of the honorary staff, and had outgrown the old structure with its single point of administrative authority, a situation not conducive to effective communication.

The original medical contribution scheme had offended the doctors' professional principle that priority should be given to patients demonstrating the most medical need. An issue over who should decide medical appointments to the Mater had been brewing since 1931 and erupted into a much more bitter dispute in 1935. In this high-stakes game, Mother Alban was determined to keep a firm hold on the winning hand. The doctors' victory in achieving the revision of health insurance to incorporate their views may have given them a false sense of their authority in the hospital. Mother Alban never wavered from her clear view of the role of medical boards in privately owned hospitals. She believed that, rather than merely retaining a power of veto over the Mater's Medical Advisory Board's recommendations, the Congregation had the right to appoint honorary staff against the recommendations of the Board. The Sisters drew up new rules making it perfectly clear that the Board's choice of doctors to fill appointments would be recommendations only – the Sisters would make the decisions.[19]

Although the Medical Advisory Board was wary of the apparent change from the Sisters' power of veto to a power of appointment,

Mother Alban had good reason to be assured of the Board's compliance with her views. Dr Edward Ahern, Dr W F Taylor's successor as president of the Board, said:

> Given the undoubted good faith of both the Staff and the Management there should be no room for anything but amicable association and therefore, although he could not admire the change, he felt that such alterations in the terms of appointments . . . were acceptable conditions under which they could carry out their duties.[20]

Depression conditions made those duties more difficult to perform. Patients flooded the outpatients department instead of attending their private doctors; the hospital was too short of money to appoint additional resident medical officers; and the increasing cost of drugs was a persistent worry. The Board decided to spread its wings and, in 1933 and 1934, appointed subcommittees to investigate ways of increasing the staff and containing the cost of drugs, even though, as Dr Ahern said, it was the Board's policy not to interfere with the actual running of the hospital.[21]

Mother Alban maintained the custom of acceding to Board recommendations wherever possible, and agreed that members of the honorary relieving staff would be appointed by the Board and, after one year's service, be on the same standing as the permanent honoraries when it came to reappointments. This measure of security for relieving staff was important during the Depression, particularly as it coincided with the upheaval arising from the proposal to eliminate the honorary staff system at the Brisbane General Hospital. The whole honorary staff issue became more acute in 1936, when the long-dreaded new *Hospitals Act* was passed.

The Minister, E M Hanlon, had very definite views about the deficiencies of the honorary staff system. He castigated Brisbane General Hospital honoraries in Parliament for their inability to cope with the patient load and their inefficiency in tying up valuable facilities. Some honoraries spent only four hours each week at the hospital, leaving operating theatres idle for much of the remaining time. Hanlon seemed little impressed by the willingness of specialists to give their time free of charge. Instead, he thought that the doctors benefited from the system more than the hospital, through the experience they gained which enabled them to charge large fees to private patients. His remark that there 'is no profession or calling in the world that owes so much to the poor as the medical profession' was particularly wounding.[22]

Hanlon made it clear that he wanted a paid part-time staff so that doctors could be 'sacked if they did not turn up for work on time'. Hanlon's accusation that the doctors at the Brisbane General Hospital ran a closed shop, as evidenced by complaints from young doctors that they could not secure an honorary appointment, put the doctors on red alert. Any thought that the government would exert even more power in the hospital world was anathema to the doctors. They were well aware that the Minister was supported by his new director-general, Sir Raphael Cilento. Cilento, a doctor of formidable intellect who was a strong advocate of centralist departmental control over hospitals, was convinced that there was no room for unpaid staff in a modern hospital.[23] At that time, the medical profession in Brisbane was not large. Most doctors, wherever they worked, knew one another, and their networking was further facilitated by the British Medical Association. Mother Alban stepped into this highly charged atmosphere with another decision: to appoint a small board to advise her directly and to act as a conduit between the Sisters' administration and the honorary staff. This small group would replace both the older, larger Medical Board and the separate board established when the Children's Hospital opened in 1931. The doctors were appalled that at the Mater as well as at the Brisbane General Hospital their influence on hospital management was further curtailed.

Four influential members of the honorary staff were appointed to the new board: Dr P J Kelly, president of the Medical Board, Dr Ellis Murphy, former Board secretary, the orthopaedic surgeon Dr A V Meehan, and Dr H J Windsor, president of the Children's Hospital Board.[24] The honorary staff, however, wanted nothing less than an advisory board elected by and from their own membership. Doctors Kelly and Meehan arranged to meet Mother Alban to put the proposal which, they said, would 'prevent the honorary medical staff from feeling that they are completely cut off from the Administration'. Mother Alban,

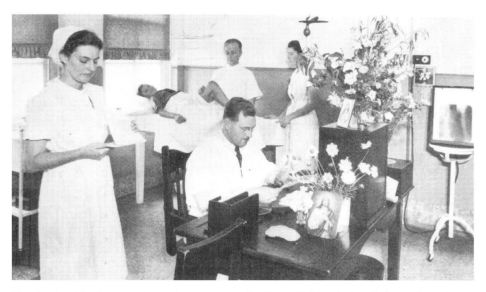

Working hard in the outpatients department at the Mater Children's Hospital. Dr John Lahz sits at the desk while an orderly and a nurse attend the patient on the examination bed behind him. MHHC

in her usual direct and forthright manner, put her objection that 'if this were done it may happen that someone quite unsuitable might be elected'. She was convinced that Board members should be 'practical Catholics' so that the hospitals could be 'Catholic in atmosphere'.[25]

Her major concern was the developing specialty of gynaecology. It was becoming clear that the addition of further specialties to the Mater Public's honorary staff could not be deferred indefinitely. The development of birth-control methods, and the view among some doctors that pregnancies could be terminated in exceptional circumstances, brought medical science into conflict with church law. Non-Catholic doctors could be exempt from church law; a Catholic hospital could not. This was one of many issues, which grew in number in the second half of the twentieth century, in which the junction between medicine and the Church could be difficult to navigate.

Any suggestion of sectarianism was destined to become a hot issue. The old spectre of the strict separation of church and state in Queensland also emerged. A E Moore, leader of the Opposition, contended in Parliament that a hospital which received even a modicum of government funding should be blind to religious adherence.[26]

Moore read from a letter in which the honorary staff addressed their complaints to the Reverend Dr John English who, as administrator of the Archdiocese, was Archbishop Duhig's right-hand man. Mother Alban was suffering from the horror of any administrator in contentious times – an appeal from disgruntled staff to a higher authority!

The new Advisory Board pressed on, agreeing with Mother Alban's proposal that orthopaedics should be established in the Public Hospital with an allocation of ten beds. This brought the Mater Public into alignment with the Mater Children's, where A V Meehan had been appointed honorary orthopaedic surgeon when the hospital opened in 1931. The honoraries were enraged that a department of orthopaedics would be created without prior consultation. They also rejected Board endorsement of Mother Alban's suggestion that honorary staff should retire at 60 in order to make way for younger doctors.[27]

It became quite clear that the staff had never accepted the Advisory Board concept, its constitution, or its role in representing both the Mater Public and the Mater Children's hospitals. In this, the Mater followed the model established by the Brisbane and South Coasts Hospitals Board when it amalgamated the administration of all hospitals under one board on which government representatives held sway. Any idea that management matters should be discussed with the full medical staff was regarded by Mother Alban as hopelesssly inefficient; any suggestion that the Sisters should relinquish control of appointments or, for that matter, full decision-making power, she resisted absolutely:

> Members [of the honorary staff] must realise that the Sisters of Mercy have interests and duties (not always of a temporal nature) which might not be understood by all members of the Staff, and for this reason alone, it is necessary that these interests be adequately safeguarded by an Advisory Board on which the Sisters are fully represented.[28]

The medical staff representatives on the Advisory Board resigned, an action Mother Alban found 'incomprehensible', and one she described in a letter to all members of the medical staff as likely to be the result of 'some grave misunderstanding'.[29]

These troubled waters needed much oil. Mother Alban conceded two important points. She delegated administrative authority while she was overseas in 1937 to the Reverend Dr John English, on the strict understanding that the Sisters' line on honorary appointments and control of the hospital would be maintained. Dr English relayed her promise that the 'monster of sectarianism' would be expunged in future appointments, and that the Advisory Board would be enlarged to include more elected representatives, four from the Mater Public and two from the Mater Children's. There would not, however, be separate boards for the two public hospitals and the Advisory Board would remain strictly advisory. In a move the Sisters saw as facilitating 'a complete and abiding understanding', this refashioned seven-member board was, however, to have a lay chairman.[30] The doctors, perhaps with the Brisbane General Hospital example of a lay chairman at the forefront of their consciousness, regarded these concessions as completely inadequate.

Mother Alban pressed ahead: the new Advisory Board was appointed in 1938. The honorary staff unsheathed their ultimate weapon. They resigned. In doing this, they went a step further than the medical staff at the Brisbane General Hospital, who had threatened resignation in their contest with the government in 1936.[31] But Mother Alban had not come this far only to retreat. The new Board met for the first time on 25 March 1938, with a formidable task on its agenda: processing applications to fill the vacant positions. This it somehow accomplished within a few months. Mother Alban accepted all the Board's recommendations.[32]

The dispute did not end without public controversy. There were reports in the press in Brisbane and Sydney, further discussion in Parliament, and a need to reassure the Apostolic Delegate in Sydney that Archbishop Duhig had been kept fully informed and had counselled her to maintain control. If they conceded authority over the hospital, the Sisters would be, Mother Alban said, 'failing in our first duty to the Institute of the Sisters of Mercy and the Catholic Church'.[33] The Apostolic Delegate was reassuring:

I completely approve of the course of action which you have outlined in your letter; and I congratulate you on the stand that you have taken . . . God will bless your work and make it prosper, despite opposition.[34]

In the end, the honoraries' resignations were an ill wind. Many highly respected doctors disappeared, but considerable good did come to the Mater with the new appointees. They included doctors who became very important in the hospitals' future development: the orthopaedic surgeons Dr A V Meehan (who reapplied) and Dr John Lahz, the obstetrician and gynaecologist Dr M J Eakin, and a resident medical officer, Dr H W Noble, a future Minister for Health. Perhaps most importantly of all, the Mater under challenge has always seemed able to produce remarkable people. One of the most memorable in its first century was a Brisbane solicitor J P Kelly, the layman appointed to chair the new Advisory Board, a position he held for decades with courage and decisiveness, wisdom and geniality.

The clash between the Sisters and the honorary medical staff was, in many ways, a great shame. In addition to their individual expertise in treating patients, the Mater's honorary staff had made substantial contributions to the hospitals' medical reputation, with, as Sister Gertrude Mary later remarked, 'only the prayers of the Sisters for remuneration'.[35] Clinical meetings were held regularly, the medical records systems at both hospitals had been modernised and refined, plans were laid in the 1930s for a blood bank, and a postgraduate committee had assisted in training young doctors in the specialties. The doctors and the Mater had, as a young paediatrician later recounted, a 'sort of love–hate relationship with love triumphant in the end'.[36]

It is likely that this prolonged controversy had sorely tested Mother Alban. The less serious dispute over the medical insurance scheme had left a wound so deep that Mother Alban later revealed that, in 1935, the Sisters had considered relinquishing the hospitals to lay control.[37] In 1938, Mother Alban had to face the additional strain of concern among the Sisters at the Mater. Through their daily work they had come to admire many of the doctors who resigned. Mother Alban sought to explain the position in an open letter to the Sisters, revealing that the situation had been referred to ecclesiastical authority, and to three separate sources of lay opinion. All had been of one mind that 'the Sisters of Mercy must decide between keeping control of their institution or handing it over to the medical staff'.[38] It had not really been a choice.

Sisters in departments and wards had helped to steady the ship during the storms of conflict. While disputes raged, the work of the hospitals continued and developed. Many of the Sisters of Mercy of this era were among the longest serving and most remarkable of the Mater Sisters. In many ways, it was still a very Irish community. Superiors from the All Hallows' Congregation frequently made the trip to Ireland to inspire young aspirants to the religious life to join them in Brisbane. Many groups of Irish postulants arrived.

Sister Mary Cletus Gibney arrived from Ireland in 1915, after having completed nine months' nursing at Mullingar hospital. She completed her training at the Mater. Always quiet and unassuming, Sister Mary Cletus held a variety of positions in her nursing career. She worked as a ward sister and in the laboratory with Sister Mary Chanel, and became Tutor Sister in 1947 when Sister Mary Chanel died. She never saw her beloved Ireland again, and remarked wistfully that 'I

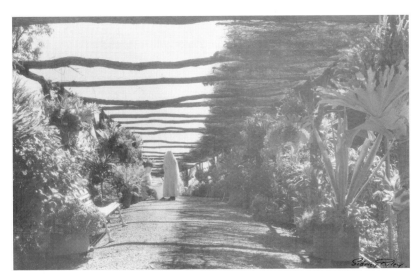

The hill on the St Laurence's College side of the Mater grounds was beautifully landscaped through the hard physical effort of the early Sisters, particularly Mother de Chantal James and Sister Mary Chanel. This lovely walkway was an appropriate place for quiet reflection. SOMCA

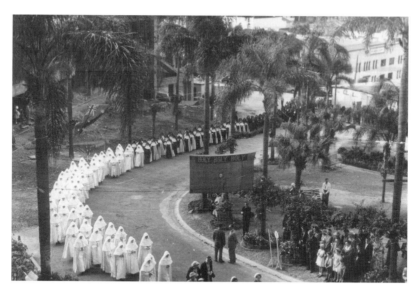

Important Church festivals were celebrated at the Mater. This Corpus Christi procession winds its way up the main drive in the 1950s, with the site works for the Mater Mothers' Hospital visible at left rear, and the old Army huts where nurses on night duty slept visible at right rear. MHHC

won't be travelling but my soul will pass through old Ireland on its way to heaven'.[39] Sister Gertrude Mary Lyons wanted to be a teacher, not a nurse. She was born in Roscommon in 1906. Feeling that she was going to the end of the world, Sister Gertrude Mary arrived in Brisbane in 1924 with forty-eight other postulants. In 1927, she was sent to the Mater to train as a nurse, a direction which did not appeal to her at all. Nevertheless, she responded to Matron Sister Mary Dominica Phelan's excellent training at the Mater Private and became a first-rate theatre sister for thirty years. Always known as 'Gertie', she was much admired by the surgeons. Sister Mary Bride, born in Ireland in 1901, was another identity at the Mater Private Hospital, where she reigned over Ward 1. She was highly regarded as a head injury nurse and set up the first intensive care unit in a small area of Ward 1.[40]

Many of the Queensland-born Sisters of this era were country girls. Sister Mary Winifrede, a Mater identity for fifty-three years, was born in Winton; Sister Mary Christopher Weidmann from Warwick was one of the North Quay nurses who moved with the Mater to South Brisbane. She managed Outpatients for almost forty years, between 1925 and

1963. Sister Mary St Roch, born in Roma, had a varied career. She was a tutor in nursing and a relieving Matron, but was most remembered for helping to develop electrocardiograph and electro-encepholograph services, and medical photography.

Many sections of the hospitals were expanded and improved during the 1930s, despite the Depression and the hospital's administrative conflicts. At Mother Alban's request, the radiologist Dr B L W Clarke examined new equipment for the over-strained X-ray department. He recommended a four-valve Solus outfit with an electric refrigerator connected to the drying rack to ensure the control of temperature of the chemical solutions necessary to produce a first-class X-ray film. This, Dr Clarke thought, would eliminate scratching on the films, which occurred when ice in a tank was used.[41]

As well as developments in pharmacy, pathology and radiology, the hospital underwent physical expansion during the 1930s. The convent was extended in 1932 to accommodate growing numbers of Sisters and, in major extensions between 1934 and 1937, a new wing was added to the eastern end of the Private Hospital. This provided additional private rooms, twenty-four ward beds, another lift, a nurses' station, a pantry, a utility room, bathrooms, toilets, storage, and staff dining rooms on the ground floor. This major extension required considerable rearrangements. The operating theatres were demolished, and two grand new theatres were completed by August 1937. The new patient accommodation was modern and comfortable with built-in wardrobes, fluorescent lighting and windows to floor level. All the new rooms opened to balconies with beautiful views of the city.[42] The Mater Private had become Brisbane's largest private hospital and, under Matron Sister Mary Dominica Phelan's exacting regime, highly respected by both patients and admitting doctors, particularly the surgeons.

Surgery and pathology benefited from innovations at the Mater Public in the late 1930s. A new three-storey wing was linked to the main building by its ground and sub-ground floors which accommodated, at long last, a larger laboratory. One of the new operating theatres was air-conditioned and contained a students' observation gallery, claimed to be the first of its kind in Australia. The surgeons

SISTER MERCIA MARY HIGGINS helped to pioneer new directions. A doctor's daughter, she was a trained pharmacist when she
entered the Sisters of Mercy in 1926. She was a devoted reader
of history, whodunits and P G Wodehouse, and was originally
sent to work as a biochemist in the laboratory with Sister Mary
Chanel. However, she always wanted to develop pharmaceutical services at the hospital and to train young Sisters in hospital
pharmacy, a lofty aim as there was no training course in Australia
for this sub-specialty in the early 1930s. With the company of
her pet cats Izzy and Sammy, she worked more or less patiently
in the laboratory, biding her time. Mother Alban, with her characteristic eye on the future, supported the idea, but it did not
became a reality until 1941 when Sisters Mary Conrad and Mary
Agnese became fully trained hospital pharmacists.

wore microphones on their coats to broadcast to observers in the
gallery.[43]

The new theatre was a key part of another of Mother Alban's plans
for the future. She was determined that the Mater would become a clinical school for the University of Queensland's new Faculty of Medicine.
After abortive attempts to establish a medical school in Queensland,
dating back to the 1880s, Dr W N Robertson chaired the University
Committee which finally established the medical school. The Mater's
old friend, Dr J V Duhig, was a committee member. The medical course
began in 1936. Fully supported by the honorary medical staff on this
occasion, Mother Alban put her pitch to the registrar of the university
with a comprehensive report on the hospital's facilities. In the Mater
Public and Mater Children's, there were, she said, 250 beds, shortly
to be increased to 300, with fifty gynaecological beds. In 1935, 4,554
patients had passed through the hospital, 3,818 operations had been
performed, and 10,101 outpatients and 2,611 casualties were treated.
Mother Alban also pointed out that the Mater had Queensland's first
hospital pathology department and the first cancer clinic.

In Mother Alban's view, there was no reason why a privately owned
public hospital could not be a clinical school in Queensland in the

same way as had Mercy hospitals in southern states, particularly as her hospitals were 'supported with a minimum of cost to the people of the State, and, in fact, the continual expansion . . . has been carried out largely with monies from profits earned by the Mater Misericordiae Private Hospital'.[44] Teaching needs could be easily accommodated. In addition to the splendid new operating theatre, pathology facilities were already available to conduct post-mortem examinations, and lecture rooms were being modified to accommodate seventy students.[45] Despite these preparations, clinical teaching was confined to state hospitals until 1949. The Mater finally achieved its goal at this time and began clinical teaching because the Brisbane General Hospital could not cope with the large numbers of students in the post-war boom.

The government had readily spent taxpayer funds on the long-delayed University of Queensland medical school but was far less enthusiastic about improving the education of nurses. The ninety trainees at the Mater during the 1930s shared with trainees in other hospitals the experience of a restricted academic syllabus, and only 112 hours of formal lectures spread over four years. Long working hours in the wards certainly provided excellent practical experience, but it was very much like apprenticeship training rather than education for a profession. However, there were compensations. The experience of living together in the nurses' home, with its strictly enforced curfew and mandatory standards of behaviour, developed a strong sense of camaraderie cemented by long-lasting friendships. Many trainees were former students at Sisters of Mercy schools. The Mercy 'family spirit' remained strong in the Mater Past Nurses Association.[46]

Plans to improve nurse education generally had to wait until after the Second World War. Japan's entry into the war signalled danger to the Queensland public and changes were made at the Mater to accommodate the emergency. The top floor at the Mater Children's was vacated and prepared for war casualties. Lists of patients who could be discharged at a moment's notice were rigorously maintained in case the hospitals were suddenly inundated with casualties. In all three hospitals, windows were blacked out with paper, blast-proof walls were erected and the precious stained-glass windows in the chapel were removed and stored safely. The obligatory sand-bagging around the buildings obscured the noble architecture, and hastily erected air-raid shelters replaced the tennis courts at the back of the Private Hospital. Many of the doctors – honoraries at the two public hospitals and private practitioners at the private hospital – disappeared on war service. Many Sisters also found their lives changed. Sister Mercia Mary Higgins was enlisted to teach chemistry at All Hallows' and sick Sisters were evacuated to Gympie with Sister Gertrude Mary dispatched to care for them.

Even the most trying conditions generate benefits. The new pathology laboratory, opened in 1941, was reasonably spacious. There was even a special animal house for Sister Mary Chanel's guinea pigs. Work in the pharmacy and the laboratory became as hectic as patient care in the wards. Sister Mary Chanel and Sister Mercia Mary continually pressed Mother Alban for more staff, but staff shortages were widespread. Sister Mercia Mary later commented that, 'if we had £1 for every time we have been thrown out of Rev Mother's office, we would have enough money to build the lab'.[47]

Somehow they managed not only the laboratory work but also the new blood transfusion service. Once a week, donors gathered in the late afternoons at a special unit set up in the former ear, nose and throat area of the Mater Children's. Laboratory and nursing staff processed the donations under Dr George Taylor's watchful eye, and the blood was dispatched to the soldiers in New Guinea during the night.[48] The Mater laboratory staff also benefited from the American 42nd General Hospital which had taken over the Yeerongpilly experimental station, not far away. Its modern laboratories included facilities for serology research. There, Dr Merkel trained Sisters Mary Chanel and Mercia Mary and helped to set up modern testing at the Mater.

The end of the war brought a very special group of patients to the Mater: repatriated prisoners of war from Japanese prison camps. The untimely deaths of friends and relatives had brought the tragedy of war to Mater people, and the strain on the hospitals had made wartime difficulties an ever-present challenge, but the presence of these soldiers reinforced the reality that the costs of war are a long-term legacy.

Many plans for development were deferred during the war. By the end of 1945, the Mater was moving from a very difficult fifteen years into a hectic period. Mother Alban had a saying for testing times: 'There's a great big God in Heaven and the birds will sing again'.[49] The Mater was fortunate that, in the post-war era, J P Kelly was there to help orchestrate the chorus.

PART TWO

GROWING UP

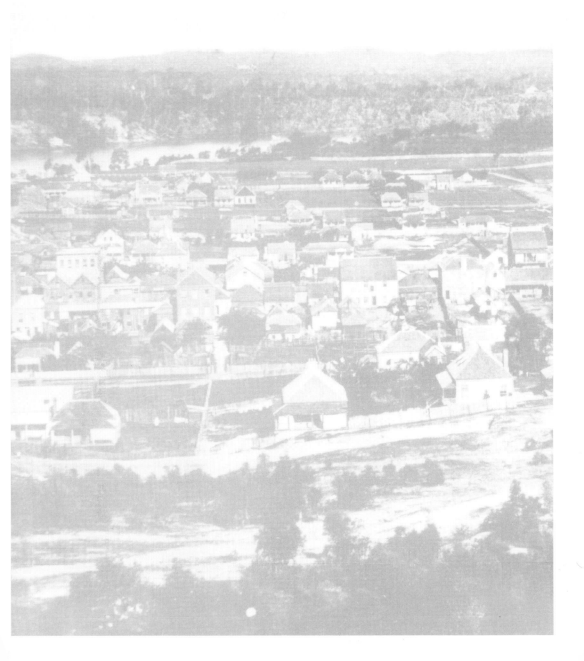

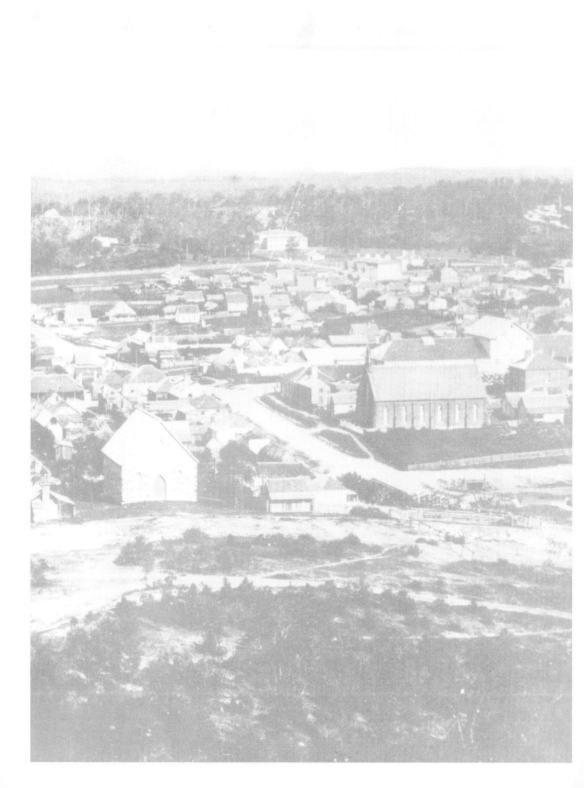

CHAPTER FOUR

MAKING A LARGE BRICK STATEMENT

I have already intimated to you (and I now renew the intimation) that our Catholic people will be prepared to stand by you in any financial obligations you incur to give Brisbane a first class maternity hospital. All that is needed is to establish and put into action an organisation for the collecting of funds for so worthy a purpose.[1]

Archbishop Duhig, 1946

In making this bold assertion to Mother Alban, Archbishop Duhig put his stamp on an exciting and innovative period in the Mater's history. As a strategic platform, the ambitious maternity hospital proposal offered several important opportunities to enlarge the Mater's presence. It would round out the services available on Mater Hill to provide care from birth to death; in an era when building families was a widely promoted community value, it could increase the Mater's popularity in the community generally; it was a valuable means of ensuring that Catholic values would be visibly expressed in the sensitive areas of conception and fertility; and it would make a bold statement that a private organisation offering public hospital services should be supported by government. The downside to this investment in the future was the Archbishop's statement that financing a new maternity hospital would be the responsibility of the Sisters of Mercy. Building the Mater Mothers' Hospital was a high-risk venture. Raising the necessary finance made the period between the end of the Second World War and the admission of the first patients to the Mater Mothers' early in 1961 an extremely difficult and, in many ways, dangerous era for both the Mater and the Sisters of Mercy.

The maternity hospital idea was at least a decade older than its public announcement in 1946. Mother Alban, who had directed Mater affairs since 1927, had a clear vision of the way in which Mercy ideals could be furthered and was an able strategist in putting the necessary steps in place. Good strategists always plan ahead. As early as 1935, Mother Alban wrote to the Queensland government, pointing out the need for a maternity hospital on Brisbane's growing south-side. The new hospital would, she said, also provide training in obstetrics for the Mater's resident medical officers. In this, Mother Alban anticipated the requirements of the 1943 amendments to the *Hospitals Act 1936* which required all graduating doctors to spend their year as resident medical officers in public hospitals with obstetric beds.[2] This focus on medical education was entirely consistent with the Mater's efforts before the war to be a clinical school for the University of Queensland's new medical course. To be a 'university' hospital would, of course, further entrench the Mater as a necessary part of Queensland's hospital network. Mother Alban even had a location in mind – the area where an additional wing for the Mater Children's had been planned but not constructed because of tight finances during the Depression.[3]

During the war, expansionist plans had to take a backseat to keeping the existing hospitals going. Local politics indicated that the climate after the war would not be easy for the Mater: there were worrying signs that the Queensland government was becoming even firmer in its determination that it alone would own and manage public hospitals. On a visit to the hospital during the war, the Health Minister, T A Foley, told Mother Alban that the government was 'entirely opposed' to public hospitals owned by private organisations.[4] This determination to maintain the nationalisation of health services was, to the Catholic

Church, a deeply worrying sign, made worse by unsettling signs from the Commonwealth government.

The Commonwealth government acquired the power to tax income during the war to finance the war effort. In peacetime, income taxation gave the Commonwealth the financial clout to intrude in fields reserved for the states under the Australian federal Constitution. At the end of the war, the Chifley Labor government acted on its platform to extend Commonwealth control into spheres ranging from banking to health care. New Commonwealth medical benefits legislation effectively ensured that treatment in public hospitals would be free of charge.[5] Until the Commonwealth Hospital Benefits Scheme came into effect, treatment in Queensland public hospitals was not free. All patients were 'means tested' to assess the fee they should pay. The Queensland government paid a small maintenance grant, one shilling per public patient per day, for public patients at the Mater; remaining costs were met from Sisters of Mercy funds. The Commonwealth benefit for public hospital patients was much larger – six shillings per day – which covered all costs, thus introducing free public hospitals to Australia, a concept that rapidly became a sacred cow in Queensland.

In its negotiations with the Commonwealth over the new arrangements, the Queensland government did not acknowledge the Mater's status as Queensland's second largest public hospital. Indeed, the Health Minister informed the Commonwealth that all public hospitals in Queensland were owned and managed by the government. J P Kelly later recalled his emergency dash to the Brisbane General Post Office on 31 December 1945 to telegraph the prime minister, Ben Chifley, and all members of the federal Cabinet, to set the record straight. To the Queensland government's chagrin, Chifley stepped in on 27 January 1946 and instructed the Queensland government to recognise the Mater public hospitals and ensure that the Commonwealth benefit scheme applied to them.[6]

Nevertheless, government control of health services at both federal and state level alarmed the Mater. 'Socialisation' appeared to indicate that private enterprise would be reduced or eliminated in a variety of areas, and raised more fundamental ideological issues. In many ways, the Second World War had been a contest of ideologies. The western democracies waged their battle against fascism in an atmosphere of fear that the Communist Soviet Union, a convenient and necessary ally during the war, would become a foe during the peace. The end of the war did not, therefore, bring any cessation to ideological conflict. The Roman Catholic Church interpreted the Communist threat in a much wider and somewhat insidious context: the godlessness of socialism pervading many aspects of life in the free world. As far as the Mater was concerned, socialism's most worrying and dangerous manifestation was the increasing trend towards the nationalisation of health services. The Sisters saw themselves as having a role in demonstrating that private organisations could be players in public health care. It was also a means of keeping Christian, specifically Catholic, values to the forefront. The idea of a Mater maternity hospital was a key to success in this area. Dr Matthew Eakin, chairman of the Mater Mothers Appeal, referred more than once to contemporary social and political conditions which threatened to 'undermine the sacredness of Christian motherhood'.[7]

The state government was certainly taking motherhood seriously. Maternity care had been one of its priorities since 1922. Maternity wings at district hospitals, and maternity wards in smaller hospitals, were built all over Queensland. The Brisbane Women's Hospital, which opened in 1938 to replace the old Lady Bowen Hospital on Wickham Terrace, was the ninety-fifth new maternity facility. Competition from the government's new hospital had severely affected the network of small, private maternity hospitals dotted through Brisbane's suburbs. One by one they began to close. Although the quality of these hospitals varied considerably, they had provided much of the city's maternity care in an era when the local general practitioner, rather than a specialist obstetrician, delivered most of the babies. The new Brisbane Women's Hospital had no hope of coping with the gap left by the demise of the small hospitals, let alone the baby boom that began as soon as the war was over. By 1945, the last year of the war, the daily average of patients at the Women's Hospital was 216, in a hospital with a bed capacity of 160.[8] Another hospital was badly needed.

The Mater's maternity hospital proposal resurfaced very shortly after the war. Early in 1946, Mother Alban sought the advice of the specialist hospital architects Stephenson and Turner on the pre-requisites for a maternity hospital. They reported that appropriate accommodation for babies was particularly important. The hospital would need four different types of nurseries – one for healthy babies, another for babies who were ill, a third for babies with infections, and a fourth for premature infants. Mothers were not forgotten: the architects recommended that they have an entirely separate entrance.[9] The Mater's long-standing, trusted architects, Hall and Phillips, accompanied by Sister Mary Marcelline, studied facilities in maternity hospitals in Sydney and Melbourne in the middle months of 1946.

Quite apart from design and structural requirements, Hall and Phillips' report confirmed that the baby business was booming in post-war Australia. In the 1940s, Queensland's birth rate, 23.5 per 1,000 of the population, was its highest since the 1911–1920 decade, only to rise to 24 per 1,000 in the 1950s.[10] The Mercy Maternity Hospital in Melbourne, originally designed for 22 patients, was very overcrowded with 45 patients, and the North Sydney Mater was struggling to cope with 70 patients and 150 deliveries each month in accommodation designed for 49. Hall and Phillips recommended that any new hospital in Brisbane include ample antenatal accommodation, public beds in four-bed units rather than Nightingale wards, soundproofing in the nurseries, and a separate milk-preparation area where the highest standards of hygiene could be maintained. A separate laundry was also recommended for the babies' washing.[11]

With preliminary planning for the new hospital well in hand, Archbishop Duhig stepped in. He was concerned that Brisbane was the only Australian capital city without a Catholic maternity hospital and was well aware that the Mater's ambition to be a clinical training school was in jeopardy if it could not provide obstetric training. The Archbishop dismissed Mother Alban's concern that the projected cost of the hospital, thought to be well over £100,000, was beyond the Sisters of Mercy. He commanded: 'This obstacle must not be allowed to stand in the way of a work so urgently needed'.[12] Archbishop Duhig had a fundraising plan. Clergy would not be represented on the appeal committee. This would be a project for the laity because it 'was not a matter for the priest or the pulpit', and too vast a project

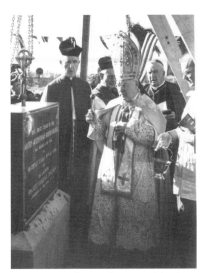

Cardinal Spellman of New York laying the foundation stone of the Mater Mothers' Hospital on 16 May 1948, supported by Monsignor Molony (left) and Monsignor Jordan (right). MHHC

to be managed at parish level. The women's organisation, the Catholic United Services Auxiliary (CUSA), which had raised funds for comforts for the troops and to support soldiers' families, seemed an appropriate model. In October 1946, immediately after Archbishop Duhig and Mother Alban had met to confirm that the Sisters would build the hospital, CUSA was to be disbanded at a meeting in the Brisbane City Hall, leaving experienced fundraisers available for the new project. In assigning a large role to the laity, Archbishop Duhig hoped to reinforce the point that this would be a hospital for the whole community and not just for the Catholic faithful.[13]

The organisation for raising funds was one of the most innovative aspects of the Mater Mothers' project. The fundraising plan achieved several important goals, in addition to its

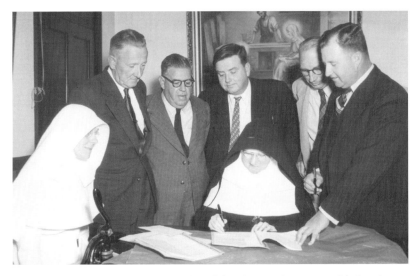

At last, Mother Norbert Byrne, Superior of the Sisters of Mercy, could sign the Mater Mothers' construction contract, surrounded by, from left, Sister Mary St Margaret, Mr Charles Butcher (the builder), Mr K D Morris, Mr John P Kelly, and the architects, Mr Lionel Phillips and Mr Noel Wilson. MHHC

DR MATTHEW EAKIN was appointed Honorary Assistant Gynaecologist to the Mater Public Hospital in 1938. He resigned his appointment at the Brisbane Women's Hospital to accept the position at the Mater. Dr Eakin had been a general practitioner before becoming an obstetrician and gynaecologist. He became a member of the Mater's Medical Advisory Board and the Advisory Management Board. He had wider community interests as co-founder of the Xavier Society for Crippled Children and a member of the Queensland Branch of the United Services Auxiliary. He chaired the Mater Appeal for more than fourteen years. The Sisters of Mercy commissioned a portrait of Dr Eakin by the renowned Australian artist Sir William Dargie, in recognition of Dr Eakin's selfless service to the Mater Appeal. Dr Eakin was supported in his work by his wife Mrs Eakin, particularly during her term as publicity officer for the Mater Public Hospital's Ladies Auxiliary.

obvious aim of making the new hospital possible. The Mater Mothers' Appeal made the Mater more widely known in the general community and consolidated esprit de corps among Mater people, particularly the various voluntary auxiliary committees. Events moved quickly. In November 1946, a public meeting to open fundraising was held at All Hallows'. At this meeting, two of the Mater Mothers' Appeal's most successful appointments were revealed. The gynaecologist Dr Matthew Eakin was appointed to chair the appeal,[14] and Mr John Ohlrich was appointed organising secretary. In Ohlrich's capable hands, the appeal reached widely into Queensland cities and towns.

A grand foundation stone ceremony on 16 May 1948 put the prospect of a new maternity hospital squarely before the public. Cardinal Spellman of New York performed the ceremony with Archbishop Duhig. Even E M Hanlon, by then the Queensland premier, appeared to swallow governmental pride to support the appeal. 'Providing hospitals is not an easy task,' he stated at the ceremony, and continued, 'You may ask, "can we afford them?" I ask myself, "can we afford to do without them?" There is nothing more important to this country than providing accommodation for mothers.'[15] Like the Archbishop, however, Hanlon was only too happy for others to fund the new hospital.

Despite the public fanfare which opened the appeal, the going was slow in the first few years, notwithstanding the huge commitment of voluntary work, spread among a range of activities, which attracted a wide support base. Although art unions eventually dominated public perceptions of Mater fundraising, the success of voluntary and less prominent fundraising activities can be measured both by the significant levels of money they raised – it was reported in 1966 that these activities had raised more money than the art unions – and by the breadth of the support they achieved.[16] The long queue for tickets for the first fashion parade at the Princes Café in 1948 caused a traffic jam in Queen Street; bottle and rag drives reached a different section of the community; social functions in people's homes reached others; a Younger Set concentrated on party-going youth; the Green Shop was established in a corner of a verandah at St Mary's Nurses Home to sell gifts and refreshments; the Mater fetes brought people to the hospital grounds; chocolate wheels and raffles were taken to country shows; and there were many, many street collections.[17]

These activities raised the initial target of £100,000 within the first three years, but, at that rate, £1,000,000 – a more realistic costing than the £100,000 estimated in 1946 – would take years to accumulate. There were even some rumblings of concern about where the funds had gone when nothing more tangible than a foundation stone had appeared.[18] Clearly, something more had to be done if the public was not to lose confidence in the project, particularly as the ill-fated scheme to build the Holy Name Cathedral was still fresh in the minds of Brisbane Catholics. Finally, on 30 April 1952, a few months after Mother Alban's death, a contract was signed with the builders K D Morris. The financial situation dictated that it be a cost-plus contract, with the shell of the building to be completed first, and each storey fitted out as funds became available.

The brick shell slowly rose in a prominent position facing Stanley Street with its back intruding into the Sisters' garden. It was soon clear that much more than £1,000,000 would be needed, but the government steadfastly refused to offer any form of subsidy for capital works.

Late in 1952, shortly after the contract was signed, ready money totalled £66,000 in bonds, a total of £34,000 in fixed deposits, £22,000 in the Mater Mothers' Hospital public hospital general account, with a balance of £4,313.15.6 in the Green Shop account.[19] The Mater Appeal obviously needed a bright new look. Art unions, which had been successful in raising funds for the first hospitals at Mater Hill, seemed to provide the answer.

John McCann was appointed to direct this major means of raising funds. He came from a background in advertising and the media and had used an art union to raise £80,000 to build a memorial hall for the Southport Sub-branch of the Returned Servicemen's League.[20] McCann's background, experience and flair for public relations were important in the art unions' public relations success, scarcely less important than the money they raised. Mater art unions became widely known in Queensland; the urge to buy tickets even percolated into other states, doubtless helped by a number of interstate winners. The first art unions offered cars, caravans and boats as prizes. Australia's own car, the Holden, featured prominently in the prizes in the early 1950s. Humour was frequently used. In one advertisement in 1955, an ersatz headline proclaimed: 'Art Union will cause traffic problems in Brisbane'. In brief, punchy text, the advertisement claimed that cars would be falling into the laps of Brisbane people. The SPCL – revealed as the Society for the Prevention of Cruelty to Laps – was 'interviewed' about the consequences of three Holden cars landing in people's laps.[21] At a mere two shillings a ticket, Brisbane flocked to the call to be in it to win it.

If the cars were a success, better was to come. Ownership of a Holden car, the first motor vehicle to be mass-produced in Australia, was an aspiration shared by most Australians in the early post-war era, but home ownership was an even larger and more widely shared dream. For many, a home of their own appeared an impossible goal. Personal finances were not usually the problem. Although few ex-servicemen left the military with any significant level of savings, employment was easy to find whether in the cities or the country. The real difficulty was the backlog in house building which had accumulated during the Depression and war. This deficit was aggravated by a shortage of building materials, which took more than a decade after the war to clear. Many young post-war couples began married life living with relatives or in unsatisfactory rental accommodation. When the baby boom was in full swing, existing housing was bursting at the seams.

Older houses, many of which were dilapidated after the Depression and war, had little appeal. The mood was modern. Many Australians had acquired a taste for things American from their encounter with American troops on the home front during the war and from their love affair with American movies. From the mid-1950s, the lifestyle of American families in their fresh, up-to-date houses, with built-in kitchens and sleek labour-saving appliances, entered the consciousness of young Australians through their television screens. Portrayals of happy parents and children in comfortable suburban houses suited the family formation mood of the 1950s and inserted a subliminal message which supported the aim of the Mater art unions – a sparkling modern hospital where the children could be born and the mothers well cared for.

The Mater appeal hit on a winning formula. The art unions would offer as first prize a fully furnished home, equipped with everything from a brand new washing machine to a packet of porridge. Even better, those who purchased an entire book of tickets would be eligible for the ticket-seller's prize, usually a car to put in the new home's beautiful new garage. In a decade of domestic fantasy, these would be dreams come true. The Mater Prize Home Art Union chalked up another first for the Mater – it was Queensland's first real estate art union. The first Mater Home Art Union in 1954 tested the water. The house in Birt Street, Surfers Paradise, was a modest two-bedroom fibro house valued at £4,150. The organisation for selling the tickets was anything but sophisticated. There was no real mailing list; sixty door-to-door salesmen were employed to door-knock. The innovative home art union concept then hit a hitch. The Queensland legislation regulating art unions made no provision for real estate prizes. There was no such prohibition in other Australian states and the Queensland Act was quickly amended with bipartisan support on 1 April 1954.[22] Although the government was determined not to provide any capital subsidy towards building the new hospital, it was very supportive of the Mater art unions, perhaps regarding them as a way of dissipating requests for government support.

With legal obstacles overcome, Mater Prize Homes were an instant hit. The appeal committee realised that ticket buyers would best be attracted by a really good house with a spectacular new feature not previously seen in Brisbane. Architectural innovation was not the aim. The Mater homes deliberately provided features sought by people hoping to settle in the city's newer suburbs. As the years went by, such features included double garages, cocktail bars, en suite bathrooms and rumpus rooms. The developers of new suburbs were deliberately targeted by the Mater appeal organisers. They drove a hard bargain in securing donations of land, building materials and all necessary fittings. In return for their gifts, donors' company names were prominently featured in extensive advertising for each art union.

The Mater Home program was intensive. At least three houses were offered each year. By the mid-1960s, an average of 90,000 people visited each prize home. Between 200,000 and 300,000 tickets were sold in each art union, and about 40 per cent of all winners came from

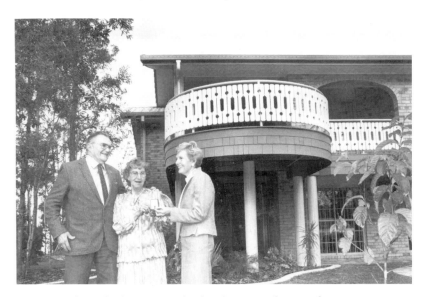

Mater art union prize homes remained an important feature of Mater fundraising. Here, Mrs Andrea Ahern, the Premier's wife (at right) presents the keys to the 150th Mater prize home to the lucky winners, Mr and Mrs Dorst. MHHC

interstate. This was deep market penetration. So popular did tours of the homes become that in the mid-1960s a tour of a Mater Home was Brisbane's third most popular weekend activity following visits to Mt Coot-tha and Lone Pine. Some prize winners were a marketer's dream. Prize Home Number 15 in Fernlea Street, Chermside, was won by a widow with seven children, another house was won by a homeless man, and another by a recently arrived immigrant from Ethiopia who moved his wife and children from immigrant accommodation into the large prize home.[23] These stories and the exciting features of each house made good copy for newspapers and alluring film for television.

This level of community acceptance was irresistible to politicians. A steady stream of Cabinet ministers presented Prize Home keys to happy winners. Their willingness to be present for the cameras did not, however, translate into increased subsidies. There was little change in Queensland's health and hospital policies when the longstanding Labor government lost power in 1957. Many Catholic politicians and voters had deserted the Labor party which they suspected had come under the influence of Communist trade unionists. However, the Country Party–Liberal Party coalition government showed no softening of governmental determination not to fund the new hospital. Shortly after the new government took office, Dr H W Noble, Minister for Health and Home Affairs and a former Mater resident medical officer, informed the Sisters that there would be no increase in subsidy, with the soothing but vague promise that the Mater's request would be reconsidered when the state's budgetary position improved.[24]

The Sisters had to turn elsewhere. The art unions and other fundraising had harvested £800,000 by 1956, well short of the daunting sum – by then estimated at £2,000,000 – needed to complete the Mater Mothers'. The Mater's bankers, the Commercial Banking Company of Sydney, refused the Sisters' request for loan funding to complete the hospital and the government made the situation even more serious by refusing to guarantee a loan.[25] A frantic search for financial accommodation ensued. The ANZ Bank at last came to the party and, what was more, offered very favourable terms. Mother Damian Duncombe,

Mother Alban's successor, was less than pleased with the previous bank's performance and closed the Sisters' accounts:

> Our decision to close the account in your bank arises solely from our need to borrow a substantial sum of money for the completion of the Mater Mothers' Hospital . . . Application was made to your own principals first, as the CBC, Fortitude Valley Branch, had handled the whole of our Appeal Funds . . . we have raised and spent over £800,000 to date. The application was refused and in the intervening two years we have kept negotiating in other quarters. Now that we are to be accommodated without mortgage, in common justice we should channel as much of our business as possible to the Bank undertaking to make the loan.[26]

But even this was not enough. With Archbishop Duhig's support, the Sisters asked the Apostolic Delegate for permission to approach the Sacred Congregation of Religious to borrow £500,000 to complete the Mater Mothers', offering the whole of the existing hospital as security for the loan. It appeared very likely that art unions and other fundraising would raise £150,000 each year, so the Sisters undertook to repay the loan within four years.[27] This was only one of the challenges Mother Damian tackled head-on in the 1950s and 1960s.

Government intransigence in refusing to provide any form of capital subsidy was politically risky. The Mater's own fundraising efforts were widely popular with the community and were disseminating the 'Mater message' ever more widely. J P Kelly, chairman of the Advisory Board,

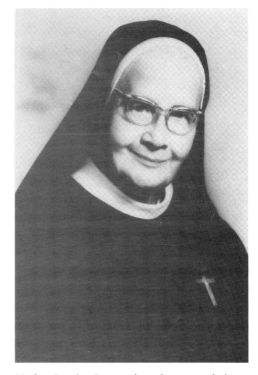

Mother Damian Duncombe, who succeeded Mother Alban Salmon and oversaw the completion of the Mater Mothers' Hospital. SOMCA

MARY ELIZABETH DUNCOMBE, CBE, was born in Hughenden in 1899. When her father died in 1907, her mother bought and managed the Royal Hotel in Hughenden. The young Molly Duncombe was sent to St Mary's School in Ipswich where she became the school's first State Scholarship candidate, making her secondary education at All Hallows' possible. She won a teacher's scholarship to the University of Queensland, but wanted to enter the Sisters of Mercy. Her mother thought she was too young, so her entry was postponed until 1927. The young Sister Mary Damian taught at All Hallows' until 1944 when she became Mother Superior at the Mater, and in 1950 its first Sister Administrator. She was passionately interested in the Mater Mothers' Hospital, and continued to take a close interest in it after she was elected Superior of the Brisbane Congregation. Mother Damian broke new ground. She started the McAuley Teachers' College, reflecting her determination that the young Sisters would be educated, established the Sisters' mission in New Guinea, and built cottage homes at St Vincent's orphanage. She was a shrewd, able administrator, with a keen interest in new ideas and new methods. She became the first Mother General of the Sisters of Mercy in 1954, and first president of the Australian Federation of Sisters of Mercy in 1957. Mother Damian had some very human traits: she was known to keep international aircraft waiting, and she loved photography and tape-recording. On her death in 1980, a successor remembered her as, in many ways, 'our Pope John XXIII . . . she broke the manacles of time-honoured habits and customs and freed us to grow to full stature as religious women . . . she could think no thoughts but big thoughts'. She was, however, usually very strict and always intolerant of the fearful and faint-hearted.

continued to broadcast the simple proposition that the Mater Hospitals were essential facilities for the whole community and deserved the support of the government as well as of the public. Kelly was not a man to pull his punches. He was a sage and shrewd advisor in legal,

JOHN PATRICK KELLY, OBE, LLB, was born in Brisbane on 15 February 1907. He received his primary education first from the Sisters of Mercy on Thursday Island when his policeman father was stationed there, and then from the Christian Brothers at St James' School, Fortitude Valley, and St Joseph's College, Gregory Terrace. He became school captain and captain of the cricket and football teams, as well as representing 'Terrace' in swimming and athletics. He went on to play rugby league for Wests for several years and to represent Queensland in rugby union. J P Kelly graduated in Law at the University of Queensland in 1930 and was admitted as a barrister in 1932. He was admitted as a solicitor in 1934 and established his own firm, J P Kelly and Co., in 1939. Archbishop Duhig invited Kelly to his residence, Wynberg, to encourage him to accept the Sisters' invitation to chair the Medical Advisory Board at the Mater. Kelly went on to chair the new management Advisory Board established in 1958. His commitment of time to the Mater was very generous, taking at least one day each week. By 1963, for instance, he attended twelve meetings each month, provided legal advice, and conducted negotiations for finance and property acquisitions.

Kelly retained a broad interest in community life. He contributed articles to legal journals, was president of the Christian Brothers' Old Boys Association, founder of the Aquinas Library, a foundation member of the Queensland Literature Board of Review in 1954, and its chairman in 1958. Kelly demonstrated his belief in the lay apostolate through his involvement in lay activities and his support for Catholic Action. He was awarded the OBE in 1966. He was a large man, usually presenting a serious demeanour, but known to have a wry, understated sense of humour. He often chaired board meetings sitting with his arms folded across his chest, eyes closed, apparently asleep, only to open his eyes and sum up the discussion in one short statement.

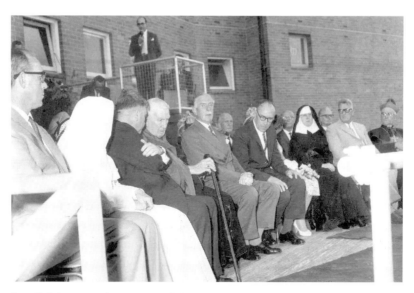

The official party at the opening of the Mater Mothers' Hospital: from left, the Lord Mayor of Brisbane, Sir Reginald Groom, Mother de Chantal James, Mr John P Kelly, chairman of the Mater Advisory Board, Archbishop Sir James Duhig, the Governor, Sir Henry Abel Smith, Dr M J Eakin, Lady May Abel Smith (obscured), Mother Marcella McCormick, the Premier of Queensland, Sir Francis Nicklin, and Archbishop Patrick O'Donnell. MHHC

administrative and business affairs and an ardent advocate for the Mater at all times and in all quarters.[28]

Kelly's speech at the Mater Mothers' opening ceremony in December 1960, and the special booklet commemorating the opening, provided ideal platforms for Kelly to expound his views before a general audience.[29] Kelly stated his belief that the Queensland government's determination to maintain a free hospital service – the other states had abandoned the idea in the early 1950s – had an inevitable consequence: Queensland state hospitals were languishing behind modern hospital standards. They were under-funded, under-staffed, under-developed, under-equipped, and inundated with patients.

Times were certainly grim at the Brisbane Women's Hospital in the early 1960s. The hospital had been gravely overcrowded since the war. The labour ward, where only curtains separated the patients, had come to be known as the 'stables' and the wards as the 'paddocks'; paint was peeling off the walls, floor coverings were buckling.[30] In contrast, the Mater Mothers' Hospital was modern and sparkling when it admitted its first patients on 2 February 1961, exactly fifty years since the first patients were admitted to the Mater adult Public Hospital. Nineteen sixty-one was also the centenary of the Sisters' arrival in Queensland.

The Mater Mothers' building was designed to capture breezes and to allow sweeping views of the city from the balconies on the upper floors. There was accommodation for 140 mothers, and the necessary ancillary departments such as physiotherapy, pathology and X-ray. The special laundry for the babies' washing, foreshadowed in the earliest plans, was included. The Green Shop had its own space on the ground floor, near the main entrance and the lifts. The physiotherapy department, the records store, the nurses' recreation room and the plant room were on the first floor. Antenatal and postnatal care, pathology and X-ray were installed on the second floor, with the kitchen, cold rooms, nurses' dining rooms, staff room, mortuary, and special laundry for babies' clothes. The third floor accommodated service functions such as the central enquiry desk and administrative offices, the nurses' lecture room, the Sisters' refectory, as well as four-bed wards, nurseries and the Chapel. On the fourth floor, there were several two-bed wards, nurseries, a pantry, sterilising rooms and bathrooms. Single private hospital rooms, isolation wards, labour

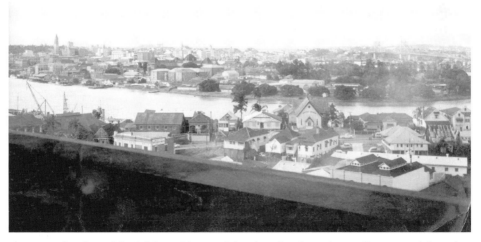

A spectacular view of the Brisbane River and the city taken from the top-floor verandah as the shell of the Mater Mothers' Hospital neared completion in the late 1950s. The Story Bridge can been seen at centre right, and the Brisbane City Hall tower at centre left. MHHC

wards and nurseries were on the fifth floor. There were more labour wards on the sixth floor, with preparation rooms, operating theatres, a special transfusion room, two special nurseries for premature and frail babies, change and rest rooms for doctors and sleeping accommodation for fourteen Sisters of Mercy. The seventh floor housed the lay nursing staff.[31] The hospital was designed to accommodate seventy public and seventy private patients and to cater for their needs with eight delivery rooms and two operating theatres.

The new hospital was greeted warmly by the public and the press. A large press photograph of the first baby born at the Mater Mothers', Maree Cathleen Carr, began a series of supportive articles about mothers and babies, portraying the facilities and the work at the Mater Mothers' Hospital very positively. The new hospital helped the Mater to elevate its clinical and research profile. This up-to-date image was essential. The world-wide growth in demand for hospital services, discernible before the Second World War, accelerated in the post-war decades. Public perception of hospitals had changed and people had come to regard hospital care as a right. As Queensland government 'free

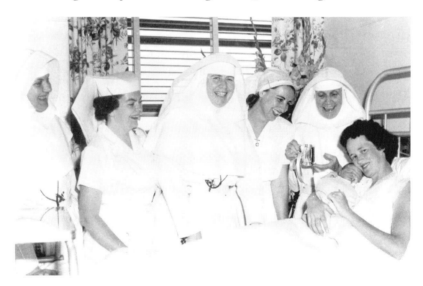

A proud and happy day. Maree Cathleen Carr, the first baby born at the Mater Mothers' Hospital, at 1.15 am on 2 February 1961, pictured with her mother, Mrs D H Carr of Graceville and, next to her, Sister Mary Audrey Lucy who presented a silver christening mug to Maree, with Sister Mary Romauld Johnson, centre, Sister Magdalen Mary Slack, at left, and two of the midwifery staff. MHHC

hospitals' policy reflected, public hospitals were regarded as public utilities rather than charitable enterprises.

New techniques based on science and technology affected health care from diagnosis to cure and introduced more sophisticated and expensive health services. Health care became more centralised and many of the services, such as obstetric care and some general surgery, previously provided by general practitioners in their surgeries, became based on specialist practice in hospitals. Ratios of patients to staff rose, with consequent pressure on nursing and medical staffs and, of course, on costs. The status of the medical profession rose when medical practice became more sophisticated.

The Sisters of Mercy planned to staff the new hospital with Sisters who had completed their midwifery qualifications, as well as lay midwives. Several Sisters acquired those qualifications in the years immediately preceding the opening of the new hospital. Sister Josephine Crawford, for instance, underwent Maternal and Child Welfare training in Brisbane. Practical work at the Inala clinic demonstrated to her how much the population in the Mater's catchment area, Brisbane's southern and south-eastern suburbs, had grown.[32] Sister Josephine and Sister Jacinta Weidmann then undertook midwifery training in Sydney with Sister Peg Slack, who was refreshing her qualifications. Sister Jill Stringer had completed her midwifery training at the Royal Women's Hospital in Melbourne before entering the Sisters of Mercy in 1959. A midwifery training program under Sister Josephine Flynn as nurse educator was introduced; forty-three graduates from the Mater training school were the first to enter midwifery training.[33]

The Matron, Sister Mary Audrey, presided over a very busy first year at the new hospital. Although many of the staff felt 'pretty raw', they supported each other and a family atmosphere rapidly developed. When Sister Jill Stringer was posted to the Mothers' hospital in 1963 to replace the highly experienced Sister Mary St Margaret, for instance, she was conscious that about five years had elapsed since she had worked in a maternity hospital. She was joined by two junior midwives, Sister Madonna Josey and Sister Fay McMeniman.[34] There was plenty of opportunity to become very experienced indeed – 2,996 babies were born in the first year, and the pace did not slacken. A

Sister of Mercy attended each birth. The junior religious Sisters also relieved Sisters of Mercy in their wards – the third floor one day, the fourth the next and so on – it was 'a good way of learning'.[35] All the nursing staff, religious and lay alike, and the medical staff, eight honorary medical officers and the first two registrars, Gresley Lukin and Clem Marrinan, were run off their feet.

The hospital soon recorded significant achievements and began to carve out a reputation for exceptional neonatal care. On Christmas Eve 1963, Antonina Vecchio was born weighing just 1 lb 10½ oz (750 grams) and needed blood transfusions to survive. She was only one of many frail babies whose astonishing stories captivated the newspaper-reading public. A tiny baby girl won the hearts of Sisters Peg Slack and Josephine Crawford. They called her 'Millie', for milligram. 'Millie' was born at about twenty-six weeks gestation, at that time thought to be too early to survive. She weighed 1 lb 1 oz and, much to everyone's amazement, was ready to start on Kate Campbell's condensed-milk feeding regime. 'Millie' slowly grew. Each week the doctors had a small wager on her weight gain. Eventually, 'Millie' was strong enough to leave hospital, but returned to visit the Sisters at various times as she was growing up.[36] Such achievements do not rest only on the skill of the medical and nursing staff. A culture valuing research and innovation, both in the exercise of techniques and in the adoption of new technologies, is even more important.

The problems which arise when a baby's Rhesus positive blood conflicts with the mother's Rhesus negative blood stimulated an early research interest. In 1961, the hospital's first year, Dr John Dique made his private laboratory available for research projects and began to train the staff in the difficult and risky procedure of exchanging a baby's entire blood supply.[37] This technique brought some startling results. In 1968, twin boys, Leonardo and Eduardo Scalione, both affected by Rh incompatibility, had fifteen complete blood transfusions in the first five days after they were born eight weeks prematurely in March; two months later, they both weighed more than 2.5 kilograms and were able to leave hospital. Exchange transfusions were also used for other purposes. In 1964, for instance, three premature babies suffering from jaundice were successfully treated by transfusion. All weighed less than

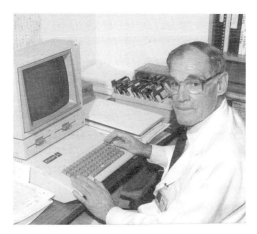

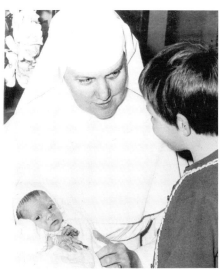

Dr Edwin Esler, first medical superintendent of the Mater Mothers' Hospital. A prisoner of the Japanese during the Second World War, Dr Esler became a consultant obstetrician at the Mater Mothers' Hospital when it opened, and was appointed Medical Superintendent twelve years later. MHHC

Sister Magdalen Mary with John Cuskelly, first baby to survive an inter-uterine transfusion at the Mater Mothers' Hospital, and his proud older sister. MHHC

one kilogram and needed exchange transfusions to remove dangerous bile pigments because their organs were not sufficiently developed.[38]

Blood transfusions before birth were a startling development. In 1967, John Cuskelly made history by needing three blood transfusions *in utero* to defeat the consequences of Rh incompatibility, a process helped not only by sophisticated pathology but also by the new image intensifier in the hospital's X-ray department.[39] He was the first baby in Queensland to benefit from the procedure. Specialised equipment, sophisticated pathology and X-ray procedures in neonatal medicine were expensive. However, donations of equipment, such as the Isolette in 1964, an intensive-care infant incubator with controlled air circulation, continued the vital voluntary fundraising work of the Ladies Auxiliary.

Research was emphasised in the hospital's early days, stimulated by its agreement to be a teaching hospital for the University of Queensland. Each section at the Mater Mothers' Hospital was encouraged to undertake its own research projects. In 1964–65, for instance, a survey examining the incidence of anaemia in pregnancy was underway, as well as studies of placental function by urinary oestriol assay and the use of Isoxuprine Hydrochloride in preventing and treating premature labour.[40]

The Mater Mothers' was under pressure almost from the moment it opened its doors. Within three months of the first birth, the third-floor nursery was overcrowded; between eighty and one hundred patients were seen in the antenatal clinics, and the ward treating women with complications of pregnancy was struggling to keep up with demand. The Mater Mothers' was not alone in dealing with these pressures. In a growing city with only two public maternity hospitals, keeping up with the demands of a high birth rate was always a challenge. In 1961, a sub-committee appointed by the Health Department to report on antenatal care in the Brisbane metropolitan area found that, in growing suburbs at some distance from the city centre, there was a need for antenatal centres staffed by the hospital to which the patient would be admitted.[41]

This was only one of the schemes devised during the 1960s and 1970s to deal with the medical needs of a rapidly growing city, which for many years had been serviced by only two public hospital groups, the large state 'base' hospital on the north side of the river, and the

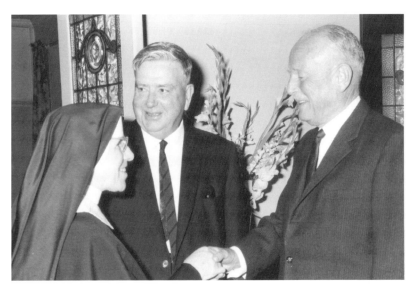

A happy occasion at the Mater Mothers' Hospital in the 1960s. Mother Benigna Burke shakes hands with the Governor of Queensland, Sir Alan Mansfield, while Mr John P Kelly looks on. SOMCA

Mater on its southern side. The opening of the Mater Mothers' Hospital elevated the Mater campus into a large and complex hospital system providing 232 adult public beds, outpatient clinics in almost all medical specialties, a 103-bed children's hospital, a maternity hospital with seventy public and seventy private beds, and a private general hospital with 135 beds. The Mater Mothers' was both a medical and a public relations triumph which elevated the Mater in public estimation and began to wear down the government's hospital policy. However, the three older Mater hospitals had been in the shadow of the new hospital during the 1950s and early 1960s. Cracks were beginning to show in their fabric, imperilling the standard of care they could deliver.

CHAPTER FIVE

NAVIGATING TURBULENCE

The Sisters of Mercy record at the Mater, plus the story of the Mater Mothers, puts us not in the position of mendicants, but of co-partners with the government in the provision of vital public hospital services. In the matter of capital expenditure, we feel that one of the partners has not made its share of proper contributions.[1]

Sister Angela Mary Doyle, 1971

In that blunt statement in a letter to the Health Minister, Sister Angela Mary summed up an old argument the Mater was determined to win. Striving to build a new Mater Adult Hospital and to extend the Mater Children's Hospital, the two projects which dominated the 1960s and 1970s, required great resolve in persuading the government to accept the Mater's argument that it should fund all capital expenditure on public hospitals. It also required shrewdness in balancing competing demands and adroitness in walking financial tightropes. These difficult times brought to the fore many of the characteristics that had moulded the history of the hospitals since the early years of the century. This period of rebuilding, restructuring and repositioning required tenacity in maintaining the Sisters of Mercy's mission to the needy, courage in taking enormous risks in achieving goals, imagination in devising ways and means, and flexibility in accepting compromise when all other avenues were exhausted. In navigating these choppy waters, Sister Angela Mary and J P Kelly made a formidable team.

Tumult in both the Church and the wider society did not make these difficult times at the Mater any easier. The decades immediately after the war have often been dismissed as bland, unimaginative, peaceful and prosperous years in Australia, a time when culture and invention languished and political debate was predictable, even uninteresting. If this were ever true, the dull years were certainly over by the mid-1960s. Even though stability and prosperity appeared to be national keynotes, the Australian population had not been standing still. The earliest of the post-war baby-boom children reached their late teenage and young adult years in the mid-1960s, just in time to be sent to fight in Vietnam, or to stay at home to protest against the war. This generation of Australians was the most highly educated in the nation's history. The baby boomers grew up in a climate of almost full employment, with every expectation that the job of their choice would be available. Family prosperity had been translated into the steady acquisition of material goods, including motor cars that took increasing numbers of people in the pursuit of recreation at the end of the working week rather than to religious observances. Australia, like most of the rest of the world, was rapidly becoming an ever-more secular society.[2]

Unlike the depression and war generations, most baby boomers were supported by the security of a comfortable domestic world and had the time and the freedom to question the assumptions of the national milieu. Young Australians were not alone in challenging the status quo. People of all ages in the democracies were becoming more vocal, challenging everything from unsatisfactory consumer goods to racial discrimination, inequalities affecting women in the workforce and government policies. 'People power' was rapidly growing and, in its more extreme forms, developing a head of steam soon to be released in upheavals around the western world. Notions of human rights were expressed not only in the general sense of social justice but also in the individual realm of personal rights. The Mater was as much affected by this mood of challenge and questioning as any other institution. The Sisters of Mercy, however, were also affected by winds of change in the Catholic Church which permanently changed church life and the lives of all priests and religious.

In many ways the Second Vatican Council called by Pope John XXIII in 1959 reflected the tenor of its times. Religious orders had changed little in either their internal organisation or their external appearance from the nineteenth century until the 1950s when Pope Pius XII exhorted them to adapt their ways to the conditions of modern life. American women religious needed little encouragement and had called for further opportunities for education in the professions before the Second Vatican Council met. A compromise between reform and the conservatism that pulled against the tide of modernism is discernible in the Decree on the Appropriate Renewal of Religious Life approved by the Council on 28 October 1965.[3]

Religious orders embraced enthusiastically the five principles of the decree, which called them to return to scripture, to embrace the charism of their founders, to be integrated fully into the church's renewal and mission, to be equipped to interact prophetically with the contemporary world and to ensure that religious life is always primarily ordered to the following of Christ.[4] These pronouncements emerged at the same time as the women's movement demanded greater opportunities for women in higher education, the workforce and all secular power structures. Some women Religious became leaders of women's movements; others took their place in the leadership of the professions; many became increasingly engaged in social justice issues ranging from racism to the amelioration of poverty; and some left their orders altogether. In a world of burgeoning career opportunities, many young women who might once have entered religious orders found worthwhile paths in the secular world.

Leadership by women had been a fact of life at the Mater since the establishment of the first hospital in 1906. In 1966, when the draughts from Vatican II were beginning to gust, Mother Damian chose the young, Irish-born Sister Angela Mary Doyle to succeed Sister Mary St Gabriel as Sister Administrator of the Mater hospitals. Sister Angela Mary had high hopes of a teaching career when she left

Ireland in 1946. She had no desire whatever to be a nurse, but, as was the practice in all religious orders in the 1940s, the wishes of her then Superior, Mother Alban Salmon, were unquestioned and immediately obeyed. Similarly, Sister Angela Mary obeyed Mother Damian's request that she succeed Sister Mary St Gabriel.

SISTER ANGELA MARY DOYLE, AO, FCNA, FAIM, B. Bus, was born in County Clare, Ireland, in 1925, one of a large family growing up on a farm during the Second World War. She was a young novice in 1946 when she responded to a call for more Sisters of Mercy to come to Brisbane. Although she had trained as a teacher in 1948 she was despatched to the Mater to train as a nurse. After completing her training in the early 1950s, Sister Angela Mary spent most of her nursing years in the adult hospital, including stimulating times in the operating theatres.

Sister Angela Mary completed her Diploma in Nursing Administration at the College of Nursing in Brisbane in 1964. However, hospital administration, rather than nursing administration, was to be her forté. She was Administrator of the Mater hospitals for twenty-two years. Sister Angela Mary realised that she needed education in business management and, after part-time study, graduated with a Bachelor of Business from the Queensland University of Technology. She retired from the chief executive position at the Mater in 1987 and became Senior Director of Health Services for the Brisbane Congregation of the Sisters of Mercy. In this role she developed many community outreach services and became president of the Catholic Health Care Association in 1988. In response to the continuing need to raise funds for research and new health care services, she became executive director of the Mater Trust between 1993 and 1997, and served on the Trust board.

In recognition of her achievements at the Mater, her leadership in hospital administration and her pioneering work in the care of AIDS patients and support for their families, Sister Angela Mary was awarded an honorary doctorate degree by Griffith

University in 1991 and the Queensland University of Technology in 1997. She was a member of the Council of Griffith University as well as an advisor to its School of Social and Industrial Administration and its School of Nursing. Sister Angela Mary's advocacy for the Mater, and her flair for public relations, made her a well-known figure in Queensland, in demand for speaking engagements and radio interviews. She was made Queenslander of the Year in 1989 and Queensland Woman of the 80s in 1992, and won an Advance Australia award in 1993 and a Queensland Premier's Millenium Award for Excellence. Sister Angela Mary was awarded the Order of Australia in 1994, and became one of the five inaugural Queensland 'Greats'.

During all her years of service, Sister Angela Mary was impelled by a strong sense of the Sisters of Mercy's mission to the disadvantaged and the suffering, and by the Mercy vision of the goal of health care, which, as she once expressed it, is to 'treat each patient as a unique composite, a unity of spirit and matter, soul and body, fashioned in the image of God and destined to live forever'. Her strong sense of the Mercy mission embraces all creeds. Attracted by its philosophy that differences between people should be reconciled by loving action rather than useless talk, Sister Angela Mary became a member of the Buddhist Tzu Chi foundation and in 2002 visited Master Cheng Yan of Tzu Chi in Hualien, eastern Taiwan. The relationship between the Mater and the Tzu Chi foundation extended to hosting Tzu Chi Collegiate Youth Foundation training camps at the Mater to provide young members with practical experience.

Sister Angela Mary's small slight figure, bright blue eyes, happy smile and ready wit are seen and appreciated at the Mater in the twenty-first century.

In being appointed Sister Administrator, Sister Angela Mary had been plucked from familiar work in the Mater Adult Hospital, where she was remembered as a quiet, almost retiring person, and deposited on a precipitous learning curve. It was, in many ways, a terrifying slope, perhaps made even more so by the isolation she felt in a lonely office on the third floor of the Mater Mothers' Hospital. She realised almost immediately that she had very little idea of what she was expected to do, let alone how to do it. The new Sister Administrator had many anguished moments during the subsequent two decades, but realised she had to convey the sense that she knew where the hospital was going so that others would be confident.[5] In her long term as Administrator, Sister Angela Mary demonstrated that she was an able and willing inheritor of her predecessors' determination to guide the Mater in the Mercy way. She was innovative in facing change and grasping opportunities; she was willing to take advice; she was courageous in taking huge risks in forging new directions; she was resolute in holding her ground when governments sought to shake it, and even to try to take it. Above all, she was prepared to face dispute in her own community, and in the hospital at large, when unpopular decisions had to be made.

First, however, Sister Angela Mary had to come to grips with managing a hospital system that was under pressure everywhere she looked. The enormous commitment of time, energy and resources that had produced the Mater Mothers' Hospital had rather tended to put the three earlier Mater hospitals in the shade. The Mater Private was in great demand and needed to expand its services, particularly for surgical patients, but of more serious concern was the fact that the two public hospitals were, like the state public hospitals, overcrowded and facing a real threat that the rapidly modernising medical world might pass them by. The urgent need to deal with the deficiencies at the Adult and Children's hospitals was paramount.

The difficulties facing the older Mater hospitals had been squarely on the table before the Mothers' Hospital opened its doors in 1961. In 1959, there were 232 beds, including thirty-five intermediate beds in the Adult Hospital, and 103 beds and a few intermediate beds in the Children's Hospital.[6] Both hospitals ran outpatient clinics and casualty departments. Each hospital had its own medical and surgical departments, and there were joint orthopaedic, neurology, urology, dermatology, psychiatry and ear, nose and throat departments and, at the Adult Hospital, gynaecology and ophthalmology. The hospitals shared

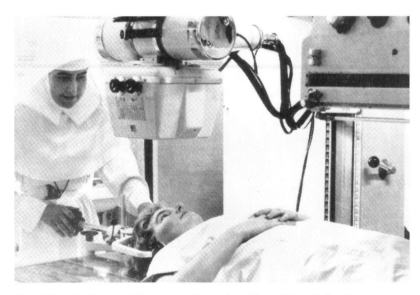

Sister Eileen Pollard working as a radiographer. Sister Eileen Pollard became an agent for change in nurse education and, in the 1980s, managed the accreditation process for the Mater Private Hospital. MHHC

speech therapy, pathology, pharmacy, radiology and anaesthetics, with some additional honorary anaesthetists at the Adult Hospital.

All wards, all departments and all ancillary services were always flat out. Conditions were far from ideal. Ironically, the new Mothers' Hospital added to the strain at the Mater Children's which received babies needing medical and surgical treatment. Stretchers, or temporary beds, were frequently used. Ever since the war, the turnover of patients had been as rapid as possible in both public hospitals, partly due to improved techniques and therapies, but mainly to enable Mater people to keep their 'heads above water' and accept all patients needing admission.[7] Honorary specialists competed for bed allocations, and many wards were shared between specialties. In Ward 8 at the Adult Hospital, for instance, growing numbers of ophthalmology patients shared the space with patients using Queensland's first neurosurgery and neurology service.

Accommodation, even for essential services, was also far from adequate. The Sisters recognised that the efficiency of the hospital would be inhibited unless basic services could be urgently upgraded. The pathology department, still in the 'new' laboratory area opened in 1941, was identified as the department suffering most from lack of space and shortage of staff. The possibilities for improved treatment offered by advances in haematology, biochemistry, microbiology and histology were exciting, but imposed great demands on staff, equip-

ment and accommodation. By the mid-1960s, the pathology department, in many ways the engine room of modern medicine, was 'cramped beyond description'.[8] New developments in everything from 'pap' smear tests for cervical cancer to more detailed analyses of blood had become routine, vastly increasing the workload.

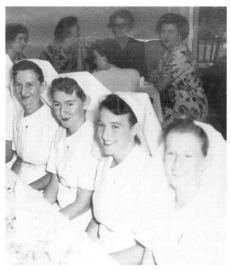

1949 nursing graduates, from right, Betty Kennedy, Madge Bowers (Sister Mary Gregory), Audrey Cronin, Val Percival. MHHC

The qualified staff had also grown. As early as 1949, when married women found life in the workforce far from easy, the Mater demonstrated that it was more than willing to employ qualified women in appointing Dr Margaret Mead as assistant clinical pathologist

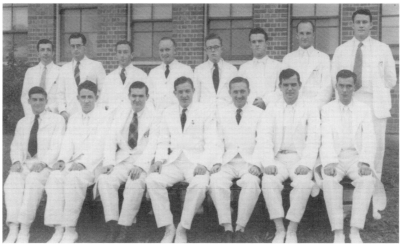

Mater resident medical officers, 1949–1950. Back row, from left, Ian Chester, Rod Meyers, Des McGuckin, John Buckley, Bill Hickey, unknown, Gary Groves, Ted McGuinness. Front row, from left, Remo Cantamessa, Hugh Tighe, Bill Shea, Geoffrey Toakley, Frank McDonald, Paddy Kelly, Peter Gill. MHHC

while she was a nursing mother; her baby was cared for at the Children's Hospital while she worked.[9] Sisters Regis Mary Dunne and Mary Athanasius Reordan joined the laboratory in 1949. Both completed their university degrees and became Fellows of the Australasian Institute of Medical Laboratory Technology. During the 1950s, three additional Sisters, Sisters Mary Benjamin, Rosaleen Mary Carroll and Judith Mary Gardiner, joined a department busy with new and exciting work. Rapid improvements in diagnosis and treatment were based on a growing understanding of the human body at the level of individual cells. Sister Mary St Rita won her Fellowship of the Australasian Institute of Medical Laboratory Technology for her published thesis on the cytology of blood fluids. Sister Regis Mary, who had already published papers on a variety of subjects, including pathogenic fungi, was pioneering an exciting new area, cytogenetics.

The pharmacy was also struggling. It occupied a cramped corner of the old Queenslander house adjacent to the Mater Children's Hospital which accommodated the outpatient department. The pharmacists had been asked to pare expenditure to the bone ever since the war, partly as a side-effect of the free hospitals scheme. The Commonwealth's hospital benefits scheme required public hospitals to treat patients free of charge but did not finance the large quantities of drugs required for modern treatments. New therapeutic wonders, such as penicillin and the sulpha drugs, were expensive; resident medical officers and honoraries alike chafed under the requirement to use them as sparingly as possible.[10] The pharmacy practised rigid economies in, for example, recycling medicine bottles, used for both tablets and liquid medicines in the post-war era. The bottles were expensive. The government's payment for National Health Service prescriptions – the cost of the drug plus 2 per cent – did not cover the cost of bottles, let alone staff and new equipment. Outpatients were encouraged to return their bottles, which the Sisters boiled in a huge copper vat under the house and re-filled.[11] Sister Mercia Mary continued to reign over the pharmacy which was always short of staff, even though Sister Marie Therese Rosenberg and Sister Mary Margarita Shannon had completed their training and joined the staff in the early 1950s.

Should largesse ever come its way, the Mater knew exactly what was required to alleviate multiple deficiencies at the Adult and Children's hospitals. The most urgent priorities were larger pharmacy, radiology and pathology departments, an additional operating theatre at the Children's Hospital as well as an extension of the babies' ward, and, at the Adult Hospital, 105 additional beds and a new operating theatre block. Next in line was another new hospital, this time for convalescent and terminally ill patients on the old St Mary's convent land at South Brisbane, bounded by Peel, Boundary and Cordelia streets. The nursing staff was not to be forgotten – a swimming pool and a squash court were planned to improve staff amenities.

Doctors in various specialties had been pressing for immediate improvements, sometimes highlighting alarming situations. In 1962, for instance, three young registrars wrote to the Director of Medical Services about the 'untoward large number of tragedies, near tragedies and an occasional last minute aversion of tragedy associated with surgery and anaesthetics in this hospital group in recent months'. This, they believed, arose from staff shortages and a consequent need for 'junior and inexperienced resident medical officers' to give anaesthetics, an unsatisfactory situation because 'modern anaesthesia required a large selection of anaesthetic agents and drugs, a wide range of equipment and a choice of technique'.[12] The solution, the appointment of a full-time director of anaesthetics, could not be solved by money alone. Even in 1965, the shortage of specialists delayed the Mater's plan to ensure that it would appoint only experienced anaesthetists who had attained their Fellowships of the college, or their two-part diplomas at the very least.[13]

There were also signs of internal disagreements. Competing views on who should be responsible for babies admitted to the Children's Hospital for medical or surgical care highlighted deeper organisational issues. The Children's Hospital's medical advisory committee recommended that all babies admitted for surgery be placed under the care of the receiving physician as well as under the admitting honorary specialist.[14] The surgeons strongly opposed putting surgical cases in the nursery under a physician. This argument brought out the fundamental issue of whether or not the Mater Children's was a children's hospital in the Mater grounds or part of the Mater hospitals as a group. If the latter

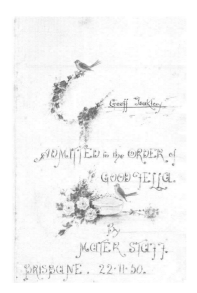

This beautifully hand-painted card was a special honour for the neurosurgeon, Dr Geoffrey Toakley.
MHHC

view prevailed, it was logical to amalgamate the separate adult and children's medical and surgical departments. Amalgamation could also reduce the effect of a practical problem. Children could not be admitted to the Children's Hospital once they reached the age of 12 years, yet, as Dr Geoff Toakley put it, 'a specialty does not end at age 12 and then start again at 12 years and 1 month'. Departmental amalgamation would at least make it easier for the same specialist to treat the child after transfer to the adult hospital.

The inaugural University of Queensland professor of Child Health, T J Rendle-Short, had his own views on the requirements for a modern paediatric hospital.[15] He differed in many respects on the amalgamation issue. Rendle-Short advocated a separate radiology department because in his view it was undesirable to transfer very sick and very young patients some distance to the existing department. He also opposed the upper age limit of 12 for admission to the Children's Hospital. Admitting young people to adult wards was, he thought, quite unsuitable, and disrupted the follow-up of patients with diseases such as rheumatic fever and coeliac disease. Rendle-Short also saw other important differences in the needs of adult and child patients. The existing outpatient area was completely insufficient to cope with the thousands of children who presented for treatment, yet the trend in modern paediatrics was to treat children as outpatients whenever possible, rather than admit them to hospital. The paediatrician Dr David Jackson had emphasised the importance of the outpatient department in 1949, believing that it was 'through the outpatient service that the hospital makes its greatest contact with the community and therefore the standard of that service is of vital importance to the hospital's reputation'.[16] Rendle-Short was perturbed that the alterations to the casualty department, already underway when he made his assessment, made no provision for an operating theatre for minor surgery which would enable children to be treated, cared for in a day ward, and then returned to their homes.

Modern paediatrics also regarded close involvement of parents as a key to improved outcomes for children. Open visiting hours were becoming commonplace in modern children's hospitals, so Rendle-Short recommended adequate space for parents, including breast-feeding mothers, to be near their children and, in the case of babies, to be admitted to the hospital with the baby. The advent of the Mater Mothers' had increased the demand for nursery beds at the Mater Children's. Improved diagnostic and surgical techniques and developments in anaesthetics had improved the outlook for sick babies and Rendle-Short saw a need to double the accommodation from twelve to twenty-four beds, including four insul-cots, with the aim of eventually providing single-cubicle accommodation for babies. Treatment of older children in hospital had also changed. The professor wrote that the 'desirability of having children out of bed and mobile . . . needs stronger emphasis in the hospital's practice than is the case at present'. For this to be practical, play areas adjacent to wards, a garden or outdoor play area, and a school for long-stay patients were necessary. At least one of the professor's dreams came true almost immediately – a teacher was appointed to begin work at the Mater from the beginning of the 1963 school year in a school room made by partitioning a verandah corner.[17]

Professor Rendle-Short also focused on requirements for paediatric teaching. He regarded as essential the provision of separate teaching areas adjacent to the medical and surgical wards, a library, and efficient record-keeping because 'the contribution that sick children make to medical progress lies in their records . . . These must be of the highest order, must conform to standards of nomenclature of disease, and must be readily available for research'.[18] Rendle-Short's identification of teaching needs touched a tender nerve at the Mater, as the hospital was getting a raw deal from the Commonwealth government which supported the clinical training of medical students through the Australian Universities Commission (AUC). The Queensland allocations for the 1961–64 triennial granting period were inequitable. The Brisbane General Hospital received £530,710, the Brisbane Children's

Hospital, £84,210 and the Women's Hospital, £1,550 – a total of more than £600,000 to the Herston campus, with a further £31,600 to the state's new Princess Alexandra Hospital, only a few kilometres from the Mater's doorstep. In contrast, the Mater's allocation was only £3,000. Even worse, it appeared that the final Queensland submission, prepared by a committee of which J P Kelly was a member, had been altered between Brisbane and Canberra without Kelly's knowledge, so that the Mater's funding was reduced from £69,000 to £3,000.[19] This seemed particularly unjust when the Mater's overloaded facilities were coping with eighty-one students in five medical areas, whereas the Princess Alexandra was teaching eighty-three students in only three clinical fields.

The AUC seemed to have based its decision on an erroneous belief that the Mater had applied for retrospective payment for the cost of residential student accommodation completed in 1953. The application was actually for obstetric and gynaecological teaching accommodation at the Mater Mothers'. Kelly was furious. He regarded this inequity as scant thanks for the Mater's accepting medical students in 1949 when the university

The Mater Revue has been a valuable means of fostering *esprit de corps* and of letting off steam in tense, exhausting times, as in the 1950s when the public Adult and Children's hospitals were struggling to meet the demand for their services. This program from the 1952 revue 'Getting Away With It' features well-known Mater people, such as the paediatric surgeon Dr Des McGuckin. MHHC

was struggling to find sufficient training places.[20] He suspected that the University of Queensland and the government were attempting to concentrate clinical training at the Princess Alexandra, even though it did not offer paediatric or obstetric services. The funding anomaly was addressed in the mid-1960s. New teaching units were built at the Children's and Mothers' hospitals. By 1966, double-storeyed annexes had been added to four of the wards in the Adult Hospital for student teaching and seminar discussions, student laboratories and offices. It was at last possible for students and their instructors to examine patients in completely private surroundings at both the Adult and the Children's hospitals.

These improvements could not disguise the strains in clinical areas at the Children's Hospital which became even more severe as the 1960s progressed. Dr David Jackson reported that, in the 1966–67 year, with 5,029 inpatients, 28,368 outpatients, and 58,589 patients in its casualty department, 'it is a matter of some wonder that these staggering increases in patient load have been accommodated and efficiently treated with so little structural alteration to one small building'.[21] By 1967, the nursery had at last been expanded to twenty-four beds, and the long-awaited new operating theatres were completed, but the hospital was still trying to provide wards for the adolescent age group, an intensive care unit, and accommodation for the mothers of sick babies. The great hope was that the Children's Hospital could expand with the completion of its second wing, deferred in 1931 because of the Depression. Shorter stays and the trend towards treating children at home whenever possible had eased the pressure on beds but aggravated crowding in the outpatient and casualty departments.

Financial incapacity, not administrative unwillingness, had been responsible for the delay in remedying the problems of the two older Mater public hospitals. The Mater was not, however, unique in its struggle. The state system had its own problems. In the early 1960s, an independent authority described one of the major state public hospitals as the worst he had come across. In Kelly's view, the root of the problem in the state system was similar to the Mater's – scarce financial resources:

Some time or other, somebody will have sufficient courage to let the people of Queensland know that those who are in a position to pay for public hospital services must pay for them in so far as their means will allow . . . The true fact is that the ideal of a free public hospital bed for every person is an ideal beyond the financial capacity of this State if a free public hospital bed is to mean a free public hospital bed of the highest standards which a country can offer.[22]

The health benefits system, designed to assist contributors to enter private hospitals, was, Kelly thought, counter-productive. Contributors to private health benefit funds could enter a public hospital, pay no fees, and receive a cheque from the hospital benefits fund at the rate of £10.10.0 per week for each week of hospitalisation. This apparent fraud occurred with the knowledge of the private health funds, which actually saved money because the payment to their members as public patients was lower than the benefit that would have been payable to those same members if they had chosen to enter a private hospital. Kelly's description of this situation as 'Gilbertian' masked a deep concern: generous payments to health fund contributors as public patients reduced the attraction of the Mater Private.[23]

As if this were not enough, the phenomenon of 'intermediate beds' in public hospitals added to the Mater Private Hospital's problems. Patients admitted to intermediate beds were entitled to the specialists of their choice, but paid a lower fee for this service than private hospital charges. In state hospitals, intermediate beds were heavily subsidised by the government, but the Mater had to subsidise intermediate beds from its own resources. In this sense, the Mater subsidised competition with its own private hospital. The community perception that private hospitals were very expensive and existed to make profits to enrich their owners was even more dangerous. Nothing could have been further from the truth at the Mater, where profits from the Private Hospital – if any remained when its own needs were met – still subsidised the Mater public hospitals. Government suggestions that the Mater Mothers' should include some intermediate beds provoked Kelly's testy rejoinder that intermediate beds would be provided if the state subsidised them at the same rate as its own intermediate beds.

Even more galling, the fees charged for private beds in the Mater Mothers' were less than it cost the state to provide intermediate beds in its Women's Hospital.[24]

Things began to look up in the mid-1960s. There was, at last, some softening in the government's attitude. In May 1965, the rate of capital subsidy for new beds rose to 50 per cent of the cost, provided that did not exceed £3,500. The government also agreed to subsidise the purchase of essential equipment used by public patients and to provide a subsidy of £1,000 on new beds for chronically ill patients. The Mater took a large leap of faith and, in 1968, announced plans for a major development – a new Adult Hospital to be built at a cost of $9,000,000, including $2,500,000 for nurses' education and accommodation. Subsidies would contribute $2,453,333 towards the total cost, and the Mater's own resources could provide $2,000,000, but a huge gap of $6,500,000 remained to complete 'the largest charitable undertaking ever assumed by a private body in Queensland'.[25] It would, however, come at a price: there was no chance that the planned hospital for the chronically ill could be built.

In this combination of circumstances – urgent needs, restive staff and a commitment to a huge project – the most efficient management was essential, particularly if there were to be any hope of finding the money needed for the huge new project. The decision to engage management consultants in 1969 began a period of intense scrutiny of the Mater's management, its financial capacity and its clinical services. The reports of formal reviews and less formal assessments of the Mater's clinical profile provide important insights into conditions at the Mater in the late 1960s and early 1970s. The management consultants, W D Scott and Co. were given a wide brief 'to consider, evaluate and report on all matters affecting the administration of the hospitals so that a full appreciation could be gained of the situation facing the Sisters of Mercy'.[26] The evaluation was a searching investigation of all aspects of all the hospitals. The report was frank, almost harsh, in highlighting the Mater's problems. It was not, as the Congregational Superior, Mother Damian Duncombe, was informed, a matter of overlooking the 'bright side', but more a matter of identifying the issues which urgently needed addressing.[27]

Finance was critical. The Scott report recommended debt financing for capital improvements, arguing that the gap between needs and cash resources would only grow if the Mater continued to finance major projects with government grants and accumulated savings.[28] Scott recommended debenture loans geared to attract banks, investment companies, insurance companies, the government and the public. Such loans could be serviced by government subsidies, the Mater art unions and other traditional fundraising sources. This scheme, the report suggested, could be attractive to government, which might increase its contributions if they were spread over the forty years of a loan rather than two to three years of a project. Perhaps most importantly of all, such a scheme would allow future generations to pay their share of the improvements from which they became the main beneficiaries. The *Hospitals Act* allowed debt financing for hospitals, but, at the Mater, any such suggestion revived the old nightmare of years of trying to finance the Mater Mothers'.[29]

It was quite clear that the Mater Mothers' project had been nerve-wracking. Late in 1961, J P Kelly revealed that the total cost of the Mothers' Hospital was £1,650,000 – more than £500,000 over the original worst-case scenario. He wrote to Mother Damian:

> We have only been saved from disaster . . . by the use of £250,000 from other hospital sources and by the Bank not requiring any reduction in the overdraft for the period from 1 October 1960 to October 1961 . . . It is quite clear that the situation in which the hospital found itself in regard to the Mater Mothers' project should never be repeated and that no large scale operation should again be attempted without a completely planned project and firm prices obtained on all aspects before the project proceeds.[30]

Never optimistic that the Queensland government would reform its policy and fund all capital expenditure on public hospital facilities, and unconvinced that the risks of debt financing were worth taking, the Mater sought expert advice on ways to raise large sums from the public and the corporate sector. The corporate fundraising firm Compton and Associates was asked for its assessment of the Mater's prospects of bridging the formidable gap between the estimated cost of the new Adult Hospital building ($9,000,000) and the available resources (less than half that amount).

The Compton report was frank – and frightening. Raising such a large sum, Compton wrote, 'represents one of the greatest challenges ever placed before the people of Queensland'.[31] Even the modest target of raising $1,000,000 by direct giving had been achieved only once before in Queensland. The Compton team surveyed more than 5,000 previous patients, doctors, politicians, public servants and members of the business community to assess their views of the Mater and their willingness to help. In view of the sacred place the concept of free hospitals had achieved in Queensland, it is surprising that very few of the people interviewed actually believed that public hospital care should be exempt from means testing.

There were some comforting findings in the Compton report. Compton thought it was 'quite staggering' that 98.8 per cent of past patients favoured the existence of non-government hospitals in the community, when 80 per cent would have been an outstanding result. Most held the Mater in very high esteem: more than 85 per cent of previous patients reported that they would choose the Mater again, and 76 per cent of the doctors said that the Mater's standards were as good as other Australian hospitals. However, there were some

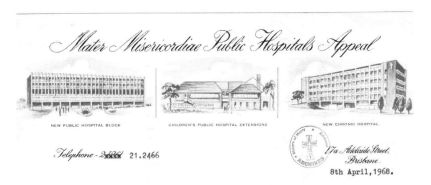

A letterhead which tells the poignant tale of the long struggle in the 1960s and 1970s to build a new Public Hospital: the hospital which was opened in 1981 did not resemble the model at the left of the letterhead; the second wing added to the Children's Hospital in the mid-1970s was very different from the sketch in the centre; financial stringency in the post-war decades put the planned hospital for the chronically ill, at right, completely out of reach. SOMCA

frightening revelations: 54 per cent of doctors said that existing plans for the extensions did not provide all the facilities they wanted. The Children's Hospital was found to be most in need of attention. Some doctors said the Children's Hospital was 'so disgraceful it should be closed down immediately' and many others believed that, by 1980, the Mater would have to spend $29,000,000, rather than $9,000,000, to create first-class adult and children's public hospitals.

The Mater would have to be more open about its difficulties to attract large sums from business. Compton discovered that the business community thought that the Mater's financial situation was 'shrouded in mystery'. However, with decades of government refusal to allow 'outsiders' on the boards of any of its public hospitals, the Queensland business community had had little opportunity to participate in any hospital's administration and, therefore, would be unlikely to have much idea of the high cost of providing hospital services. Compton found that many in the wider community thought the Mater was affluent because of the high standard of the Mater Mothers': photographs of the old sections of the hospital might startle the public into reality, and improve the public relations potential of the project to extend it. The waiting area for adult emergency patients, for instance, was in the open outside the main entrance; patients sat or stood for hours, exposed to the sun, the wind and the rain, or clustered inside the cramped foyer.

Compton had several suggestions to improve the Mater's public image. The internal newsletters 'The Mater' and 'Hospital Happenings' could, for instance, be much more widely distributed to business, industry and the professions with items slanted towards a variety of readers and a two-way flow of communication. 'Hospital Happenings', which catered mainly for hospital executives, could become more representative of all sections of the hospital community and thus help with communications within the hospital. The Mater's generally good coverage in the press could be improved with, for instance, lavishly illustrated sponsored segments on television and in the newspapers. A documentary with some controversial elements to attract public attention was also recommended. Suitable controversy would not be difficult to find. A visit to outpatients any morning would, Compton

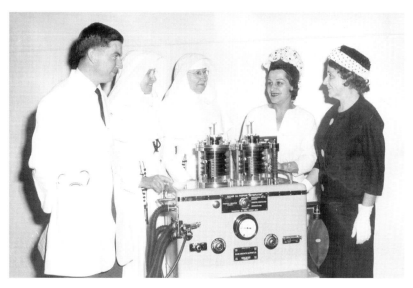

The work of ladies auxiliary committees at the Mater public hospitals was always important in raising funds for badly needed facilities. This Blease Pulmoflator respirator was presented to the Adult Hospital by its ladies auxiliary in 1962. Dr Des O'Callaghan is pictured on left with Sister Mary Virginia Boothby, Sister Mary St Gabriel Corbett, the Vice-President of the Ladies Auxiliary, Mrs Nell George, and the President, Mrs John P Kelly. MHHC

thought, be 'a real shocker to most businessmen'. The Mater also had an invaluable public relations asset – the Sisters of Mercy, the Mater's most distinguishing feature. If there was to be any hope of raising $1,000,000, the Sisters would have to become public figures in a public education program explaining precisely why the community should give generously to the Mater.

The Mater Mothers' project had given the Mater valuable experience in combining fundraising with public relations. By 1970, cash in hand from the art unions and various appeals stood at $2,000,000.[32] The volunteers again set to with a will. During the 1960s and into the 1970s, there were several fundraising committees – the Mater Mothers' Ladies Committee, the Green Shop Committee, the Mater Public Committee, the Mater Children's Committee, the Mater Ball Committee, the Nurses Amenities Committee, the Past Nurses Association, the Younger Set and a Bargain Bazaar committee. The committees worked hard to raise funds for new items of equipment which the government still refused to subsidise, and to improve conditions for nurses, as well as eliminating the debt on the Mothers' Hospital. Finally, when the profits from the 33rd Art Union in July 1966 were calculated, the entire Mater Mothers' debt was paid.[33]

Competition to Mater fundraising loomed in the early 1960s. The Brisbane Children's Hospital established a Foundation to raise funds for a hospital which, in the Mater's view, was already richly endowed by the state. However, the results of the new Foundation's public appeals tended to be rather disappointing. J P Kelly suggested that the best possible public hospital services could only be provided to the community through a partnership between the state and the Mater. He recognised that:

> . . . no government today is in the happy position of being able to provide all necessary equipment in its public hospitals. Charitably minded people must continue to supplement the efforts of governments to provide those things which mean so much to the health and well being of patients in our public hospitals.[34]

The ending of unproductive competition might, Kelly thought, encourage both the government and the community to a greater spirit of generosity. Victoria provided a useful example. The Victorian government had given £10,000 to the Sisters of Mercy appeal to build a new maternity hospital, on top of a £3,000,000 state subsidy; the Sisters' fundraising was required to produce only £490,000.[35] The Victorian government's vote of confidence in the Melbourne Mercy Maternity Hospital project had the happy result of convincing the corporate sector to donate generously – a goal which the Mater in Queensland had yet to achieve.

In 1970, the opening of a special appeal office in Clarence Street heralded renewed fundraising vigour. Channel 7 offered its services for broad publicity, and an article on the 'hopelessly congested' Children's Hospital, including an interview with the matron, Sister Mary St Pierre, appeared in the *Sunday Mail* in 1970.[36] A group of leading business figures were brought together to promote the cause. They included Sir William Gunn of the Wool Board, doctors Clive Uhr and Charles Roe, Eric Robinson, the owner of a number of well-known sports stores, George Purcy, the managing director of the Myer store in Fortitude Valley, the barrister Raymund Smith, D E Rossell of the ANZ bank, George Lovejoy from the radio station 4BH, and Peter Bell, president of the United Graziers' Association.[37] There was, however, discernible internal reluctance to appoint professional fundraisers to manage a direct appeal because the 'hospital now knows the principles of direct giving campaigns and can do it without professionals', and disquiet about appointing 'outsiders' to the appeal board. Many initiatives reflected Compton's recommendations. Though his firm was not appointed, Compton continued to write to J P Kelly with useful suggestions.[38]

Despite these preparations, however, there was confusion late in 1970 about which priorities should be addressed first. A master planning process, recommended in the Scott report, had not been systematically implemented. There were those who felt that 'we know what we want and we are determined to get it', but J P Kelly had a more realistic view. He felt that, rather than knowing what it wanted, the Mater was 'in a state of crisis re its future'.[39] The project to rebuild the Adult Hospital and improve the Children's Hospital, announced in 1968, was deferred while the future of the Mater was evaluated. J P Kelly and Sister Angela Mary – indeed the whole Mater administration – were well aware that years of delaying the extensions, no matter how good the financial reasons, had created morale problems internally and public relations muddles externally. Patients, doctors and staff had been well and truly warmed up to the thought that the planned ten-storey extension to the Adult Hospital would proceed. For years, the cleared frontage in Stanley Street had promised better things to come and church and secular media had publicised the project. In April 1970 the *Catholic Leader* prematurely announced that the project was about to begin. Kelly issued a press release stating that the tender process had revealed that the costs would be far beyond the Hospital's financial capacity.[40] This was no panacea in the climate of rising frustration among the staff on Mater Hill.

The Scott report's recommendations for debt financing were not on the table even at this desperate stage. J P Kelly and Sister Angela Mary were trying something rather more daring. Overtly, Kelly and the

Mater maintained the position that the government should take greater responsibility for capital works at the Mater and treat the Mater 'as a partner, rather than a Quixotic follower'; privately, they had decided that their best tactic would be 'a major confrontation with the Minister and Director General of Health'.[41] Sister Angela Mary had one weapon at hand: the reaction of the prominent business leaders she had appointed to the appeal committee. She told the Health Minister bluntly that:

> There was almost a unanimous reaction of dismay and incredulity that we were attempting to raise from public charity the amount of approximately $9,000,000 for a minimum capital development necessary to cope with the pressing demands by the public on the health facilities provided by our hospital. These men were highly appreciative of the work carried on at our hospitals, and were most sympathetic and willing to help in a reasonable project, but firmly reached their own conclusion that the major part of this development was the responsibility of the government.[42]

This salvo reinforced an earlier assault on the government's policy of providing subsidies for new beds but not for equipment or ancillary services: 'The present parlous condition of the adult and children's hospitals is a direct result of this regrettable policy . . . pursued over many years'.[43]

A completely unforeseeable event turned the tide of the Mater's anguish into constructive and far-sighted plans for the future. The fire at the Mater Children's Hospital on 12 May 1971 could have been an appalling disaster. Instead, the calm, purposeful, successful evacuation of all 119 children concentrated public attention on the needs of Brisbane's only southside children's hospital and the community's dependence on it. The fire erupted in the ceiling and roof structure of the university section at the rear of the hospital, close to the babies' ward. The newspapers provided extensive coverage of nurses carrying children out of the hospital. Some of the children had drips attached, others were carried in special beds and insul-cots. There were stories of real heroism. Sister Mary Lea risked her life by returning to the nursery and, in the dense smoke, put her hand into each cot to make

sure that no baby had been left behind. In one of the operating theatres, Dr Des McGuckin was operating on a child with oesophageal
atresia, accompanied by the anaesthetist, Dr Tess Brophy. Their work
continued in the theatre's ante-room.

The fire occurred before fire drills became standard practice in
modern hospitals. Sister Angela Mary later attributed the successful
evacuation to common sense, good leadership and trust in key people.
Although there was great relief that the evacuation had succeeded,
there was one tragedy. Stan Anderson, the Mater's Superintendent of
Works for many years, died the next day from a heart attack, thought
to have resulted from his horror at a fire in his domain. As Sister Angela
Mary said, he 'had a position of great responsibility and trust, and the
Sisters placed great faith in him, and relied on him heavily'. Many
Sisters of Mercy formed a guard of honour at his funeral at the South
Brisbane Baptist Church.[44]

The fire highlighted the affectionate place the Mater Children's

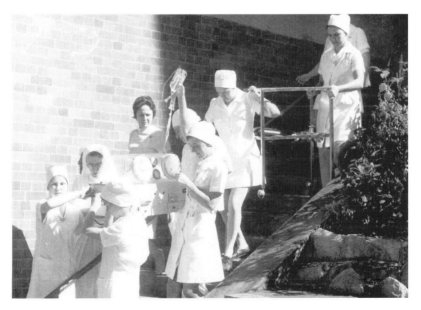

A delicate evacuation. The baby in the insul-cot weighed only 2 kilograms and
had just come from the operating theatre after surgery for oesophageal atresia.
The anaesthetist, Dr Tess Brophy, can be seen at left, and below her, wearing
spectacles, is Sister Angela Mary Doyle, and, below her, Sister Dorothy Byrne.
Mr T Hendry is behind the crib with nurses Lynette Bowen and Kathy Ryan.
Sister J Boyle is in front. MHHC

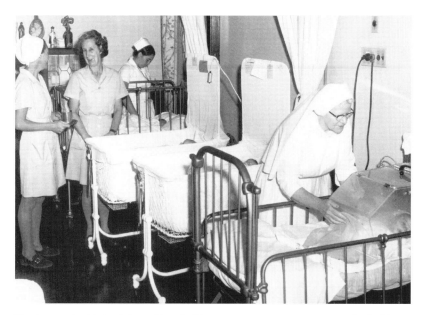

Ward 23 at the Mater Private Hospital became an emergency nursery for babies evacuated from the Children's Hospital. Sister Mary Lea, who risked her life to return to the babies' ward in thick smoke to ensure that no baby had been left behind, is pictured at right watching over one of her charges. MHHC

had claimed in Brisbane hearts. The fire damage was repaired and those children too sick to recuperate at home were returned from the Royal Children's Hospital on the north side of the river. Extensive press coverage of the hospital's difficult situation inspired the community, which rallied around, as is always the case in times of disaster. Donations and offers of help flowed in. Queensland Newspapers, particularly its chairman, Reg Leonard, began to take a close interest in the needs of Brisbane's two children's hospitals. The first step was to make the hospitals beneficiaries of the Good Friday appeal conducted by radio station 4BK, owned by the newspaper group. This initiative was modelled on the successful joint appeals conducted in Melbourne for several years by the *Melbourne Herald* and a local radio station. General fundraising was also more successful following the fire. The net income from the Mater door-to-door appeal reached almost $460,000 and art union proceeds rose by $30,000 in 1971.[45]

It was a perfect time to present a major submission to the government on the precarious situation and urgent needs of both the Adult Hospital and the Children's Hospital. Sister Angela Mary's letter to the Minister was very direct. She upped the stakes by stating that the 'hospital was at a crossroads as to its future' with real consideration being given to reducing its adult public hospital services or vacating the field altogether.[46] Sister Angela Mary also called in old debts by reminding the government that, until the Princess Alexandra Hospital opened in the late 1950s, the Mater was the only hospital offering public hospital care and casualty services on the southside of the river, a factor which would have been of no small importance during the Second World War if the cross-river bridges had been destroyed. Further, Sister Angela Mary informed the Minister, the Mater had voluntarily given up its right to charge fees in order to cooperate with the government's free hospital policy.[47]

The Health Minister, the Honourable Douglas Tooth, responded immediately. He telephoned Sister Angela Mary and agreed to take the submission to Cabinet in July 1971. This phone call was a perfect opportunity to put some additional points to the Minister about the Mater's vision of its future role, particularly in obstetrics, possibly gynaecology, certainly paediatrics, with a limited, but definite, role in adult public hospital medicine.[48] Sister Angela Mary did not waste the opportunity to acquaint the Minister with some of the difficulties in working harmoniously with the state system. The Mater had had great difficulties in accommodating children suffering from infectious diseases, but no longer transferred them to the Royal Children's Hospital because 'they were unhappy about taking any patients that they felt belonged to us'. This reluctance extended to items of expensive equipment. Sister Angela Mary told the Minister about needing a special piece of equipment to remove a foreign body from a ten-month old baby – an instrument the government had refused to provide – only to find that the Royal Children's Hospital refused the loan, forcing the Mater to borrow it from a private doctor. She noted: 'Mr Tooth remarked that these are the things that never come to his ears. We have, subsequently, made a further appeal for this essential equipment'.[49]

The Minister wanted to see the Mater 'integrated into the State system' with a 'greater rationalisation of services between the Mater and the Princess Alexandra Hospital', because 'it was ridiculous to have two hospitals within a mile of each other, one duplicating the services of the other'. Sister Angela Mary assured him that duplication was not the Mater's intention. Rather, in proposing that the government provide $14,000,000 to replace the Adult Hospital, with any excess cost financed by the Mater, the Sisters were planning 'not to build an empire but . . . merely to preserve the integrity of institutions which exist only to serve God and humanity'.[50] This lack of empire building, the Minister assured Sister Angela Mary, would strengthen the chances of Cabinet's approval of the submission for substantial capital assistance.

Mr Tooth convinced Cabinet that if, as Sister Angela Mary's letter attached to the submission threatened, the Mater stopped providing adult public hospital services, 'the impact on the State hospital system would be extremely serious'. Cabinet had become well aware of deficiencies in diagnostic facilities at the Mater and, more seriously, knew that 'some of the ward buildings are considered to be a risk factor to patients and staff'.[51] The Mater's submission was not entirely successful, but there were welcome indications that, at long last, the policy grounds were shifting. Cabinet decided to tell the Mater that the government recognised that it filled an important role in the free public hospital system of Queensland and in teaching medical students. The government was, therefore, prepared to review its policy on capital assistance to church and charitable institutions providing public hospital services. In future, capital subsidy at the rate of $2 for each $3 of approved expenditure would include the whole range of accommodation and services associated with the conduct of public hospital and outpatient services, and no longer be confined to the provision of additional public beds. Nevertheless, Cabinet baulked at the request for $14,000,000 towards completely rebuilding the Adult Hospital, offering as its reason a reluctance to bind future governments. A staged program was preferable, with Stage 1 to cost no more than $5,000,000. This stage should be the most urgent work and should be a complete entity. Further subsidy for subsequent stages would be considered towards the end of Stage 1.

This compromise solution was not without a rational basis. The Queensland government had its own problems in raising money to finance state hospitals in 1970. It was really feeling the pressure of trying to provide essential public hospital services throughout a rapidly developing state entirely free of charge when other states were charging fees. As if this was not sufficient challenge, changes in the entire financing of Australia's hospitals were in the wind. New Commonwealth government policies were emerging which would affect all public hospitals, all patients and all doctors for decades to come. Costs of hospitalisation everywhere in the nation had been rising at an alarming rate ever since the war; consequently, the Commonwealth's costs in providing bed subsidies were mounting steadily. The enthusiasm of both patients and doctors to take up the opportunities provided by technological and scientific advances increased demand for expensive treatments.[52] Health costs had risen from 0.38 per cent of gross domestic product in 1900–01 to 2.68 per cent in 1969–70. The Commonwealth was meeting 55 per cent of total expenditure in 1969, a huge increase from its 25 per cent contribution in 1945–46.

The late 1960s were peppered by debates on health costs, quality of life issues and criticisms of private health insurance. The federal government established the Nimmo enquiry to report on hospital and medical benefit schemes. At the same time, Scotton and Deeble published their proposals for a compulsory national health insurance scheme. Their scheme to provide free public hospital care was to be financed by a levy on all taxpayers and a matching Commonwealth grant, but Scotton and Deeble did not intend that all services would be free of charge to all users. They foreshadowed the continuation of private health insurance for private hospital care with freedom of choice of doctor. The fee-for-service mode of medical remuneration was to be continued, but would be restricted to a guaranteed payment of 85 per cent of a standard fee established by the government. Both the Deeble and Scotton and Nimmo reports recommended the establishment of a Commonwealth Health Insurance Commission to oversee the system. Many doctors feared that the 'common fee' idea would introduce nationalisation of medical services, a prospect they had dreaded for decades.[53]

The new health scheme came into force under the Gorton coalition government on 1 July 1970. It was refined, but not substantially altered in principle, by the Labor government which succeeded it. The Labor 'Medibank' scheme sparked vigorous debate in the 1970s between those who thought health care was a right and should be a communal responsibility and those who thought health care was an individual responsibility with patients making a contribution to the costs of their care. The debate over the future of the Mater hospitals was conducted against this heady background of cost challenges and policy changes.

In Queensland, new public hospitals were being planned to cater for rising demand in areas of rapid population growth. The government's investigation of the suburbs of Mt Gravatt and Sunnybank as possible locations for a new public hospital was only in its preliminary stages in 1971 when the Mater crisis was at its height. As the Health Minister told Cabinet, if the Mater ceased to provide adult public hospital care, the new hospital would have to be brought on stream immediately at a cost of $30,000,000.[54] The Mater's submission for $14,000,000 should have been considered a very good deal, particularly if the Mater fulfilled its undertaking to integrate its services with other metropolitan public hospitals.

Support from the Health Minister had been an important gain, but as far as everyday negotiations were concerned, the unfailing assistance of Dick Strutton, Under Secretary for Health, was critically important at this stage, and for years to come. Dick Strutton attended a crucial meeting in August 1971 with Dr Peter Livingstone, Deputy Director-General of Health. Sister Angela Mary, Pat Maguire (Assistant Administrator) and Dr O'Callaghan (Director of Medical Services) represented the Mater, and emphasised that the Mater hospitals saw themselves as 'participants in the comprehensive delivery of medicine on the south side of the river'. They offered to reduce the number of beds in the Adult Hospital by between sixty-five and seventy to appease the government, but were gratified to find that the state did not want to lose any public hospital beds. Instead, the Health Department asked the Mater to continue to look after the whole of the ear, nose and throat work on the southside.[55] A sketch of the completed Mater Children's Hospital, prepared by the Mater's architect, H L Chapman, was accepted, as was the concept of eventually building an entirely new Mater Children's Hospital, closely linked to both the Mater Mothers' and the Adult Hospital, thus allowing essential services to be shared.

This was progress at last. Late in 1971, Cabinet approved the construction of the first stage of the Mater redevelopment – a new adult outpatient department and pharmacy, and a three-floor extension to the Mater Children's. A new eight-storey building, called the 'podium', was also planned to link the existing hospital buildings to a future redevelopment of the Adult Hospital. The podium was to contain sixty beds, central sterilising facilities, an intensive care unit, a recovery ward close to the theatres, accommodation for medical records and a kitchen to service the public hospitals.[56]

The new wing at the Mater Children's Hospital would complete a plan more than forty years old. The second wing had always been planned, but could not be built in the 1930–31 stage when there was no government subsidy and the Great Depression had dried up the flow of public donations. The old wooden Queenslander house, the home of the children's outpatient department and the pharmacy, was demolished, so that the new wing could be built at the eastern end of the existing hospital. A contract with the builder, K D Morris and Co., was signed on 24 July 1973 for building work costing $1,642,987. The new wing was expected to open in January 1975.[57] But construction did not proceed smoothly. In 1974, when the work was well under way, Australia again suffered economic problems. An inflationary spiral was followed by high interest rates and a credit squeeze designed to quash inflationary pressures in the economy. Many businesses felt the pressure, including K D Morris and Co. The firm went into liquidation in October 1974: it seemed that it would be a very long time before the work would be completed. Fortunately, J P Kelly had ensured that the contract provided for a very large contingency sum and another contractor, Underwood, took over the work very quickly; no subcontractor went unpaid or lost work, which greatly impressed the unions.[58] The new wing was ready to receive patients only a year later. There were more wards on the upper floors, and a completely new outpatient department, casualty section and pharmacy on the ground level.

The Children's Hospitals' Appeal was also an important player in improving the Children's Hospital. The Appeal supported the construction of a flyover linking the Children's and Adult hospitals which was opened in October 1973. The link, named in honour of Reg Leonard, the force behind the Appeal, provided an additional fire escape from the Children's Hospital and a convenient site for two important clinics – Sister Mary St Roch's electroencephalography department and Sister Regis Mary Dunne's cytogenetics clinic. The link also facilitated the shared used of core specialist services and expensive equipment, the first step in the larger picture of integrating the Mater Hospitals.[59]

The excitement over the construction of the new wing at the Children's Hospital may have given some hope to Mater staff that the Adult Hospital's day was coming. Certainly, the administration was steadily working on the government while the new children's wing was rising above Annerley Road. In April 1972, the Mater had at long last achieved some equity in the matter of intermediate hospital beds. Cabinet finally recognised that the Sisters of Mercy had provided intermediate beds in the Adult Hospital at no cost to the government for decades. The Health Minister, Doug Tooth, was again the Mater's advocate, convincing Cabinet that there was a shortage of intermediate beds in the metropolitan area and the government could ill afford to lose the intermediate beds at the Mater. The government agreed to meet operational losses on the Mater's intermediate beds. In doing this, the government had reversed an article of faith held dear by Queensland governments for decades.[60] At the 1972 rate of $10 a day, this victory was insubstantial from a financial point of view, but very substantial indeed from the overall perspective of policy and principle.

The Mater's plans for the Adult Hospital were further elucidated in 1973. Sister Angela Mary presented to the Health Department a document evaluating its current situation, its needs and the Sisters' intentions for the hospital.[61] Limitations and inadequacies were desperate in the adult casualty department, in radiology and pathology, both of which carried the load for the whole complex, and in the operating theatres. Conditions in radiology had deteriorated to such an extent by 1974 that the Mater's planning committee thought that patients were at risk and the College of Radiologists had described the conditions as the worst in Australia.[62]

Urgently needed new facilities also included an intensive care unit, a post-operative recovery ward, a central sterilising department, a new medical records system and rehabilitation facilities. Behind-the-scenes facilities were also seriously inadequate. Shower and toilet amenities originally designed for ten patients were coping with forty-two, a daily difficulty when more and more patients were up and about much sooner after surgery than once had been the case. More seriously, the Adult Hospital building did not meet fire standards. 'In general,' Sister Angela Mary wrote, 'the building is a tired old building with inadequate means for patient escape and failing services such as gas, steam, water, and sewerage.' No matter what was spent on the original hospital, 'we will still be left with an old building lacking flexibility'.[63] The Mater's push for an entirely new Adult Hospital was on!

CHAPTER SIX

BREAKING THROUGH

In view of the fact that the Mater Public Hospitals will be providing over 450 public beds when completed and that the entire services of the hospital and all the facilities provided therein are made available to the public free of charge without means test, it cannot be denied that the Mater Public Hospitals is part of the Public Hospital system in this state.[1]

Dr Llew Edwards, Minister for Health, 1975

Dr Edwards' announcement represented two of the most significant achievements in the Mater's history: first, the government had at last accepted the Mater Public Hospitals as part of Queensland's hospital system and, second, the government would fund a completely new Mater Adult Hospital. This was a complete reversal of the situation only a year earlier. In those dark days, Mater administrators knew that the old Adult Hospital could not be resuscitated, even with the planned 'podium'. Even more worrying, there was no assurance that this stage would be funded in the 1974–75 state budget. Years of planning and re-planning and a great deal of emotional and physical effort had been invested in the Mater Adult Hospital. It was time for real

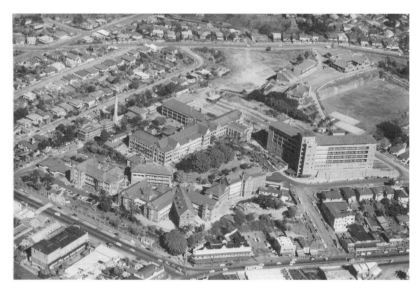

This aerial view of the Mater campus, photographed on 24 October 1977, shows the completed wing at the Mater Children's at left, and at centre right is the cleared ground where the new Mater Adult Hospital was to be constructed. The laundry building can be seen behind the Mater Private Hospital at top right. MHHC

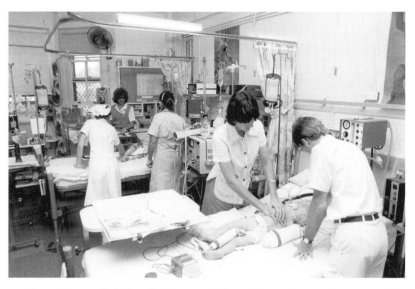

Members of many clinical professions worked together in the intensive care ward at the Mater Children's, a very crowded space before the new wing was built. Here, a physiotherapist at centre right is performing chest percussion on a small child and three nurses are caring for a patient at far left. MHHC

brinkmanship, not mere risk taking. Sister Angela Mary drafted a letter to Dick Strutton, Under Secretary for Health. She wrote from the heart:

> I believe that we have not received fair treatment in the area of capital subsidy for any section of our hospital . . . We have not been able to ascertain what our role ought to be in relation to other metropolitan hospitals. We have not been informed of decisions that affect our future in the public hospital field.[2]

The Mater, Sister Angela Mary continued, could not embark on any major building development without an assurance of 100 per cent capital subsidy: 'Given these circumstances, there seems no alternative but for the Mater to withdraw completely from adult acute public hospital work on the Mater site'.

Sister Angela Mary did not actually post her letter, but conveyed its contents verbally and very frankly to Dick Strutton, at that time a patient in the Princess Alexandra Hospital, a captive audience. Strutton was dismayed that the Mater had even considered such a possibility.[3] At this point, the Queensland government had nowhere to run. Population was increasing rapidly in Brisbane's southern suburbs and south-eastern outskirts. The Mater Adult Hospital was badly needed. Some governmental sleight of hand was called for. Much as the Queensland government of Joh Bjelke-Petersen resisted cooperation with a federal government of any political complexion, it was quite prepared to take advantage of new Commonwealth policies for financing public hospitals.

The Whitlam government, which had won the 1972 federal election, intended to shift resources into the public sector to redistribute hospital services more equally. Geographic distribution was an important consideration. The federal government was well aware that many of the nation's public hospitals were located in the centres of cities rather than in outlying suburbs where the great post-war suburban sprawl had placed most of the younger sections of the population. Mt Gravatt in Brisbane, previously considered by the state as an area needing a new hospital, had been identified as a site for a new

Commonwealth hospital to address inequality in the geographic distribution of health services. The Queensland government suggested to the Commonwealth that $20,000,000 be diverted from the Mt Gravatt project to the Mater.[4]

Perhaps because of the prominence of large privately owned hospitals such as the St Vincent's hospitals in Sydney and Melbourne, and the Mater in Brisbane, the Commonwealth government was not in the least afraid of accepting Catholic public hospitals as just as worthy of funding as public hospitals owned by state governments; further, it agreed to allow the Catholic public hospitals to maintain independent admission, treatment and administration policies. The state Health Minister explained to Parliament that the Commonwealth's suggestion that it should start to build a new Commonwealth hospital early in 1975 was a decision made in 'indecent haste' and one that would interfere with the state government's forward planning. This would have been news to the Mater which had been considerably frustrated at the apparent lack of any centralised health planning in Queensland.[5]

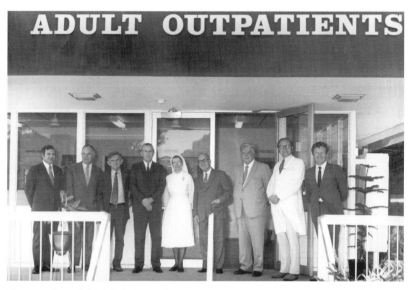

The opening of the Adult Outpatients Department on 2 January 1973 marked a significant achievement. With Sister Angela Mary Doyle after the ceremony are, from left, an official from the Queensland Health Department, Mr Jack O'Brien, Executive Officer of the Mater Public Hospitals, Mr Dick Strutton, Under Secretary of the Queensland Health Department, the Honourable Douglas Tooth, Minister for Health, Mr J P Kelly, Dr John Eckert and Mr Pat Maguire. MHHC

Nevertheless, the Mater welcomed the proposal that Commonwealth money be diverted to the Mater.

The hospital had already told the state that the total redevelopment costs at the Mater would be $19,000,000, plus $3,000,000 for furnishings and fittings; additional space required by the university would add to the total cost. A meeting between the Mater and officials of the Commonwealth government and the state government was scheduled for March. This would be a make or break opportunity. Dick Strutton offered to assist the Mater in preparing a submission, to be based on a few key, wide-ranging points.[6] The Mater argued that, because there was overwhelming support for continuing the Adult Hospital at South Brisbane, the total number of beds should be increased from 210 to 280–300. Existing specialties would be maintained, but the 'super-specialties' such as renal transplantation and cardiac surgery would be avoided, and, because the Princess Alexandra Hospital was developing a major psychiatric care department, the Mater would not duplicate this service. Instead, the Mater would try to excel in a speciality not yet developed in Brisbane. Rheumatology was cited as a pertinent example.

Next came a Mater proposal designed to appeal to the Commonwealth, which was planning to integrate acute hospital services with community health services: 'There is a growing realisation that the hospital has many of the qualities of a community hospital and that this is desirable and ought to be developed'. The Mater would, therefore, try to establish a family care centre to which people with social problems could be referred. This, the Mater asserted, would fill a gap because 'at present, these patients are passed through to casualty and fare worst of all in the process. No one adverts to the fact that they may have come for personal problems under the guise of a minor medical complaint'.[7] Rehabilitation services would also be developed further and coordinated so that physiotherapy, occupational therapy, speech therapy and social work would be coordinated as soon as the patient was admitted and not, as was often the practice, when surgical and medical treatments were almost complete.

There was also a proposal designed to satisfy the state government. The Mater would be prepared to be involved with the community health centre the government had proposed at the outer suburb of

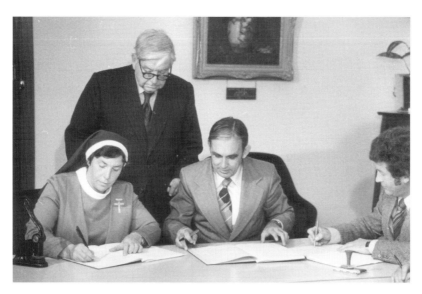

Sister Catharine Courtney, Superior General of the Sisters of Mercy, signs the contract for the new Mater Adult Hospital. The Health Minister, the Hon. Sir Llew Edwards looks on at right, with Mr John P Kelly (standing) and Mr Graham French of Leighton's contractors. MHHC

Inala, a lower socioeconomic area. The government had been planning this centre ever since it acquired land there in 1971.[8] The Inala initiative would be very satisfying to the Sisters of Mercy as it would directly link their acute health services to the care of the poor in their own community. A family centre at Inala would include care for antenatal and post-operative patients as well as casualty, outpatient and rehabilitation services. A variety of welfare projects funded by the Commonwealth could also be coordinated at Inala. The Commonwealth wanted to upgrade the status and role of the community nurse and the general practitioner, ensuring that there was a strong link between acute hospital services and medical care at the community level. This was a substantially broader focus. Before 1972, the Commonwealth had subsidised private expenditures, rather than deliberately expanding public services.[9] The Mater's Inala proposal was not devoid of self-interest: 'Involvement with Inala could ensure that patients will continue to be directed to the Mater, even if a major general hospital is provided at Mt Gravatt'.[10]

The Mater's carefully refined proposals and unrelenting pressure at last had a result. In October 1975, the Queensland Health Minister, Dr Llew Edwards, announced that the government would fund the new Mater adult public hospital at a cost of $18,000,000, a project that would increase bed numbers to 275 and take four years to complete. Most gratifying of all, the Health Minister proclaimed that the Mater had a vital role in Queensland's health system. After decades of effort, the Mater's place in public health services had at last been recognised. It was time for profound thankfulness. Sister Angela Mary rang Dick Strutton to thank him for his support in 'our long struggle for recognition in the public hospital field'. She reminded him of the time only three years earlier when the Mater could not obtain secure state or federal funding and had wondered if its public adult hospital was really needed. Strutton remained very comforting, confirming that 'the Mater was most certainly needed . . . [and] gave a quality of personal caring that was not always possible in state hospitals . . . the Mater would always be needed'.[11]

In deciding to fund the hospital, the government had had to take a great deal on trust. It was a large government investment on private

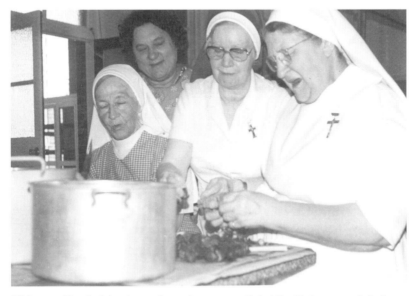

All forms of fundraising have always been essential at the Mater, especially in the tense 1970s. These busy hands making jam for the Mater fete were, from left, Sister Mary Winifrede Patterson, Peg, a member of the Convent kitchen staff, Sister Mary Genevieve McGill and Sister Mary John Patch. SOMCA

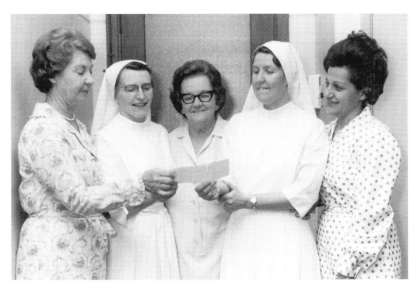

The ladies auxiliaries at the various Mater public hospitals raised significant sums for the hospitals and helped spread the Mater message throughout the community. Here, from left, Mrs Edna Byrne, Sister Angela Mary Doyle, Mrs Cath Schmidt, Sister Rita Pugh and Mrs Nell George are shown at the presentation of a cheque in March 1970. MHHC

land, something which Queensland governments had been very nervous about for at least fifty years. After all, as Dick Strutton pointed out to J P Kelly, a great deal of public investment would be lost if the owners of the land, the Sisters of Mercy, decided to close the hospitals and sell the land. Kelly, ever adroit in argument and well aware that the Mater's reputation for ethical business conduct was unquestioned, reassured Strutton that the Sisters regarded their acceptance of government finance as a trust which they would at all times fulfil. He did not, however, cede the point that the government was building a hospital on Sisters of Mercy land. He successfully reversed that notion – the Sisters of Mercy were building the hospital with the government's assistance. Kelly also sought Strutton's assurance that further development of the Princess Alexandra Hospital would not imperil the Mater's future role. Strutton was forthright: 'The notion of the Mater as an adjunct to the Princess Alexandra Hospital could not possibly be entertained'.[12]

Government agreement to finance the entire cost of the new Adult Hospital did not come without risk to the Mater's independence. There was considerable concern about the consequences of acceding to the government's demand that a project group composed of government and hospital representatives manage the construction phase. Sister Angela Mary was concerned that this system could mean that the project would lose the personal touch that had characterised all earlier Mater building projects. The Mater also wanted to retain the services of its loyal and trusted architect, H L Chapman, of the firm Hall Phillips and Wilson, which continued the practice of the Mater's original architects. However, there was pressure to start the work because the Queensland government was becoming increasingly concerned at the nation's deteriorating financial situation. Health Department budgets were cut in 1976, which gave the Mater great problems in carrying on its usual public hospital services on a reduced operational allocation. The Health Minister had, in fact, assured the Commonwealth early in 1976 that the Mater project was ready to proceed. For this reason, and to ensure that the Commonwealth did not withdraw, the government regarded it as essential that the work begin by 30 June 1976.[13] The pressure was on again. Fortunately, common sense prevailed and further detailed planning proceeded before a brick was laid.

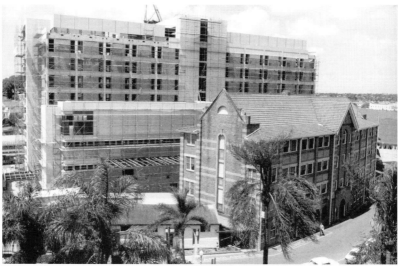

A view of the nearly completed new hospital from the top of the hill, just before St Mary's Nurse's Home was demolished. The old Army huts, moved to the Mater from the Beenleigh Showgrounds in 1946 to accommodate growing numbers of nurses, can be seen at left. MHHC

In the end, fears that the Mater's personal touch would be lost in the building process were not realised. Leighton's, as project manager, assigned a design analyst to spend 1,000 hours processing the results of staff discussions. These discussions allowed the staff – administrative, maintenance and catering staff as well as the medical and nursing staff – to contribute the benefit of their experience and their ideas for an efficient, effective hospital to the design process. This level of consultation, including feedback regarding which ideas would be used, and the reasons why, and which could not be used, and the reasons why not, helped to develop in the staff a strong sense of ownership and a sense of teamwork which carried over into everyday work in the new hospital.[14] However, the project did not proceed without sacrifices. The beloved but somewhat decrepit St Mary's Nurse's Home had to be demolished to make way for the new building. By then, however, more nurses were living outside the hospital, a concept which would have appalled Sister Alphonsus Mary, known affectionately as 'Alfie', during her long tenure as Home Sister. Camaraderie continued to be strong among nurses who had lived at St Mary's. The past nurses donated a statue of Our Lady, placed near the new Adult Hospital, to commemorate the home of their training days.

There was also a nasty scare. In 1978, inflation had taken its toll and Cabinet had to be asked to approve a higher sum. However, it was too late to look back and Cabinet approved the new cost of $28,000,000.[15] The new Adult Hospital was completed in September 1981, after just three years of construction from the turning of the first sod. There were nine levels of hospital functions sandwiched between two additional levels accommodating the plant and machinery necessary to run the air-conditioning system and the lifts. The entry level facing Raymond Terrace accommodated the chapel and an integrated rehabilitation department combining physiotherapy, occupational therapy, speech and hearing, dietetics and social work, as well as the admissions office and the medical records department. There was also a coffee shop, a necessary adjunct for the comfort of patients and visitors.

After decades of congestion in the foyer of the old hospital, where traffic jams regularly occurred around the doors of the single lift, the entrance level of the new hospital was spacious and peaceful. An

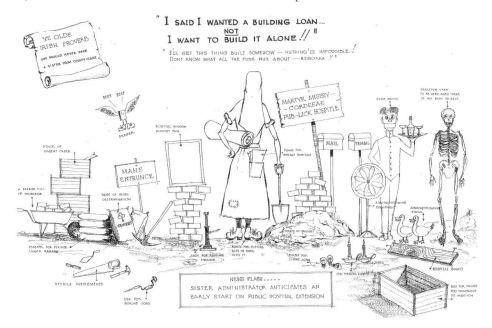

Great determination, humorously portrayed in this cartoon by Mr H L Chapman, the Mater's architect. MHHC

enormous tapestry telling the story of the Sisters of Mercy since their arrival in Queensland was mounted on one wall. The modern mood of the foyer was carried over into the spare design of the beautiful chapel. A local Brisbane artist, Nickolaus Seffrin, worked an unusual presentation of the Stations of the Cross in beaten brass. The images in the sculpture were created to enhance a religious space which would be a peaceful refuge for people of all faiths. Tradition was not forgotten – the inner doors of the chapel incorporated the stained glass from the doors to the St Mary's Nurse's Home.[16]

The next level accommodated the hospital's main office, the kitchen, the staff dining room, conference rooms, a private dining room, and the central stores department. The ambulance entry on the fourth level led directly into the accident and emergency department, with a large radiology department and specialist clinics located nearby. Operating theatres, each with its own anaesthetic room, a special theatre for day surgery, a recovery area, and the intensive care and coronary care units were located on the next floor. Two of the new operating theatres were equipped with laminar flow air distribution to reduce infection in major surgery, such as joint replacements, as much as possible. At long last the pathology department had an entire floor, adjacent to the mortuary. Four levels of wards, by then known as 'patient care units', completed the building. There was not even the remote suggestion of large, impersonal Nightingale wards on these floors. Each patient care unit comprised thirty-two beds arranged in three-bed, two-bed and single-bed units, each with its own bathroom and extensive views over the Brisbane River and the city. The new ward arrangement was not without its drawbacks. It was no longer possible for nurses to see everyone at a glance as they could in the old open wards.[17]

Integration of some costly areas was at last possible. The deficiencies in radiology facilities were largely overcome. The new department served all the public hospitals with modern equipment, including ultrasound, CAT scanners and angiography facilities. The various separate areas of the new pathology floor – haematology, cytology, microbiology, cytogenetics, histology and biochemistry – also serviced all the public hospitals, and the kitchen provided food, already on its plates, to the three public hospitals. Flexibility was enhanced through the use of lightweight plasterboard partitions so that whole areas could be re-configured comparatively easily. The hospital was linked by flyovers to the Mater Children's Hospital via the old adult hospital, to the Mater Mothers' and to a large carpark.

Winning big battles with government, building a large new hospital and planning for future health services could have been sufficient challenges for any organisation, but the Mater also needed to review its nursing and medical staffing and to modernise its management, a task bedevilled by internal stress as taxing as the pressure to provide new clinical facilities. It was, as Sister Catharine Courtney, Superior General during the second half of the 1970s, described it: a matter of dragging a cottage hospital into the modern world.[18] In many ways, the pressures and strains at the Mater in the late 1960s and 1970s reflected the tenor of stressful times in both secular and religious society. Assertions of a universal right to health care, including hospital care when necessary, long granted as a right in Queensland, became more widely expressed. The revolution in health policy and financing in the 1970s was as influential in hospital planning and the delivery of health services as the rapid development of medical science and technologies. Consumer advocacy in the late 1960s and 1970s also reached health care, with a new emphasis on communication with patients and accountability to them. The day of the 'god doctor' and the omnipotent hospital had passed. Doctors, nurses and hospital administrators were questioned searchingly. Patients questioned diagnoses and prescribed treatments and wanted to understand available options and likely outcomes. Accountability in the modern hospital meant much more than knowing how many dollars from which source were spent on what functions; accountability increasingly came to mean who took which action for what reason, and when.

Accountability required clearly understood, comprehensive procedures. However, the Scott report in 1969 and another management review by J C Kable in 1973 identified a serious structural problem at the Mater: there were no clear-cut lines of authority and responsibility. Kable found that these problems were encountered 'by <u>all</u> personnel, at <u>all</u> levels, irrespective of background or training'.[19] Fractured communications were damaging morale in areas ranging from the highest levels of administration to interactions between patients and staff to relationships between lay nursing sisters and religious sisters in the wards. Dealing with clinical issues had been more important than administrative processes, but this could not continue, especially as closer government scrutiny would be the inevitable result of long-sought state funding. There were real communication problems within various departments in each of the individual Mater hospitals, between the hospitals, and between the administration and the medical and nursing staff. The old custom of passing information and instructions informally by word of mouth could not continue. The risk of misinformation, and even damaging gossip, inherent in this custom was serious enough, but, in one respect at least, it also endangered relationships among the staff. Religious sisters regarded the hospitals as their home and their property as well as their workplace, and tended to bypass heads of departments in favour of their religious Superior at the convent when communicating information or seeking authority for particular actions, including transferring nursing staff. This confusion of the appropriate source of professional decisions with the necessary source of religious guidance increased tension between religious and secular staff.

Sorting out this difficulty was critical in clarifying lines of responsibility and authority. The 'mystery' of the convent organisation was one factor. Members of the lay staff, no matter how senior, were excluded from decisions made at the convent and found them difficult to understand, a considerable cause of irritation when the convent appeared to intrude in daily hospital administrative decisions. Sometimes, Sisters were transferred after having been trained for a position, leaving their supervisor to train someone else, often at short notice. Many doctors also thought that a distinct chain of command was needed, because it often seemed that Sisters in charge of particular sections were beyond direction from anyone. Friction was a sad by-product.

Some of these difficulties were inherent in the nature of the hospital. Unlike workers in industrial organisations or large commercial businesses, the great majority of hospital staffers were highly educated professionals who expected to have a say in decisions affecting their workplace. The challenge to effective communications in such an organisation was more difficult at the Mater because the administration was a many-tiered structure; there was a medical advisory committee, a general advisory board, and the General Council of the Sisters of Mercy. As well as the need to improve internal communications through clear lines of decision-making and, wherever possible, creating participative structures, Kable recognised that the government was becoming an important stakeholder and the Mater's structure would need to 'enhance the efficiency of the hospital' and be 'under the control of skilled managers'.[20]

A formal organisation chart showing how all important functions and positions fitted into the total Mater structure was essential. It was important in defining lines of accountability and was also a valuable means of clarifying the difference between the religious staff's professional and religious responsibilities and lines of authority. It also portrayed the Mater as a whole. Each hospital and its Matron had traditionally formed a tight world of its own; very rarely was there time or opportunity for either management or staff in one hospital to really absorb the challenges faced by the other hospitals, or to understand the problems confronting the entire Mater organisation.[21] The success of such structural changes was a matter of no small difficulty and delicacy, dependent for its success on both the diplomacy and the persistence of Mater management.

But the times were changing. By 1973, some of the Sisters were equally unhappy about peremptory transfers, but others felt that much of their work could be done by lay staff, especially duties that threatened to submerge their apostolic role as witnesses to Christ's work through service to others. Sister Angela Mary regarded allowing lay staff to compete for positions previously reserved for religious to be a matter of justice. She believed that no Sister of Mercy should be placed in charge of a department unless she had proved that she had the ability to hold the position.[22] Over the next few years, as Sisters of Mercy retired from senior positions, lay nurses succeeded them. In 1971, Jill Marshall was appointed deputy matron at the Adult Hospital, and Pat Golik and Karleen O'Reilly were successive principal nurse educators. In 1976, Sister Jill Stringer, RSM, returning after years working in Papua New Guinea, applied for the position of matron of the Mater Mothers', and won it after a rigorous selection process. The Sisters were pleased and doubtless relieved that one of their own would hold this key position.

Scrutiny by experts had raised many urgent issues. Tackling the problems and implementing a host of changes occupied the Mater administration for many years. Many solutions went to the heart of traditional Mater customs and practices and turned them on their head. No longer would the Sisters of Mercy have an unchallengeable right to senior positions; reporting through a proper structural organisation would replace hastily exchanged messages; and doctors would also be accountable. Stressed medical and nursing staff, coping with inadequate facilities, and Sisters of Mercy, coping with upheaval in the wake of Vatican II, inevitably found many of the changes hard to accept.

The people with the closest interaction with the patients – the nurses – formed the front line in the campaign to maintain compassionate professional care while new buildings were being debated and constructed, and administrative structures reviewed and changed. All Queensland nurses, including those at the Mater, shouldered high expectations, fortified by ample dedication and enthusiasm, but with little reinforcement from modern education or adequate wages. In most parts of the world, views of the nurse were somewhat idealised after the two world wars. Nurses' war service was much admired, but once the conflicts were over the nurses were expected to step back into the role of foot soldiers in the civilian hospitals. Various articles, usually written by priests or doctors, in the Mater nurses' own journal, *The Misericordian*, reflected the old-fashioned view that nurses should be selfless, dedicated, charitable women, rather than educated professionals with their own distinct role in the hospital system. Catholic nurses were supposed to demonstrate even higher moral and ethical standards. Archbishop Duhig expected Catholic nurses to carry out their professional activities in the light of the Church's doctrines and Christian morality.

The Archbishop's concept of the ideal nurse was somewhat old-fashioned, even in the mid-1940s:

> Nursing is not merely a profession: it is a vocation . . . The care of the sick is one of the corporal works of mercy recommended and praised by Christ Himself . . . [The nurse] must have a good personality, a pleasing manner, patience, tact, and whole-hearted devotion to duty. She must adapt herself to young and old, rich and poor alike. She must be patient with the troublesome persons whose dispositions are generally influenced by their illness, and whom it is difficult either to please or appease.[23]

Four years later, the Archbishop recognised at least some of the harsher realities:

> Nursing is . . . more than the handmaid of medicine; it is a full partner in the work of recovery of the patient . . . Of course the nurse must live, and therefore must have the material remuneration which she richly deserves. But I cannot visualise any nurse worthy of her profession laying more store by money than by the power and happiness of relieving human suffering and restoring the sick to health.[24]

The orthopaedic surgeon Dr John Lahz had a more realistic appreciation of a nurse's life:

She must have double the usual number of hands, feet, ears and eyes. She knows where everything is, when it is wanted, and why. She should be able to speak to two people on the telephone at once while she deals with the patient who has been waiting an hour and has to catch a train. She has to be smooth in calming doctors and soothing relatives. She sees nothing, hears less, and never repeats either. She must know what to do in emergencies, and what not to do when everyone but she is tired from the gruelling day. She must be jocular when the heart is cracking and, of course, must practise economy and at the same time use everything of the best.[25]

Despite these demands, or perhaps because of them, great *esprit de corps* developed among the nurses, even those accommodated in the temporary Army huts moved from the Beenleigh Show Grounds in 1946.[26] Nurses came from all over Queensland. Many mothers, particularly those whose children had not had the benefit of education in the Catholic school system, wanted their daughters to be taught by the nuns at the Mater. By the 1960s, there were many second-generation Mater nurses. The Mater Past Nurses Association thrived, holding reunions in Show Week so that former nurses living in the country could take part.

In the 1960s, nurses in every ward were surrounded by evidence of a medical world rapidly becoming more sophisticated and far more technical, but they were still expected to cope with these challenges on the basis of an outdated education system based on a curriculum which had changed little since 1928. Modern medicine needed more highly skilled and more highly educated nurses. In Sister Eileen Pollard's view, nurses needed to know more than 'how'; they needed to know 'why' and 'why not' and 'when'.[27] An updated curriculum was, at last, on its way. Sister Eileen Pollard took up the gauntlet in nurse education and was profoundly influential in the modernisation of the Mater in the post-war decades, and played a significant part in improving nurse education in Queensland generally.

New junior nurses at the Mater had traditionally been rostered to spend nine weeks in each ward, but there was no preliminary training system. New lecture and group study rooms and a preliminary

EILEEN POLLARD first came to the Mater when she attended the Feast of Our Lady processions during her boarding-school years at All Hallows'. She started her nurse training when she was only 15 years and 6 months and completed it before she entered the Sisters of Mercy. Much to her surprise, Mother Damian decided that Sister Eileen should become a radiographer. After several years in the X-ray department, she completed her Diploma in Nurse Education and returned to the Mater in 1964 when Sister Mary Cletus Gibney retired. She established the nurse education department, and its library, in Raymond Court, and inaugurated a new preliminary course. In 1969, she was appointed to the government committee preparing the new 1970 curriculum. Sister Eileen was Director of Nursing, overseeing all the Mater public hospitals, between 1969 and 1976. Among her achievements were the development of a course for nursing assistants, the creation of the category of Enrolled Nurses, the establishment of the Nursing Personnel Department, in-service education and an occupational health and safety unit for nurses. Sister Eileen was closely associated with the foundation of the new tertiary education course for nurses at the McAuley campus of the Australian Catholic University. After a time spent nursing in Melbourne, she returned to the Mater where she coordinated the process that achieved accreditation for the Mater Private Hospital.

training school were planned for the inauguration of the 1963 curriculum. This curriculum was, however, still very light in theoretical or scientific content. There were only 148 hours of instruction spread over three years; the fourth year continued to be a practical year. The reorganisation of nursing education in the 1960s occurred against the background of wider social changes which offered career opportunities for women in fields far broader than nursing, teaching and office work. The slowly improving nurse education system faced formidable competition for the hearts and minds of young women.

As well as the new curriculum, the drive for administrative efficiency at the Mater in the 1960s also affected the nursing staff. There

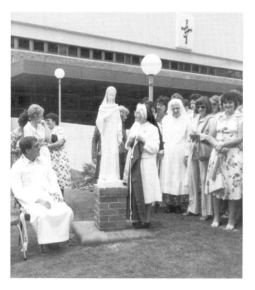

St Mary's Nurse's Home was demolished when the new Mater Adult Hospital was built. This statue of Our Lady, sculpted in Italy, was donated by the Mater Past Nurses Association and is shown being unveiled by Sister Alphonsus Mary Kennedy, always known as 'Alfie', Home Sister at St Mary's for almost twenty-five years. Sister Mary St Roch Clarke is behind her. The cairn supporting the statue was made from bricks taken from the original gateway to the hospital. MHHC

was a need for a better rostering system to accommodate the needs of both the patients and the trainees. These reforms were intended to be allied with the elimination of non-nursing duties from the nurses' workloads and with the introduction of in-service training, proposed initially to help religious sisters who had had little opportunity for further education with the requirements of nursing in an increasingly technological age. In 1970, Sister Angela Mary set up a subcommittee to suggest general organisational improvements and an appropriate structure for the nursing service.[28] Sister Eileen Pollard and the acting personnel and research officer, Sister Smyth, assisted by the Mater secretary, J J O'Brien and a management consultant, set to with a will.

Another new Queensland curriculum for nursing studies was a major influence on the subcommittee's report. The 148 hours of theoretical instruction were to be replaced by 840 teaching hours. The old fourth year, a compulsory period served by all nurses who had passed their final examinations in order to qualify for registration, would be eliminated. Busy wards would miss these senior nurses. Hospital administrations, struggling with sparse finances, would also miss them: fourth-year nurses were not paid at the level of registered nurses and, in addition, more nurses would be needed because trainees attended lectures in hospital time. With these changes approaching, the Mater committee found that uniformity in selection and training standards, as well as uniform standards of patient care, would only be possible if the nursing staff across the complex were organised under a single administrative structure which would include centralised recruiting and rostering.

This change would overturn sixty years of Mater tradition: each hospital in the Mater group had always organised its own nursing staff. A centralised roster would provide a central pool for all categories of staff, rather than individual pools for each hospital. This would ensure that available staff could be used according to each nurse's qualifications and experience, and would also enable nursing students to acquire the full range of clinical experience ready and waiting on the diverse Mater campus. For the first time, the Mater Private Hospital would be routinely included in the rotation roster for student nurses. These improvements, it was hoped, would reduce the alarming level of wastage, which reached 33 per cent of all student nurses in 1970.[29] The proposals for integration and centralised management included the religious sisters who, it was envisaged, would be rostered on an equal footing with the lay staff. This integrated approach was undoubtedly the type of system which Sister Angela Mary had foreshadowed when she appointed Sister Eileen Pollard as Director of Nursing for the three Mater public hospitals in 1969.

A new structure was devised in the 1970s to preserve the autonomy of the matrons in their own hospitals, and to create a workable system of communication between the nursing staffs of the various hospitals. The matrons would report to the Director of Nursing. There were also several new positions. A personnel and nursing research officer would also report directly to the Director of Nursing, as would the principal nurse educator, responsible for both basic and post-basic nursing courses. The subcommittee also looked to the future and recommended that the Mater plan a nursing position to be in charge of domiciliary care, an area likely to develop because the Sisters' engagement with community support was showing signs of increasing greatly. Sister Claire Irving became the first community liaison nurse employed by Queensland Health, and Sister Peter Claver, the pioneer Mater social worker appointed in 1969, was finding her work growing in both volume and breadth of involvement.[30]

The organisation of nursing work in the wards was also on the verge of great change. The new curriculum required patient-assignment nursing. Under this system, teams of nurses at different levels of education and experience would be assigned to particular groups of patients, rather than the traditional allocation of nurses to perform specific tasks for the whole ward.[31] A registered nurse, a first- or second-year nurse and a nurses' aide would comprise a typical nursing team. The team-nursing concept provided flexibility, because the number of patients assigned to any particular team would depend on the level of care those patients required. A team coordinator would be assigned to a number of teams and report to a clinical supervisor who was responsible to the matron. The days of the old ward sister as the martinet head of a hierarchy were fading fast. During her term as matron of the Adult Hospital in the 1970s and early 1980s, Sister Madonna Josey instituted weekly meetings with nurses in charge of wards and quarterly meetings with all nursing staff. Good communication, she believed, was the essential forerunner to good decisions.[32]

The old notion that trainee nurses should perform domestic tasks in the wards was abandoned. They would no longer scrub pans or disinfect beds, make morning tea for the doctors, or serve meals to the patients; in their turn, more senior staff would no longer supervise the linen supply, the ward pantry and the domestic duties, or perform routine clerical work. Hospital assistants in each of the four hospitals would take over the entire range of non-nursing duties. The assistants – known as 'blue ladies' for their distinctive blue uniforms – became highly valued members of ward teams.[33] Ward staff numbers were expanded with more highly trained nursing aides who, Sister Eileen Pollard planned, would be 'practical nurses in the wards'. A pass in the Queensland Junior certificate was required for the nursing aide course, which was open for women between the ages of 16 and 45, suitable for young girls testing the idea of nursing as a career and for married women who were increasingly joining work forces of all kinds.[34] The nurses' spiritual needs and the development of personal responsibility were not overlooked. Sister Eileen Pollard established a Student Nurses Council to help promote self-directed Christian womanhood, professionalism and improved patient care.

Reviews of the Mater's management also examined medical staffing. A redoubtable breed of senior and junior honorary specialists led

PERCY ALAN EARNSHAW, CBE, MB, ChM, FRACP, always known to his colleagues as 'PA', was born in Brisbane in 1894 and graduated in medicine at Sydney University in 1916. He was a regimental medical officer in the First World War and suffered from shrapnel wounds and the effects of poison gas. After the war, he studied at the Great Ormond Street Hospital for Sick Children under such luminaries as Sir Frederick Still. Dr Earnshaw returned to Brisbane in 1923 and became the first doctor in private practice to confine his work to the care of children. After a brief period as an outpatient physician at the Brisbane Children's Hospital, Earnshaw was appointed honorary physician to the Mater Children's Hospital when it opened in 1931, where he remained for almost thirty years. During the Second World War, he was responsible for all inpatient care. He became first president of the Paediatric Society of Queensland in 1949 and worked for the establishment of the Australian College of Paediatrics. He was chairman of the medical committee of the Royal Flying Doctor Service, and a member of the Mater's Medical Advisory Board 1946–59, Queensland's postgraduate medical education committee and the Board of the Faculty of Medicine. His influence on generations of young doctors was profound.

the various clinical departments in the post-war years. Some, like Dr P A Earnshaw, a paediatrician at the Children's Hospital, and the neurosurgeon Dr Geoffrey Toakley were Queensland pioneers in their fields.[35]

The honorary medical staff system was the focus of the first detailed investigation of the Sister Angela Mary era. A meeting of the honorary medical staff in May 1966 recommended that payment for the honorary staff should be considered. A special committee was established to review the system in 1967.[36] Chaired by J P Kelly, its membership included Sister Mary

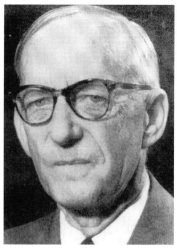

Dr P A Earnshaw, 'father' of paediatrics at the Mater Children's Hospital. MHHC

JAMES GEOFFREY TOAKLEY, CBE, FRCS, FRACS, was born in Sydney in 1921 and graduated in medicine at Sydney University where he was influenced by Sir Douglas Miller, the founding father of Australian neurosurgery. Appointed chief resident medical officer at the Mater, he came to Brisbane in 1949. He left for a short while to study neurosurgery in London. In 1954, the Mater formed Queensland's first neurosurgery department with Dr Peter Landy as physician and Geoff Toakley as surgeon. Dr Toakley worked at the Mater for forty-four years as an honorary surgeon, while maintaining a busy private practice. He was a familiar figure in the theatres at the Mater Private where his meticulous work was greatly admired. However, he retained a special love for his public patients, including those with head injuries often acquired after long sessions in South Brisbane's numerous hotels. Many aspiring young neurosurgeons were inspired and educated by Dr Toakley. 'Toak', as he was often called, became president of Australia's neurosurgeons, and somehow found time to be the doctor for the Easts Rugby Union Club.

St Gabriel, then Superior of the Mater Convent, Sister Mary St Pierre, Matron of the Children's Hospital, Sister Magdalen Mary, Matron of the Mater Mothers', and Sister Mary Owen, Matron of the Adult Hospital. The orthopaedic surgeon Dr M J Gallagher and the physician Dr I R Ferguson represented the honorary staff. Dr O'Callaghan and Sister Angela Mary were the administration's component. This was to be a broad, consultative process. The committee invited submissions from a wide range of interested parties, including the honorary medical staff, the University of Queensland, the Queensland Radium Institute, the Royal Brisbane Hospital, the Australian Medical Association, and hospitals in the other states.

At this time in the Mater's history, reviewing medical staffing was an area fraught with peril. Many doctors had been irritated by the slow progress in improving the Mater public hospitals. Queensland doctors, particularly senior specialists, had also been sensitised for decades to any possible erosion of their authority over their patients.

This authority, they believed, relied very strongly on the principle that their responsibility was always primarily to the patient, not to hospital administrations, nor to governments. The fee-for-service tradition reinforced this principle by ensuring that the 'contract' for the service was exclusively between patient and doctor. Specialists preserved this concept of responsibility, and their independence, in the public hospital system by offering their services free of charge, becoming highly valued 'honoraries' rather than employees accountable to hospital managements. In Queensland state hospitals, the government had paid visiting specialists for their hospital sessions for decades; the Mater was the last bastion of the old honorary system in Queensland, even though it continued to prevail in public hospitals in most other states.

In the perfect world of the mid-twentieth-century medical specialist, the direct employment model would be restricted to resident medical officers and slightly more senior doctors in training for the various specialties. After the Second World War, medical lobby groups, particularly the British Medical Association, the forerunner of the Australian Medical Association, gathered strength in resisting any attempt to replace the fee-for-service principle which had delivered autonomy for the doctors and increased their power in the health system.[37] This power grew during the twentieth century with the growth of advances in science and medical technology. The doctor achieved a new kind of omnipotence as a master of the scientific and technological universe, thought to be impenetrable to patients, politicians and hospital administrators.

In the late 1960s, there were eighty-eight honorary medical officers and forty-nine full-time doctors on the Mater's medical staff. This meant that at the Mater the average doctor–patient ratio was about one doctor to every fifteen patients, whereas it was one to fifty in government hospitals.[38] This plethora of 'honoraries' did not necessarily ensure efficient patient care. Some seemed to put their paid government sessions ahead of their duty to the Mater, and there was considerable concern that, even if the honoraries were paid, some would expect the same personal freedom as they enjoyed under the old system.[39] This 'personal freedom' was responsible for considerable inefficiency, particularly in the surgical area. A valuable operating theatre would lie idle if an honorary surgeon did not arrive for a planned operating session. Sister Angela Mary summed up the position:

> Many and constant complaints relating to honoraries are registered. In general, the complaint is that honoraries do not honour their obligations at outpatient, ward round and operating levels. This results in waste of man power and in frustration for nursing staff. It would seem that it is difficult to discipline non-paid staff.[40]

A way had to be found to deal with this situation without unduly regimenting the doctors. There was also a question of authority. Some longstanding honoraries thought they should control the delivery of all patient care at the Mater, a difficulty for the medical superintendent, Dr O'Callaghan. As well as clarifying the relationship between visiting medical officers and the directors of medical departments, Dr O'Callaghan was enjoined to 'feel confident and able to assume all the authority that is his and all the responsibility that is his'.[41]

Although many Mater honoraries made submissions to the 1967 review, there was no consensus on the payment issue. Many doctors saw payment as regrettable but inevitable; some favoured its immediate introduction; a few argued strongly that there was no need to change the existing system. There was, however, universal agreement that the University of Queensland should be required to remunerate honorary doctors who assisted in teaching medical students. Those who supported the existing system cited as their reason the old fear that this would be the first step to government control. Dr R P Yaxley, who favoured sessional payments, was willing to forgo them 'if this involves any interference with control of the hospital by the Sisters of Mercy'.[42] Dr W J Arnold, who supported this line, said that the honoraries' favoured position in admitting patients to intermediate beds was adequate compensation.

Dr Michael Gallagher had researched the position in South Australia where payment of visiting staff was expected within two years. The South Australian doctors thought that if honoraries were paid they would be more likely to spare more time for public hospital work. The Mater's ophthalmology department pointed out that no other professional group gave its services free of charge on such a large scale and, furthermore, higher rates of income taxation had allowed the Commonwealth to contribute financially to the public hospital system. Therefore, the eye doctors argued, those on higher incomes, including many medical specialists, were already paying to support hospital services for the less affluent. The ophthalmologists thought that private specialists in Queensland were disadvantaged because no means test was applied to admissions to public hospitals, and many patients who would otherwise opt for treatment by a private specialist in a private hospital were public patients. The eye doctors did not support full-time employment of doctors, apart from doctors in specialist training or in services such as radiology, pathology and anaesthetics, because the 'ablest doctors' were those in private practice who held honorary appointments.[43]

The Mater anaesthetists favoured payment for visiting staff, but recognised that the willingness of specialists to work without remuneration was 'probably a major factor in the esprit-de-corps which has always been evident at the Mater'.[44] The visiting staff's jaundiced view of full-time staff in hospitals was, perhaps, predictable, but none the less surprising at a time of great expansion in new specialties and innovative treatments which required hands-on supervision twenty-four hours a day. The neurologist Dr P J Landy foreshadowed the day when new specialties such as gastroenterology and endocrinology might require such expensive technological services that it would be impossible to provide them in both the public hospital and the Mater Private. This, he thought, could mean that private patients would be admitted to public hospitals where they should be charged fees. If this occurred, the distinction between public, intermediate and private hospital beds would be blurred.[45]

Dr Landy thought that payment of visiting staff was inevitable and should be made on the basis of a fixed salary for each session. This would also remove an inequality which irritated many specialists. The Commonwealth's increasing presence in the health system provided a range of opportunities for young specialists – they could examine recruits for the Army, provide part-time care for personnel in military hospitals, and do clinical sessions at the large repatriation hospital at Greenslopes, very close to the Mater. The Commonwealth's sessional salaries were higher than those provided by the state and were eagerly sought by young specialists who needed income while developing their private practices.

The Mater's medical staff association was well aware that promising young specialists were finding the Mater situation very frustrating because older honoraries tended not to retire from their hospital appointments, removing a valuable opportunity from younger specialists. More junior specialists would, incidentally, benefit most from payment, as they were not sufficiently advanced in their careers to benefit from the chance to admit patients to the Mater Private Hospital. More seriously, failing to provide opportunities for younger specialists could put an important pool of new talent out of the Mater's reach. As Dr Harry Windsor pointed out, the road to specialisation was no longer via the route of a few years in general practice where savings could be accumulated; instead, specialist training was tending to be a direct progression from resident medical officer appointments via more training on the hospital staff as a registrar.[46]

Paying the visiting specialists would, however, put pressure on the cost structure, estimated to add about $1.75 to daily bed costs, an implication in tight financial times as serious as the need to employ more nurses to accommodate changes in nurse education. Nevertheless, the die was cast. Visiting specialists at the Mater would be paid after 3 March 1974.[47] It says a great deal for the honorary staff's loyalty to the Mater that there was very little impatience over delays in bringing in the new system. The government kept up the pressure during the tense negotiations over the new Adult Hospital, and urged that some retrenchments be made from the Mater's large visiting staff to bring it more in line with the state system. The Mater, recognising that many existing honoraries had given years of service to the hospital, took a gentler approach and decided that it would be preferable to phase the system out rather than bring it to an abrupt end.[48]

The reviews of the nursing and medical staff were only part of the changes behind the scenes at the Mater during the 1970s. The administrative structure was next. Administrative restructuring reached all departments, changing the Mater perhaps as much as the rebuilding program, though much less visibly. There were several pressing issues. Complaints of poor communication between the hospital administration and the staff had waxed and waned for decades. Identification of deficiencies in lines of accountability had also revealed the need for much more internal consultation and improved communication with the community. Sister Angela Mary realised that neither the Sister Administrator nor the Sisters of Mercy as an organisational entity should be hidden from Mater patients, staff and the wider community. In 1967, therefore, Harry Summers, a well-known Queensland journalist, was appointed the Mater's first public relations specialist. Throughout the 1970s, he kept up a flow of interesting stories to keep the Mater's name in the press and in the minds of the Queensland public, and in 1979 he completed the first history of the Mater hospitals, *They crossed the river: The founding of the Mater Misericordiae Hospital, South Brisbane, by the Sisters of Mercy.*

Sister Angela Mary also communicated with the community. She began to publish her own annual report in 1969. J P Kelly no longer reported on behalf of the Sisters. This gave Sister Angela Mary the opportunity to put forward her beliefs and her vision for the Mater. The importance of communications and the personal touch was stressed: 'The Administrator must be concerned with human relations in their broadest sense, and with the needs of the individual at a personal level'. Planning for the future was also very much on her mind. Sister Angela Mary was well aware of the changes occurring in the general community:

> The effective Administrator must not only be alert for changes occurring outside the Hospital, but must constantly seek them out so that their impact on the organisation may be evaluated. Only thus can one safely plan, for planning means establishing clear definition of purpose and clear definition of technique.[49]

The Scott and Compton reports had both advocated structural change, particularly the need for leaders of commerce and industry to be included in the Advisory Board's membership, in addition to

J P Kelly, the sole board member who was not part of the hospital staff. It was believed that if this were done the whole business community would see that the Mater enjoyed high-level support, an important incentive because 'many companies make a decision on a gift solely because of who is on the board or appeal committee'.[50]

J C Kable's management review also recommended that board membership be broadened to create a more participative structure and introduce a wider range of expertise from outside the hospital. He suggested a lay chair, with a deputy who was also a suitably qualified professional, the director of administration, one representative of the medical appointments board, a representative nominated by the chief executive officer (as a means of introducing younger staff to high-level management), three lay members, and one representative of the Sister's General Council. To this last recommendation, Sister Angela Mary added the notations 'non-voting' and 'residing away from the hospital'; she deleted Kable's recommendation that the Roman Catholic Church be represented on the board.

The new Advisory Board met for the first time in 1974. It had three lay members from outside the hospital's immediate circle – J C Kable, the architect, H L Chapman, and its first lay woman member, the ardent fundraiser Mrs Nell George. J P Kelly continued in the chair, with the barrister and later Chief Justice of Australia F G Brennan QC as his deputy. Dr Tony McSweeny and Dr Ian Ferguson represented the medical staff. Sister Angela Mary and five other Sisters of Mercy, J J O'Brien, Pat Maguire and Des O'Callaghan completed the board. For the first time in the Mater's history, the Sisters of Mercy on the board could be outvoted in making recommendations to the Sisters' congregational leadership.

The Congregation was the ultimate decision-maker, but J P Kelly recognised that it was impossible for the Mother General and the Sisters' General Council to grasp the complexity of the modern Mater's management needs when they were also grappling with the schools and the Sisters' social work, as well as assisting all the Sisters to come to terms with changes in governance and administration following the Vatican Council changes. Kelly and Sister Angela Mary both agreed that there needed to be another mechanism to link the hospital to the

General Council.[51] A special Hospital Council, formed by members of the Sisters of Mercy General Council with special responsibility for the Mater, seemed to be the answer. Kable disagreed with this idea because he felt that the Mother General's representative on the Advisory Board should be sufficient communication. Sister Angela Mary, who had studied religious organisational structures in the United States, preferred the hospital council concept, even though there was a risk that many secular members of the Mater staff could think that the council was just one more secret religious organisation making decisions affecting their lives. The Hospital Council was established and congregational leaders found it to be an effective innovation, particularly as many Sisters who became part of leadership teams had had no previous acquaintance with the hospital's management needs.

J C Kable recommended that the Advisory Board concentrate on policy, and leave detailed matters to an executive committee which would manage the day-to-day running of the hospital complex and implement the Advisory Board's policies. The new executive included the Sister Administrator, Sister Angela Mary, the Director of Nursing, Sister Eileen Pollard, the Director of Medical Services, Dr Des O'Callaghan, the Secretary of the Board, Jack O'Brien, and the Director of Administration, Pat Maguire. This committee, Kable suggested, should be readily identifiable to all hospital staff to mitigate the feeling, identified in all the management reviews, that hospital administration was an impenetrable mystery. However, it was initially a somewhat uneasy committee – some doctors found it hard to accept that the nursing service would carry equal weight at executive level.[52] One of the oldest of the Mater's administrative bodies, the Medical Advisory Committee, continued to represent the interests of the visiting medical staff and, through its representative on the Advisory Board, to recommend medical appointments.

The Director of Medical Services was a key position in improving communications in the clinical areas of all the hospitals. The director of obstetrics at the Mater Mothers', the supervisor of paediatrics at the Mater Children's and the clinical supervisor at the Adult Hospital reported to him. In addition, a new medical services group advised the Director of Medical Services. This group included the heads of the clinical services, as well as the director of nursing, the directors of pathology, radiology and anaesthetics, the senior pharmacist, and representatives of the resident medical officers and the rehabilitation services. Their suggestions and recommendations were sent to the Sister Administrator. There was also an urgent need to provide more full-time staff positions in both the clinical areas and the administrative areas. Instead of the Director of Medical Services supervising the clinical practice at the Adult Hospital, J C Kable suggested that a clinical supervisor in each hospital would be a key position in improving communication with the resident medical staff. He also found that work in the laboratories and the pharmacy had grown to such an extent that the time had come to separate their administration.

The Director of Nursing position remained the most controversial. The matrons and their deputies were divided between full support for the concept of an integrated Director of Nursing position, or complete opposition to it. This was not surprising, given the Mater tradition of separation between the nursing staffs at the various hospitals, which had equipped the matrons to take full control of all nursing problems within their hospital. Any diminution of this authority was seen as an incursion into their legitimate spheres of influence. On the other hand, there was a recognition that much of the detailed administrative pressure on the matrons could be relieved by the Director of Nursing. The first Director of Nursing, Sister Eileen Pollard, recognised these oppositional tussles within senior levels of the nursing staff, a situation further complicated by the reality that the matrons effectively had two bosses – the Director of Medical Services for the care of the patients, and the Director of Nursing in nursing matters. To ensure that the matrons had a means of making their views heard, a nursing committee was created comprising the Director of Nursing, all the matrons, the principal nurse educator, the sister in charge of personnel, the Director of Medical Services and the Sister Administrator.

In the early days of Sister Angela Mary's era, there had been no administrative committees. There was now a plethora of bodies to consider issues and make recommendations. The new structure was a complex matrix linked both vertically and horizontally. The idea was to deliver more transparency in hospital administration, broader participation and more effective linkages among hospital departments. Keeping the flow of ideas, decisions and suggestions running smoothly up, down and across the matrix, and implementing policies, was the remit of a tight core of senior executives.

The role of the Sister Administrator was clear-cut. She was simultaneously managing director, chief executive officer and the public face of the Mater. Sister Angela Mary's sharp mind, honed by academic study, and her ready grasp of policy concepts and ability to absorb mountains of detail supplied the administrative fuel. She readily sought counsel – not only from the Sisters' general council and J P Kelly but also from other key Mater executives. Sorting out their roles and responsibilities was essential. J J O'Brien, as board secretary, had been a senior figure since his appointment in 1954. His portfolio of tasks had greatly expanded over the years to embrace budget and personnel management and oversight of the art unions and hospital appeals, as well as implementation of policies. By the early 1970s, he was assisted by a former bank officer, Mr Pat Maguire, who came from a managerial position at Mt Olivet Hospital to the Mater in 1969. It was essential to divide the overlapping areas of their responsibilities into clearly distinguishable functions. J C Kable suggested a new position, Director of Administration, to control administrative and financial activities and supervise hospital purchasing, the art unions, the engineering section and the medical records department. The Board Secretary would implement directions from the board and the Sisters' Hospital Council and would also supervise the budget officer, the controller of the household, the head wardsman and the personnel officer. As a final touch to managerial reorganisation, the administration was consolidated at Clarence Court in Clarence Street in 1974–75.

By the mid-1970s, there were many staff to manage: 1,440 employees in the three public hospitals. If, as the old saying goes, it takes many people to support one soldier in the field, the same can be said of a modern hospital. The medical and nursing staff have always been the most visible face of the diverse workforce needed to keep one patient in a bed. The army behind the Mater scene included the engineering section, responsible for the operation and maintenance of all the major plant – the boiler, the air-conditioning, the hot water, the plumbing, the refrigeration – as well as answering urgent calls to fix a myriad of small things. About two dozen skilled tradesmen kept the Mater running in the 1970s, a considerable task in the aging buildings. They were closely involved in planning the new Adult Hospital, which had more complex systems and services to be kept running around the clock.

Patients and staff have to be fed three meals a day, always with the complexities of special diets to add to the challenge. Before the new Adult Hospital was opened in 1981 with its streamlined kitchen catering for all the public hospitals, each Mater hospital had its own kitchen converting vast quantities of raw produce into tempting dishes, always said to be of a higher standard than those at other hospitals.[53] The food, prepared under the watchful eye of Sister Ann Marie at the Adult Hospital, Sister Mary Madeleine at the Children's, and Sister Patricia Plint at the Mater Mothers' tempted many a resident medical officer to continue at the Mater. One basic service was of more than usual importance. In the early 1980s, about 200,000 pieces of fabric – sheets, towels, theatre gowns and so on – were laundered each week. The Mater's laundry was owned by the Mater Private Hospital, and the public hospitals were charged for its services. It was, therefore, an essential service in two completely different ways. It helped the Mater Private financially and, with more than thirty full-time staff, the laundry, like the engineering services and the kitchens, was an important employer.

By the early 1980s, when the new Adult Hospital received its first patients, the Mater had been reviewed, restructured and partly rebuilt. Construction of buildings and administrative rearrangements were not, however, the only innovations at the Mater in the 1970s and 1980s. The purpose of all the turmoil – continually improving the care of the patients – had also taken on some interesting new dimensions.

CHAPTER SEVEN

FACING DIFFICULT QUESTIONS

As we move towards the year 2000 and a new society,
the Mater Hospital is challenged to a deeper level of
openness. Through its daily clinical practice and
highly-valued research it will be facing complex and
totally new medical, ethical and technological questions
about life and death: who can be born, what constitutes
human life, who decides between competing claims
for life-support?[1]

Sister Kath Burke, Congregational Leader, 1981

In 1981, when Sister Kath Burke wrote those words, all the Mater
hospitals and all departments within them were reaping the harvest
of enormous developments in scientific and technological medicine.
All sick people, from tiny premature babies in the Mater Mothers' to
elderly patients in the Adult Hospital, were part of a medical milieu in
which ethical questions raised by new forms of diagnosis and treatment
were almost as significant as the opportunities for health and happi-
ness they offered. Scientific medicine and its ancillary technologies
introduced complex machinery of all kinds into the wards, bringing
with it the possibility that patient care would be mechanical, even

dehumanised, confronting the Mater's almost eighty years of emphasis on holistic care and the dignity of the individual. Medico-moral questions centring on the meaning of life and death were accompanied by debates over the appropriate allocation of human and financial resources in the hospitals. These wider social justice questions were very much part of the ethical cocktail. In one way or another, all the Mater hospitals faced ethical dilemmas which, while they were often nothing more than old issues in new guises, nevertheless required more complex responses.

From the 1970s onwards, the nurseries at the Mater Mothers' provided a poignant arena in which the community was drawn into the drama of the life-saving potential of scientific, technological medicine and the ethical questions it raised. Steadily improving prospects for very tiny premature babies and babies born with illnesses and disabilities were, however, only one aspect of the changes which led to ethical questions concerned with the well-being of mothers and babies. Science had also revolutionised obstetrics. Women who appeared to have no chance of conceiving a child appeared to be offered a reprieve by *in vitro* fertilisation; genetic testing and new ways of monitoring

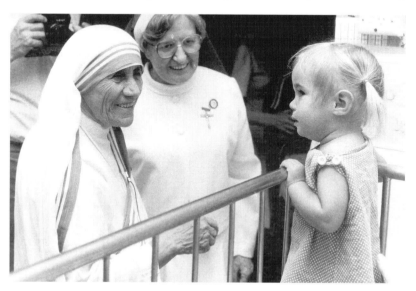

Mother Teresa of Calcutta, a special visitor in 1981, the seventieth anniversary of the Mater Adult Public Hospital, is seen here with Sister Mary Dorothea and one of the Mater's younger patients. MHHC

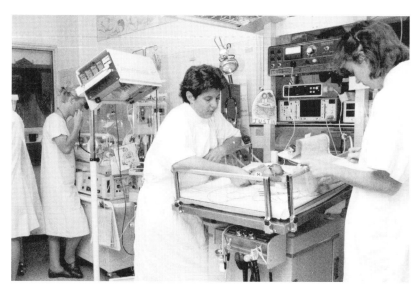

Tiny babies in the intensive care nursery at the Mater Mothers' Hospital were surrounded by high technology but retained their individuality. Note 'Justin's' name above his cot. MHHC

developing babies *in utero* promised better outcomes for babies with development disorders, but, on the other hand, provided advance warning that a baby with a permanent disability might result from the pregnancy.

Termination of pregnancy for any reason other than the likely imminent death of the mother remained forbidden, a Roman Catholic stance shared by people of many faiths, as well as by increasing numbers of secular groups motivated by humanistic moral concerns rather than by religious precepts. On the other side of the argument, the view that commencing a pregnancy, or maintaining it to term, should be a woman's own choice was increasingly expressed. This was in some ways a product of the women's movement, and in others an outcome of the promotion of individual rights, a catchcry of the late 1960s and 1970s. Loud pleas for wider availability of artificial forms of contraception imposed additional pressure. The Encyclical, *Humanae vitae*, issued by Pope Paul VI in 1968, had made the Church's prohibition of contraception, including the increasingly popular oral contraceptive, very clear. Other issues in obstetrics and the care of very premature infants raised more blurred moral and ethical challenges.

In an era of increasingly costly technologies and shrinking health care resources, the claims of immature pre-term babies for large shares of those resources thrust the morality of saving and preserving life hard against both altruistic social justice advocacy and more materialist cost-effectiveness dogmas. The visit of Mother Teresa of Calcutta to the Mater in 1981 was a potent reminder that advocacy for the poor remained a vital modern notion.

Babies are natural attention-grabbers. Exciting news items had regularly appeared in the Queensland newspapers in the 1960s featuring tiny premature babies who were surviving, and infants with Rh incompatibility saved at the Mater Mothers' by exchange blood transfusions. Paediatricians had become a common sight in all maternity hospitals, but neonatology, the care of the newly born, was a new specialty in 1961 when the first babies were born at the Mater Mothers'.[2] The Mater Mothers' first consultant neonatal paediatricians, Dr David Jackson, Dr Geoffrey Bourke and Dr Stephen Clark Ryan, supervised neonatal care at the Mater Mothers' public hospital in the 1960s and 1970s. Dr John Thearle was the first specialist in neonatology to be seen in the wards at the Mater following his appointment in 1973 to the Department of Child Health staff of his *alma mater,* the University of Queensland. John Thearle had completed his postgraduate training in Bristol where ultraviolet light as a means of combating jaundice in new babies was first used in 1958, a technique he introduced to Queensland.[3]

Advances in neonatology required new equipment and, in 1972, $50,000 was spent on intensive care equipment for babies.[4] This may have been a mere drop in the technological bucket, but was nonetheless significant, given the pressing needs of the other Mater hospitals. However, the Mater was aware that any maternity hospital registering more than 5,000 births per year should have an intensive care unit. Neonatology was further advanced at the Royal Women's Hospital at Herston, but both Brisbane maternity hospitals lagged behind international standards. The national newspaper, the *Australian*, reported in September 1972 that Brisbane was the only major Australian city without a fully equipped neonatal intensive care unit.[5] Between 1972 and 1974, Mater babies needing ventilation were transferred to the Royal Women's Hospital, giving reason to fear that only full-term, healthy

DAVID IAN TUDEHOPE, AM, MBBS, MRACP, FRACP, was born at the Brisbane Women's on 16 February 1944, and grew up in the eastern Melbourne suburb of Mont Albert. He matriculated from Scotch College to study medicine at Monash University, and completed his residency at the Alfred Hospital. During a term at the Fairfield Infectious Diseases Hospital, he greatly enjoyed working with children and completed his paediatric training at the Royal Children's Hospital where he obtained his Membership of the Royal Australian College of Physicians at the first attempt. Following a term as neonatal registrar at Hammersmith Hospital in London, where he usually worked 110 hours each week, David Tudehope was awarded a post-doctoral fellowship at McMaster University in Ontario. Dr Jack Sinclair became his mentor in neonatology and helped him achieve a post-doctoral year at the University of California, San Francisco, a position he found to be most intellectually stimulating. Nineteen seventy-five was an exciting year in neonatology in Australia – David Tudehope was offered specialist positions in Adelaide, Melbourne, Sydney and at the Mater Mothers' in Brisbane. He chose Brisbane, and was appointed Director of Neonatology in July 1977. During almost thirty years in that position, he has published textbooks and dozens of papers and been both an Associate and a full Professor in Child Health at the University of Queensland and an honorary Professor in Neonatal Paediatrics at Zhejang University in China. He has been awarded the Bancroft Medal and a Centenary of Federation Medal and was nominated three times for Queenslander of the Year. In 2002, he was awarded the Queensland Great accolade by the premier of Queensland.

babies would be nursed at the Mater unless changes were made. Sister Peg Slack was certainly doing her bit, travelling to the United States, the United Kingdom and Europe to study neonatal intensive care nursing in 1973.[6] At last, in 1974, the first ventilators were purchased for the special-care nursery, a small room on the sixth floor.

Dr David Tudehope, the first neonatologist appointed to the Mater staff, arrived in 1977. Young and enthusiastic, David Tudehope was determined to develop neonatology at the Mater Mothers' to the highest international standard.[7] He had four dreams: the development of a first-class neonatal intensive care unit, the inauguration of a neonatal emergency transport service, the establishment of a multi-disciplinary growth and development clinic, and the foundation of Queensland's first post-basic neonatal nursing training course. He set to with a will. In August 1977, only a month after Dr Tudehope's arrival, the Mater celebrated the first retrieval – baby Brad Treadwell was flown to the Mater from Charleville. Always ready to speak out for causes he believes in, David Tudehope was featured in local newspapers criticising sparse state resources for babies in remote areas. Chided by the then Director-General of Health, Dr Ross Patrick, that he should not 'bite the hand that feeds you',[8] Dr Tudehope pressed on and the Neonatal Emergency Transport Service, NETS, using its own Vickers Model 77 incubator, with a suitably modified ventilator, was formally inaugurated in April 1978, when twins were transported from Toowoomba.

The first few years were tough. Sister Jill Stringer, Director of

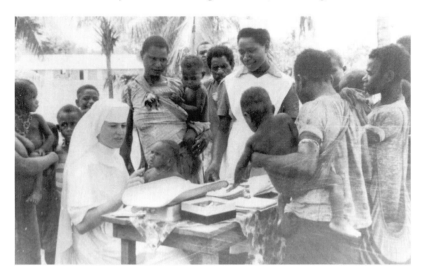

Sister Jill Stringer came from the Sisters of Mercy mission in New Guinea to be Nursing Superintendent of the Mater Mothers' Hospital. She is photographed here with her patients at Kunjingini in 1966. MHHC

Nursing at the Mothers', frequently drove a hospital vehicle at high speed to transport the retrieval team to hospitals in various parts of south-east Queensland. In the first year, forty-five babies were transported to the Mater Mothers'. Some were very ill, and it was remarkable that only three babies died.[9] It took some time to come to a satisfactory arrangement with the ambulance service, because the region was rigidly divided into ambulance districts; no ambulance vehicle dared breach a divisional border. At last, road ambulances retrieved babies from Lismore, Toowoomba, Southport and Ipswich. Air retrievals from Mackay, Longreach, Cunnamulla, Roma and as far away as New Guinea used aircraft from State Wide Air Charter and, sometimes, the Royal Australian Air Force. Helicopter retrievals commenced in 1984 when the lawn outside the Adult Hospital and the St Laurence's school oval were pressed into duty as landing pads. At St Laurence's, police car headlights guided night landings.[10] In 1989, NETS received its first dedicated vehicle, funded by the Bingo Parlour of Fortitude Valley and equipped by the MacGregor Lions Club.

Back at the hospital, much remained to be done. Although the state government had provided $284,405 for enlarged special-care nurseries, opened in December 1976, and the inimitable Joy Shields and her Ladies Auxiliary provided equipment worth $51,000 during the 1970s, standards were still considerably behind American neonatal intensive care units.[11] In 1977, when the unit was in desperate need of state-of-the-art technology, a very substantial donation from Mrs Lynette Mulcahy was a turning point for neonatal care at the Mothers'.

Changes were dramatic. The seventh-floor nursery was opened in 1979 as a recovery care unit, where mothers were encouraged to look after their babies as much as possible. Results were impressive. By 1978, Dr Tudehope could report that the Mater's neonatal survival rate was among the world's best – 84 per cent of babies born between 1,000 and 1,500 grams survived; 85–90 per cent of babies under 1,500 grams would develop normally; and only 5.5 per cent would have major handicaps. These were powerful arguments against critics, including the Australian philosopher Dr Peter Singer, who suggested that spending money on very premature babies was usually pointless because they would all need long-term care and have poor quality of life.[12]

Success was very much a team effort, enhanced by the purchase of new ventilators, and innovative treatment such as peritoneal dialysis for acute renal failure in 1979 undertaken by the nephrologist Dr John Burke.[13] The ability of Alana Barlow and Avril Robinson and their team of dedicated nurses in the special-care nurseries, the work of nurse educators, and Cathy Bagley's physiotherapy, were critical to some remarkable results in the late 1970s and early 1980s. In 1982, for instance, the Mater Mothers' reported a lower incidence of neonatal necrotising enterocolitis than anywhere else in the world.[14] A baby born in Lismore with gastroschisis (intestines outside the body) was rushed to the Mothers' and survived emergency surgery. In 1981, Rebekah Allen, born at twenty-three weeks' gestation and weighing only 650 grams, became the smallest surviving Mater baby, an achievement surpassed in 1983 by baby Aimee Santacaterina, also born at twenty-three weeks but weighing under 500 grams, who was flown to the neonatal unit from Mackay. Baby Aimee was discharged after seventeen weeks. Her story confronted those who advocated new

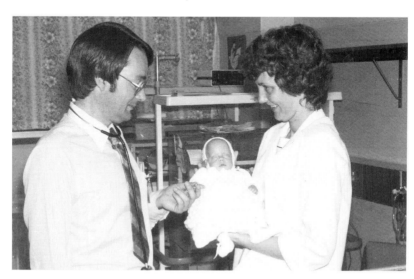

A triumph for neonatal care at the Mater Mothers' Hospital. Baby Aimee Santacaterina was born at twenty-three weeks gestation, weighing 400 grams, and was flown to the Mater from Mackay. She is shown here with her mother and Dr David Tudehope. MHHC

guidelines to allow aborted foetuses lighter than 400 grams, or less than twenty weeks' gestation, to be used in tissue research.[15]

The third Tudehope dream, a multidisciplinary growth and development clinic to evaluate the progress of infants of birthweight less than 1,500 grams, and babies whose lives had depended on a respirator, was established in 1978 under Dr Michael O'Callaghan, a paediatrician specialising in child development. This was a multidisciplinary effort. The physiotherapist, Professor Yvonne Burns, and the psychologist, Professor Heather Mohay, were essential members of the child development team. In 1982, the clinic reported that only 6 per cent of premature babies born at the Mater had handicaps, a low rate in international terms. The clinic developed broad interests, such as a project, supported by the Queensland Sudden Infant Death Syndrome (SIDS) Foundation, which investigated whether or not neonatal sleep apnoea in low birthweight infants was a factor affecting their growth and development in the first two years of life.[16] Studies of all kinds became more systematised through the Queensland Council on Obstetric and Paediatric Morbidity and Mortality, established in 1979.

Collection and analysis of statistics in obstetrics demonstrated rapid change in the management of labour and birth at the Mater Mothers'. Caesarean sections were performed more often – an increase from 2.9 per cent of births in the Mothers' public hospital in 1961 to 14 per cent in 1975 – reflecting both the increasing use of epidural anaesthesia and the finding that Caesarean delivery could improve the outcome for babies at risk.[17] At 29 per cent, the Caesarean rate was much higher in the Mothers' private hospital, a phenomenon reported in many private obstetric hospitals, giving rise to claims that Caesareans were often performed on private patients to suit the comfort of mothers or the convenience of private specialists. Technological advances enabling sophisticated fetal monitoring during labour, ultrasound scanning during pregnancy, and a wider range of pathology investigations were important features in obstetric developments in the 1980s. These also gave rise to remarkable stories. In 1980, for instance, a mother with a heart pacemaker safely delivered her second baby, and in 1982 twins were born to a woman who had undergone a kidney transplant.[18]

On the less joyful side of the ledger, many less than desirable aspects of life in the 1980s were reflected at the Mater Mothers'. Babies were born with heroin in their systems, and it was not long before there were calls for increased accommodation for mothers with infectious diseases such as hepatitis B, most commonly acquired through injecting illegal drugs. Acquired Immunity Deficiency Syndrome, known commonly as AIDS, a terrifying disease, made its presence known in Australia late in 1982 and tragically visited the nurseries at the Mater Mothers' in 1984. Three babies were infected with the virus through a blood transfusion in February and died later in the year.[19] The AIDS tragedy sparked some remarkable responses among Mater people.

The Sisters of Mercy developed a major program to care for AIDS sufferers, batting away media suggestions that this was, in some way, peculiar work for a religious order, with a pertinent reminder that the Sisters of Mercy's mission was to address need wherever they found it. At that time, people affected by either the human immunodeficiency virus or full-blown AIDS were frequently ostracised. The Sisters of Mercy provided houses for sufferers and a range of care services. On the scientific side of the Mater, a research team consisting of Dr Dick Chalmers, Prof Yee Hing Thong and Miss Judith Renouf, working on the blood of one of the AIDS babies, developed the first test for measuring enzyme levels in lymphocytes, an important indicator of the progress of AIDS sufferers. It was a breakthrough of international importance.[20]

During the 1980s, it became increasingly obvious that many pregnant women faced serious social and economic problems. Increasing rates of teenage pregnancies sparked a long-term study of attitudes to pregnancy in partnership with the University of Queensland Department of Anthropology and Sociology. There were worrying trends, with reports that girls as young as 12 were having babies, but Dr Esler, the medical superintendent, was frustrated that tight resources would not allow follow-up of very young mothers who did not live in stable relationships.[21]

Illness during pregnancy remained a matter of considerable concern. It was obvious that, despite antenatal care in community clinics at Woodridge, Kingston, Inala, and at the new Queen Elizabeth II hospital, more outreach and educational programs were needed. It was a sobering thought that complications of pregnancy and childbirth put more women in hospital in the 1980s than any other illness. This was a considerable pressure on resources, given that a mini baby boom started in 1981. In 1982, the Mater Mothers' Hospital was reported to be Australia's busiest maternity hospital, with a total of 6,342 births and almost twenty deliveries every day in September alone. The boom continued and was thought to be caused by young people coming from interstate looking for work, and a reduction in intermediate admissions at the Royal Women's Hospital as people dropped out of private health insurance.[22]

With high bed-occupancy figures, the Mothers' was struggling to cope with demand. Despite its international clinical reputation, the fabric of the Mater Mothers' Hospital lagged badly. It was over twenty years old; deterioration was everywhere. In Dr Esler's opinion, the 'appalling' state of the public antenatal clinics and the overcrowding in most areas would harm the hospital's reputation if they became public knowledge. Even in the private section, bathrooms were inadequate and most rooms needed renovation. The catalogue of needs was long: six extra labour rooms, an additional observation nursery, an infection control area for the special-care nursery, and twenty additional beds. There was a real fear that the Mothers' might have to limit private bookings, even if a new private hospital not far away at Sunnybank could accommodate 500 deliveries a year.[23] At this point, it was ironic that the Mater had succeeded in its argument in 1978, when the birth rate was lower, that the proposed Queen Elizabeth II hospital at Mt Gravatt was not needed as a maternity hospital. There was only one way of expanding the accommodation at the Mater Mothers' – converting the convent on the seventh floor of the building to patient accommodation. This reprieve allowed the Mater Mothers' to concentrate on tertiary-level care, supplemented by the state's Queen Elizabeth II hospital which would accommodate low-risk obstetric patients.[24]

Accommodating the patients was one pressure; dealing with their demands was quite another. All obstetric hospitals were under constant scrutiny and subject to repeated criticism of their clinical methods and apparent lack of personalised care for patients, fathers and families.[25] Maternity hospitals were feeling the impact of consumerism and the awareness of women who were more highly educated and more likely to demand choices. In the 1970s, the Childbirth Education Association became a popular movement, advocating the least possible intervention in natural childbirth through the use of drugs or surgery. To some extent, this trend was a reaction against the medicalisation of childbirth, and, in turn, placed a higher value on midwives. This 'return to nature' movement manifested itself in areas as diverse as preferences for food produced without chemicals and alternative medical therapies. The reaction against artificial hormones in the contraceptive pill led many women who were not conscientious Catholics to the natural family planning clinic at the Mothers'.

Satisfying consumer demands while providing safe obstetric care became a delicate balancing act. Fathers were allowed in the labour wards in the 1970s; babies were released from the nursery to 'room in' with their mothers; and greater parent access was allowed to babies in the special-care and intensive care nurseries. The plaintive cry 'When can I see my baby?' gradually faded away.[26] The next step – fathers in the operating theatre during Caesarean section procedures – was more difficult. In the mid-1980s, when this became a burning issue, the Mater Mothers' was still working with its original operating theatres, thought to be too small to accommodate the father as well as the surgical team. However, the pressure of competition had its influence. The newer Sunnybank and Queen Elizabeth II hospitals were allowing fathers this privilege, and private obstetricians were feeling pressure from their patients to bypass the Mater. The numbers of valuable private patients fell. Finally, in May 1986, fathers were permitted in the operating theatres, but only when epidural anaesthesia was used, a condition similar to the rules at the Royal Women's Hospital.[27]

These innovations placed a great deal of responsibility on the midwifery staff, both inside the hospital and in conducting educational programs at community level. As well as parenthood classes, the staff also developed educational programs for mothers of the babies in the special nurseries to develop their confidence in handling their babies, and programs for adopting parents. Postgraduate obstetric and neonatal nursing seminars on Saturday mornings became regular features, attended by midwives from country and provincial hospitals as well as from the Mater. However, David Tudehope's fourth dream did not become a reality until 1985, when the Board of Nursing Studies at last approved the post-basic course in neonatal intensive care nursing after negotiations with the state's Board of Nursing Studies had ground on since 1979.[28]

Both the nursing staff and the medical staff at the Mothers' developed additional support structures for parents. Groups such as the Childbirth Education Association and the Nursing Mothers Association had pioneered the 'self-help' concept, which was extended at the Mater with the establishment of the Preterm Infants Parents Association, PIPA, in 1980, and the Sudden and Neonatal Death Society, SANDS, in 1982. SANDS, and the Mater's world-leading inauguration of a rite for mourning a miscarried child in 1983, were part of a general recognition that miscarriage, stillbirth and neonatal death all meant the death of a child, leaving parents to mourn the loss of the future they had envisaged.[29]

Caring in the technological era still had a distinctive Mater touch.

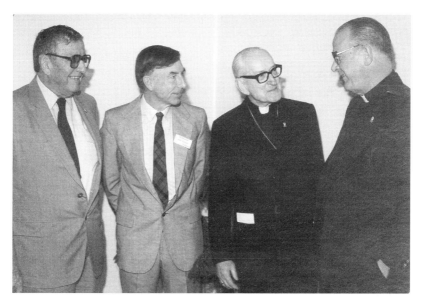

In 1985, a major seminar on ethics was part of the celebrations of the seventy-fifth anniversary of the opening of the Mater Private Hospital. Participants photographed here are the ethicist Father Richard McCormick, SJ, a speaker from the United States (far right), the Archbishop of Brisbane, Francis Rush (next right) with the Professor of Obstetrics, Eric Mackay, and Mr Kevin Cronin (left). MHHC

In 1983, the Sisters celebrated the delivery of one family's eleventh child by giving them an industrial washing machine, chosen on the advice of the Medical Superintendent, Dr Des O'Callaghan, who had eleven children of his own.[30] Care of the whole patient, clinically, spiritually and practically, was a Sisters of Mercy ethic practised since the days of Catherine McAuley. The biomedical dimension of ethical conduct was, however, the one most commonly discussed in the mid-1980s. The silver jubilee of the Mater Mothers' in 1986 was an appropriate occasion for a major seminar, 'Ethical issues in Catholic health care today'. The topics included the ethical implications of prenatal diagnosis, a medical overview of methods of prenatal diagnosis, obstetrical clinical dilemmas and their ethical resolution within the Catholic setting.

The silver jubilee marked some major milestones. The original medical superintendent, Dr Edwin Esler, retired. He had overseen the delivery of 122,000 babies, including the birth of Brisbane's first 'test tube' triplets in 1985, and seen the neonatal intensive care unit grow from a one-cot nursery in 1973 to a nursery which looked after 825 babies in one year in its forty-three cots. One of the hospital's original success stories, Robyn Allen, who had weighed only 750 grams when she was born in 1963, came back as a healthy, active adult to visit the hospital in its silver jubilee year. The hospital had much to be thankful for when it hosted the Silver Jubilee clinical meeting of the Australian Perinatal Society in September 1986.[31] It also had much to look forward to – a new medical superintendent, Dr James King, had taken up duty, and the new antenatal services department was nearly complete, at a cost of almost $1,000,000. In addition to three times the number of antenatal examination rooms, the new addition provided areas for important clinics, such as genetic counselling, and a new administration centre.

In the late 1970s and early 1980s, the 'nappy valley' extending south and west of Brisbane produced patients for the Mater Children's Hospital just as readily as it did for the Mater Mothers'. Both the inpatient and ambulatory patient services at the newly extended Mater Children's Hospital were in great demand. Social changes were also discernible in the development of paediatric services in the 1980s.

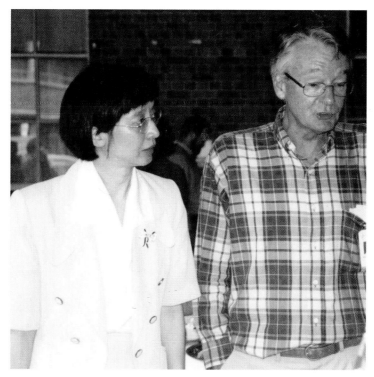

ABOVE: Dr Fung Yee Chan photographed in an informal moment with Dr David Tudehope. MATER HISTORY AND HERITAGE CENTRE

Dr Robyn Rodwell who has been at the forefront of scientific and clinical innovation in haematology at the Mater for many years photographed at work at the Cord Blood Bank.
MATER PUBLIC RELATIONS AND MARKETING

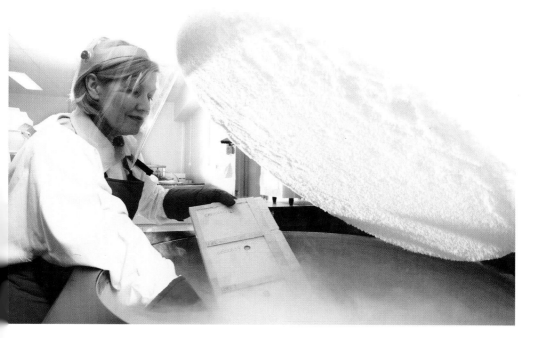

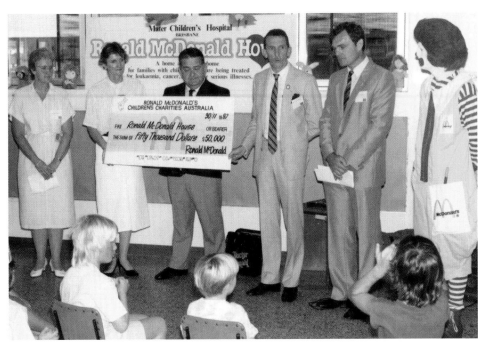

ABOVE: Ronald McDonald House was an extremely important addition to Mater facilities in the 1980s. Ronald McDonald in his clown uniform is shown here making an additional donation to the Mater from the Ronald McDonald Children's Charities Fund with, from left, Caroline Bushell, Linda Boyle, Mr J McCarthy, Under Secretary, Department of Health, Dr John McNee, Medical Superintendent, Mater Children's Hospital and Mr Lars Hedburgh of McDonald's.

MATER HISTORY AND HERITAGE CENTRE

BELOW: Dr Grace Croft, second from right, the Mater's first Assistant Director of Nursing, Research, photographed at her farewell in 2002 with from left Dr Neil Carrington, Director of the Mater Education Centre, Mrs Pat Snowden, Director of Nursing, Mater Private Hospitals, Annette Wilcox and Mrs Rosalie Lewis, formerly Director of Nursing, Mater Children's Hospital.

PHOTO COURTESY OF PROFESSOR ANNE CHANG

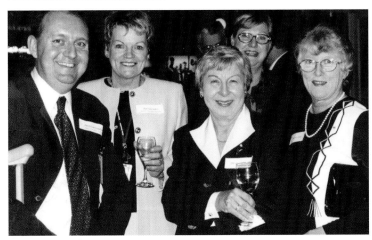

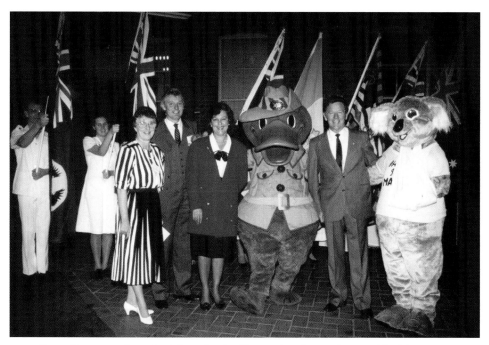

ABOVE: Expo 88 was an important time for the Mater when its services and its history were shown to visitors from all over the world. It was also an occasion for a conference on modern nursing. Here, from left, Mrs Rosalie Lewis, Nursing Superintendent of the Mater Children's Hospital, Mr Rex Ducat, Director of Nursing, the Lord Mayor of Brisbane, Sallyanne Atkinson, 'Expo Oz', the Mater chief executive officer, Mr Pat Maguire, and Matt the Bear are shown on the evening the conference opened. MATER HISTORY AND HERITAGE CENTRE

BELOW: The chief executive officer, Mark Avery, escorting the President of Ireland, Her Excellency, Mary McAleese, on the occasion of her visit to the Mater to open the Diabetic Clinic in 1998. MATER HOSPITAL MEDICAL PHOTOGRAPHY

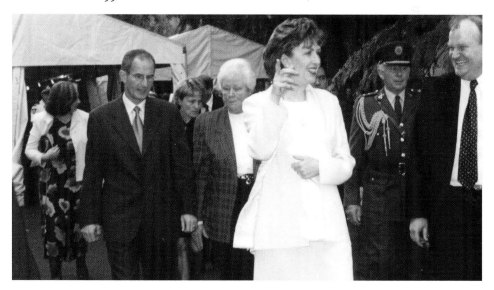

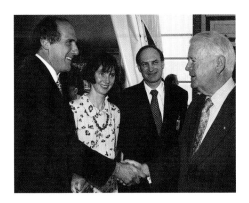

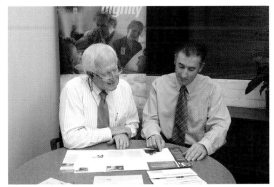

The Governor-General, Sir William Deane, opened the Mater Medical Research Institute and is pictured here, far right, shaking hands with Professor Ralph Steinman of Rockefeller University in the United States, Dr Georgina Clark and the Director of the MMRI, Professor Derek Hart. MATER MEDICAL RESEARCH INSTITUTE

The Mater Foundation supports important Mater projects with the funds it raises. Here, Mr Frank Clair QC, Chairman of the Mater Foundation Council, discusses a project with the Executive Director, Nigel Harris. MATER FOUNDATION

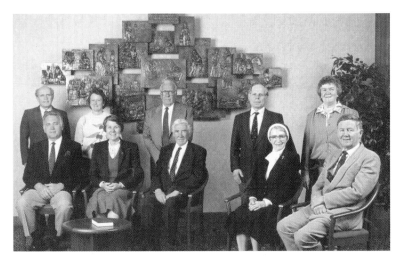

The Mater Health Services Governing Board, 1990, photographed in front of the 'Mater Bronze' sculpted by Sister Gail O'Leary. Standing, left to right, Dr John Burke, Sister Mary Tinney, Mr Colin Henshaw, Professor Colin Apelt, Ms Lesley Robinson and seated, left to right, Dr Laurence Brunello, Sister Madonna Josey, Justice Kevin Ryan, Chairman, Sister Angela Mary Doyle, Mr Pat Maguire, chief executive officer. MATER HISTORY AND HERITAGE CENTRE

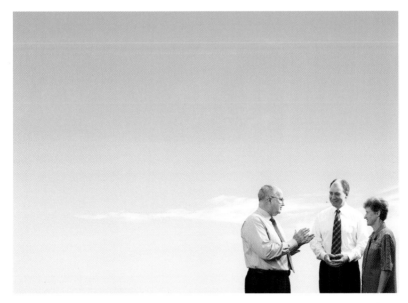

ABOVE: The chairman of the board of Mater Health Services Limited, Mr John McAuliffe, at left, with the chief executive officer, Dr John O'Donnell, and Sister Pauline Burke, Congregational Leader of the Sisters of Mercy in Brisbane. MATER PUBLIC RELATIONS AND MARKETING

BELOW: Mater Redlands hospital was officially opened on 19 November 2000. The hospital's coffee shop was named 'Nellie's Place' to honour an Aboriginal woman known to have been born on the site.
MATER PUBLIC RELATIONS AND MARKETING

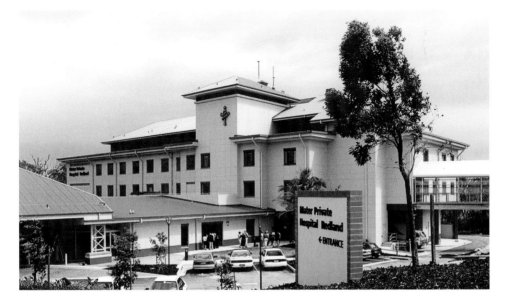

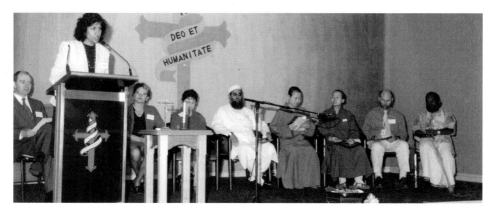

The opening of the Queensland Integrated Refugee Community Health Service in October 2002 was an opportunity for many cultures and many faiths to be recognised at the Mater. Christian, Islamic, Hindu and Buddhist clergy shared the ceremony. Ms Raelene Baker from Brisbane's Aboriginal community is shown addressing the group. Seated behind her are from left the Mater chief executive officer, Dr John O'Donnell, Ms Karen Struthers, Member of the Queensland Parliament for Algester, Sister Deirdre Gardiner, the Imam from the Mt Gravatt mosque, two Buddhist nuns, Father Martin and a Hindu priest. PHOTO: COURTESY KATE RAMSAY

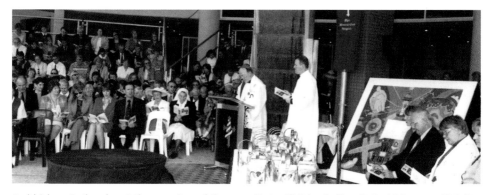

Archbishop Bathersby at the opening of the new Mater Children's Hospital which was officially performed by the Governor of Queensland, His Excellency Major General Peter Arnison.
MATER MEDICAL PHOTOGRAPHY

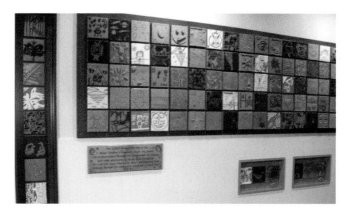

Some of the 5,000 handcrafted ceramic tiles installed in corridors at the new Mater Children's Hospital. The theme uniting the tiles is 'life in Queensland seen through the eyes of children'.
PHOTO: COURTESY DR GRACE CROFT

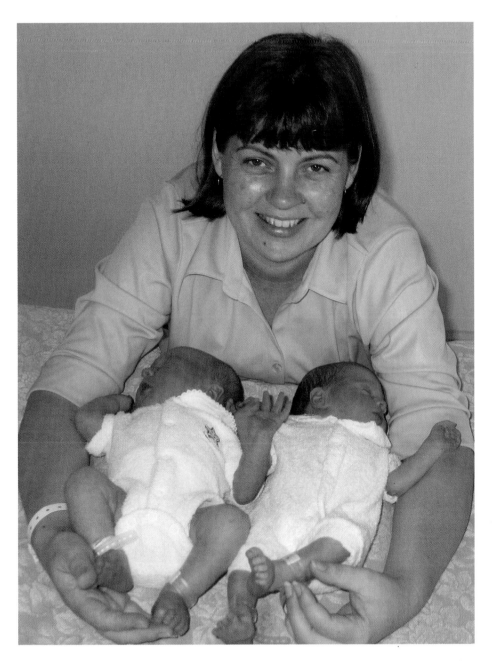

Karen Gray with her newborn twins, Thomas and Samuel. Thomas was the 250,000th baby born at the Mater Mothers' Hospital, in February 2004. MATER PUBLIC RELATIONS AND MARKETING

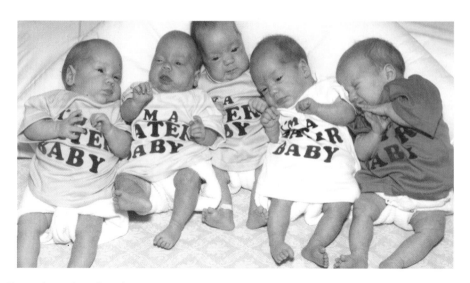

The Wales quintuplets, born in 1991, give public relations a new spin in their Mater T-shirts.

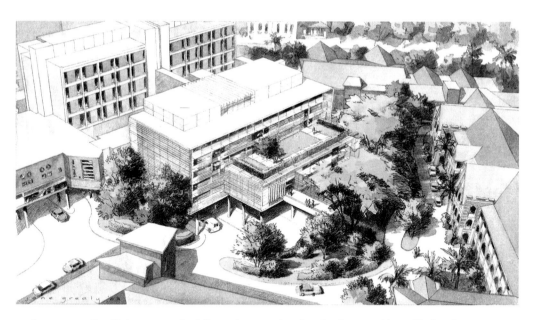

In 2005, as the Mater approached its centenary, planning for the new Mater Mothers' Hospital was in top gear and the design was evolving. This image shows the location of the new hospital, chosen to ensure that expensive services can be shared between the Adult, Children's and Mothers' hospitals, and gives an impression of the likely shape of the new building. The massive fig trees, valued by generations of Mater people, will remain.

MARY DOROTHEA SHEEHAN, MBE, was born in Warwick in 1916. She trained at the Mater, and entered the Sisters of Mercy in 1938. During the Second World War, she administered a military ward at the Mater. After some years caring for aged Sisters and children in the nursery at St Vincent's Home at Nudgee, Sister Mary Dorothea returned to the Mater as assistant matron to Sister Mary St Pierre. After completing her Diploma in Nursing Administration in 1970, she became Nursing Superintendent in 1971, a position she held until 1986. Always known to the senior staff as Dot, and Sister Dot to the more junior, she created a strong *esprit de corps* among the nursing staff. Sister Dot invariably made cups of tea to support staff working with a dying child. They felt that she respected them, as nurses and as people, with her 'listening ear and compassionate heart'. She was so highly respected by paediatricians that she received a special award from the Paediatric Society of Queensland and an Australian Medical Association award.

Sister Mary Dorothea's kindness did not reduce her capacity to be very firm in promoting high standards. Sister Dot did all she could for the Mater Children's case in hospital meetings and in the media. She was a natural performer on television, with her wide smile, happy laughter, personal poise and charm that captured the hearts of many donors on telethons. When the time came for Sister Mary Dorothea to retire, she entered another challenging area, working with AIDS patients and helping terminal sufferers to face death in dignity and peace. She was made an honorary life member of the Queensland AIDS Council. Despite the serious and difficult work she coped with all her professional life, she retained a lively sense of fun and revelled in her holidays at Tugun. She was described by one of her fellow Sisters as 'a most wonderful blend of the saint and the sinner'.

Sister Mary Dorothea Sheehan died on 9 July 1999. The Sister Dorothea Golden Jubilee Fund for Nursing Education at the Mater Children's Hospital was established in her memory.

Most general practitioners had ceased their home visits, particularly at nights and weekends, throwing a greater load on outpatient and casualty services. Medical developments were also reflected in developments at the Mater Children's. A remarkable woman, Sister Mary Dorothea Sheehan, reigned over the hospital during some very hectic years in the 1970s and early 1980s.[32]

Sister Mary Dorothea coped with a maelstrom of changes in paediatric care in the 1970s and 1980s. In 1977, for instance, the first Medical Superintendent was appointed to the hospital and the previously awesome power of a Sisters of Mercy Nursing Superintendent had to be shared, an adjustment 'Sister Dot' made graciously, keeping the interests of her hospital paramount. In 1975, the Mater Children's Hospital became a paediatric training hospital, at a time when Brisbane's demographic shift to the southern suburbs was at its height. Because Sister Dot had always believed that mature, well-educated nurses were essential in children's hospitals, the Mater retained one of the highest Registered Nurse to patient ratios in Australia.

In the 1970s, when it was clear that paediatrics was no longer a single specialty, there were few specialist clinics at either the 120-bed Mater Children's Hospital or the larger Royal Children's Hospital. Sadly, a specialist leukaemia clinic could not be established at the Mater in 1972 because the hospital was bursting at the seams before the 1975 extension was completed.[33] There were suggestions that the best option for Brisbane's paediatric hospitals would be to divide the new range of specialist services between them. The Mater was, at that stage, still hoping that it would host Brisbane's second chair in paediatrics, a dream which did not become reality until 1981, the Mater Children's Hospital's golden jubilee year.[34]

Specialist clinics became increasingly important in the 1980s. The number of Mater clinics increased from twenty-five to forty-two between 1977 and 1980 and included interdisciplinary clinics for diabetes, cleft palate and cranio-facial conditions, and cystic fibrosis, which worked closely with the cystic fibrosis clinic at Herston. In 1984, the School Function Clinic, Sister Marie Fitzgerald's Spina Bifida Clinic and the respiratory laboratory were added to the mix. Brisbane's unenviable reputation for high rates of asthma demonstrated that this

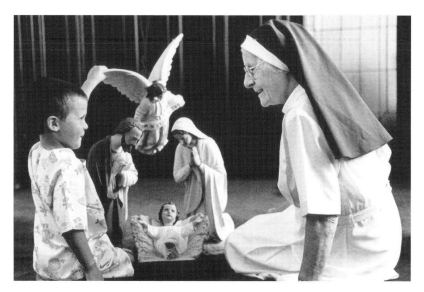

Christmas was always a special time at the Mater Children's, with decorations in the wards and visits from Santa, but the real meaning of Christmas was always emphasised. Here Sister Mary St Pierre McCormack, Matron of the Children's Hospital, and a young patient discuss the Nativity scene. SOMCA

service had been badly needed: its work grew by 450 per cent during its first year. Facilities gradually expanded. The new McAuley wing with an infants' ward and University of Queensland Department of Child Health offices was opened in March 1982. A school, built by the government on land donated by the Sisters, opened on the Clarence Street side of the hospital in 1983. By 1985, 600 children had attended the school.[35]

During the 1980s, the health problems of Aboriginal people were penetrating the consciousness of white Australians more deeply than previously. Sister Mary Dorothea wanted the Mater to assist where it could. She was well aware that Aboriginal people found the conditions at Brisbane's main immunisation clinic at the City Hall very impersonal, and in 1980 commenced a special immunisation clinic through an arrangement with Aboriginal and Islander Welfare Sisters who brought Aboriginal families to the Mater at times which suited them.[36]

Despite the development of specialist clinics and new services, many paediatricians felt that the facilities at both Brisbane's aging children's hospitals were inadequate. As in all fields of medical care, the technology required for specialties such as neurosurgery, thoracic surgery, radiotherapy and plastic surgery was extremely expensive. It was estimated in 1983 that $200,000 per year was required to support one specialist in a children's hospital. Dr Barrie Heyworth, first Medical Superintendent of the Mater Children's Hospital, was a member of the Health Minister's Paediatric Advisory Committee, the Queensland coordinating committee on child abuse and the Queensland standing committee on paediatric training. He recommended that the two hospitals be combined to eliminate duplication and competition and, if possible, an entirely new centre of paediatric excellence be created. This, he thought, might be more cost-effective than the $20,000,000 in capital works expenditure needed to bring the two existing hospitals up to date.[37]

Dr Heyworth believed that several prominent paediatricians and the Royal Australian College of Physicians favoured the creation of a Queensland Institute of Child Health combining health promotion with excellent care, research and education. More controversially, Dr Heyworth thought the only solution for the 1931 Mater Children's Hospital would be closure, because its present site could not support further development; equally, he believed that the Royal Children's Hospital should close because the cost of redeveloping it would be prohibitive. Dr Heyworth suggested that the soon-to-be-opened Mater Adult Hospital be used for combined hospital and community facilities, with day wards, family care wards, a developmental paediatric section, adolescent health facilities, and a health promotion centre. Holding beds for such a hospital could be provided at Redcliffe, Wynnum, Inala, Beenleigh or Beaudesert, the Queen Elizabeth II hospital at Mt Gravatt, and the Prince Charles Hospital at Chermside. If that occurred, the old Mater Children's Hospital could become a geriatric and rehabilitation hospital. The indication that the proposed centre could occupy the new Mater Adult Hospital incensed the doctors at the Adult Hospital, who had waited for years for urgently needed new facilities, as well as people at the Royal Children's Hospital, and even the government.[38]

Unfortunately, the Mater Advisory Board had not seen this appraisal, prepared for the Health Minister, before it was leaked to the press by a Member of Parliament who received it through a Parliamentary Committee. The press report was alarming, full of lurid claims that children were dying while the two children's hospitals fought over specialists and equipment.[39] This was a difficult situation for the Sisters and the Board. In a climate in which the Mater's relationship with the government had been improving, and it was negotiating for state funding for a new outpatient building, criticism of the Royal Children's Hospital could be seen to have Mater endorsement. The Advisory Board emphasised that these were Dr Heyworth's personal views. Dr Heyworth also stressed that the idea for a combined centre outlined in his paper was only one option among a range of possibilities.[40]

In a situation in which the press report had trumpeted an apparent criticism of both the Mater and the Royal Children's Hospital, the Board felt it had no option but to ask for Dr Heyworth's resignation. Dr Heyworth apologised for the embarrassment his suggestions had caused and the Board withdrew its request. Not long afterwards, Dr Heyworth accepted a position in the Department of Paediatrics at the National University of Malaysia, but continued to write to Sister Angela Mary and Sister Kath Burke, the Congregational Leader. While not approving of his recent activities, both thought he had achieved a great deal at the Mater in his six and a half year term, particularly in developing specialist clinics and in promoting the Children's Hospital's work with the victims of child abuse and their families.[41]

Dr Heyworth's successor, Dr John McNee, also had his mind on improvements at the Mater Children's. In consultation with the staff, Dr McNee drew up a submission on the needs of the hospital for the next ten years, the first time the Board's Master Plan Development Committee had 'a comprehensive view from the staff on the long term direction of the Children's Hospital'.[42] Nevertheless, every new facility was hard won. In 1984, the Health Minister finally announced a state grant of $1,300,00 towards a new outpatient and ancillary services building to be built on the Annerley Road–Clarence Street corner. Sisters of Mercy fundraising yielded $600,000 for the building and $400,000 came from the Children's Hospital appeal. Even this funded only the shell of the building; fittings had to wait for the next financial year. Ancillary services to be accommodated in the new building had grown far beyond physiotherapy, speech therapy and occupational therapy. Care for families was becoming increasingly important. In 1981, Sister Brigid Hirschfeld, a former nurse with training in psychodrama, commenced the Mater's grief counselling service, caring for families and Mater staff.[43]

Spacious accommodation for outpatients was essential because the trend of keeping children in hospital as little as possible had continued to accelerate. In 1979–80, for instance, a child's average stay in hospital had fallen to 2.9 days.[44] There were also increasing numbers of children suffering from a range of psychiatric illnesses and emotional disturbances. Dr Aidene Urquhart, the first child psychiatrist to be appointed to the Mater, commenced duty in 1980, in a climate of vigorous discussion about how best to expand the Mater's care of mentally ill and abused children.[45] A good while later, Sister Angela Mary complained that she had been arguing for years that a psychologist was also urgently needed at the Mater.[46] The old nursery at the Mater Children's was converted into a psychiatric care unit and, by 1990, repeated submissions had succeeded. Three part-time clinical psychologists – Elsie Harwood, Heather Mohay and Monica Emmett – were appointed.

A very old problem, child abuse, was at last taken more seriously in the late twentieth century. After years of advocacy from doctors, teachers and concerned people generally, legislation was passed compelling practitioners who suspected that a child had been abused to report the abuse. Caring for children damaged physically or psychologically became an important initiative for the Mater during the 1980s. The hospital hosted a Suspected Child Abuse and Neglect (SCAN) team, and developed a range of services to care for the children and to help their families. This was an area dear to Dr Barrie Heyworth's heart, enthusiastically developed by a staff paediatrician, Dr David Wood. The work was haunted by fears that funding could be withdrawn.

Child abuse was a tragically large and growing problem. In 1980, one-third of all notified cases of child abuse were seen at the Mater, two and a half times the cases seen at the Royal Children's Hospital. The load doubled in one year, 1984, when 474 children from

373 families were seen at the Mater; in 1985, 600 referrals were recorded.[47] Volunteers again became an integral part of family-centred care at the Mater and many voluntary 'parent aides' assisted with the families. This was no token effort. Each parent aide in Jan Hinson's team completed eight weeks' training and devoted at least 500 hours each year to child protection. They dealt with some very sad and difficult situations, including those of children referred to them by the Mater's child torture and trauma clinic, where a team from seven separate organisations within the hospital and from the community worked with young people. The government wavered in its support. The Health Minister, Brian Austin, claimed in 1985 that the Mater was not really part of the state's public hospital system and consequently the SCAN team could be withdrawn if there was any sign that the Mater was not able to cope adequately with this responsibility.[48]

Anxiety about how to provide necessary new initiatives was as old as the Mater. The Mater Children's Staff Association suggested that a Children's Hospital Foundation be established to raise funds for multitudes of emerging needs. Receipts from the Children's Hospital Appeal had begun to decline as telethons fell out of fashion. The Children's Hospital Appeal and its Chairman, Reg Leonard, had been a vital support to the Mater Children's for many years.[49] Reg Leonard House, for example, a home-unit building opened in 1979, enabled the parents of seriously ill children to stay close to the hospital. Some of the mothers who stayed at Reg Leonard House in its early years came from New Guinea, Norfolk Island and the Northern Territory; some had never previously visited Brisbane. Reg Leonard House was extended in 1982, the year Reg Leonard retired from Queensland Newspapers.

The expansion in the dimensions of clinical work and the scope of support services during the 1970s and 1980s marked the Mater Children's Hospital's development as a large tertiary-level paediatric centre. By 1990, its accident and emergency section was often the busiest in Queensland, and Dr Mansou Pabari, the director of anaesthetics, became the first full-time director of paediatric intensive care. More and more functions had been squeezed into the Mater Children's shoebox. Rosalie Lewis, the first lay Director of Nursing at the Children's, somehow always managed to rally her staff to meet new needs;

many nurses unselfishly accepted greater workloads, so that important initiatives such as Australia's first paediatric sleep studies unit could be implemented. Nurses also worked with community groups, attending Camp Quality weekends for young cancer sufferers and camps for diabetic children. Their insights were broadened through exchange visits to the Toronto Hospital for Sick Children in Canada.[50]

At the Adult Hospital, the painful 1970s process of identifying areas in which the Mater should specialise was a platform for the development of significant initiatives. Cancer treatment had been an important area ever since Queensland's first radium clinic had been established there in 1928, but many other specialties also had a long history at the Mater. The rheumatology department established by Dr Ian Ferguson celebrated its silver jubilee in 1985; it had been the only unit in Queensland for ten years. Ophthalmology was further developed when the Commonwealth government's hospital enhancement program provided $415,606 to upgrade equipment with new surgical lasers and operating microscopes. Dr Les Manning and the vitrectomy unit produced a success as widely broadcast as the Mater's establishment of eastern Australia's first eye bank in 1954. Margaret Roddick, who had been blind for fifteen years following a car accident, had never seen her husband or six children. The restoration of her sight, through removing opacities, first in one eye and then the other, made national and international news.[51]

Rapid progress in the department of medicine with the employment of five full-time specialist physicians in 1985 allowed postgraduate medical education to expand, and also opened new doors. Proposals from Dr Simon Bowler for a respiratory function laboratory and from Dr Michael Redmond and Dr Noel Saines for a brain tumour clinic exemplified a trend towards specialist clinics at the Adult Hospital, as well as at the Children's. Some had broad linkages – the endocrinology clinic was linked to both the neurosurgical and gynaecological departments, and equipment in the brain tumour clinic was used for both public and private patients.[52]

Even before the new Adult Hospital opened in 1981 with its new university section, cancer research and treatment was expanding significantly. Gynaecological malignancies were a particular interest of Dr Keith Free, the Mater's senior gynaecologist, and in the late 1970s the hospital participated in a national trial for the management of ovarian cancer.[53] However, sophisticated cancer treatment needed complex and expensive technology and in this regard the picture at the Mater in the mid-1980s was less rosy. A downturn in the Queensland economy, and less generous federal funding, raised the fear that the promised new Queensland Radium Institute development at the Mater could be deferred. With increasing linkages between the Mater public and private hospitals, the news that two linear accelerators were shortly to be installed at the Wesley private hospital only increased the tension. There was even brief discussion of the Mater making a loan to the state government to fund the new radiotherapy department.[54]

In the end, however, there was no need for the tail to wag the dog, and the Queensland Radium Institute's new Mater centre, with its own two new linear accelerators, was commissioned in November 1989. The new centre confirmed the Mater's position in cancer treatment on Brisbane's southern side; it delivered radiation oncology services to the Princess Alexandra Hospital and Gold Coast hospitals, as well as to Mater patients. At long last, sixteen beds in Ward 9B at the new Adult Hospital could be opened; a considerable increase in chemotherapy treatment, as well as radiotherapy, forced the government to fund these additional beds. Ironically, it was not the old Mater problems of shortage of space or financial resources which threatened to impede the progress of radiotherapy and diagnostic mammography; like hospitals all over the nation, the Mater was finding it very difficult to retain full-time radiologists on staff, a problem it hoped would ease with the Queensland government's decision to at last allow a right of private practice to specialists in Queensland public hospitals.[55]

Liaison between hospitals and community care agencies increased greatly during the 1970s and 1980s. Sister Fay McMeniman's stomal therapy clinic, which assisted patients to manage stomas created through surgery, was supported by the Mt Olivet Hospital and three home-nursing agencies. Self-help associations of patients with various illnesses were a feature of general medicine, as well as obstetrics, in this era. The Ostomy Association was only one of several which supported patients and lobbied hospitals for better patient care. Community services and supportive associations were increasingly necessary in the 1970s and 1980s to fill a gap in health services. Governments pressed acute-care hospitals to keep patients in beds for as short a time as possible, yet provided inadequate services to support patients needing ongoing care. The average number of days a patient spent in the Mater Adult Hospital, for example, had more than halved from 13.12 days in 1960 to 5.5 days in 1980.[56]

The care of the aged had also been a worrying problem at the Mater, ever since plans for a special hospital for the chronically ill, proposed during the 1950s, had been cancelled during the frantic push for funding to rebuild the Adult Hospital. The issue became very pressing in the 1970s and 1980s. Advances in medical science had prolonged life, increasing the incidence of various forms of dementia and physical disabilities. These patients needed long-term care, but nursing-home beds came nowhere near satisfying the demand. At a meeting with the Mater and Archdiocesan officials in 1981, the health economist Paul Gross suggested that a centre of excellence for the care of the aged and terminally ill was badly needed.[57] The management of patients with psychiatric illnesses was also a serious matter. The state had retreated in this area, closing most of its large psychiatric hospitals, but providing insufficient community services to close the gap. Pat Neely and her social work department were very important in the frustrating search for solutions for individual patients, and discharge planning became an increasingly important area for nursing research in the late 1980s.[58]

At the end of the 1980s, the Adult Hospital was in great demand. With bed-occupancy rates well over 90 per cent, finding the human resources and the equipment to meet the need was always difficult. Ancillary services, particularly speech therapy, physiotherapy and occupational therapy, were always stretched in an era of increasing focus on rehabilitation and independent living, even for seriously disabled people. For a hospital with a very long record of increasing the complexity and range of its surgery, cancelling operations because of a state-wide shortage of anaesthetists was a galling problem. In the frantic 1980s, workloads at the Mater increased by 54 per cent, but staffing increased by only 28 per cent.[59]

The Mater's aim to care humanely for all patients in this rushed and highly technological hospital world, the life and death questions emerging from rapid advances in clinical treatments, and juggling resources to cope with demand were the critical dimensions of ethical discussions and debates in the 1980s. Care of the aged, the very young and the terminally ill were at the centre of the ethical problems all modern hospitals were forced to confront. The Catholic position on some of the big questions such as abortion, fetal experimentation, euthanasia, contraception and sterilisation was clear, but establishing a definite position on other medico-moral issues, or on the allocation of resources, was much more difficult. Moral theology, as Sister Angela Mary pointed out, did not stand still: newer viewpoints sometimes came to be accepted as the mind of the Church on many moral issues.[60] Some church leaders linked social justice objectives and medico-moral concerns, and advocated coherent policies for Catholic hospitals, including clearly stated ethical codes for all health professions with detailed guidelines derived from moral precepts. However, very few doctors or nurses were trained in the intellectual foundations of Christian practice, Christian morals and the relevant theologies.[61] Developing curricula as demanding as this was a very large task.

For Brisbane's Archbishop Rush, meeting this challenge was essential. The future of mankind, he wrote, would be 'safeguarded only when science and conscience become allies; only when, in all the domains of science, respect is paid to the primacy of the ethical'.[62] Despite public attention on artificial contraception and increasing clamour for abortion to be legalised, the overriding principle at the Mater remained the dignity of the individual from the moment of conception through to death. However, in an age when new technologies could sustain life and end suffering, it was necessary to assess whether or not the Hippocratic oath and the moral law gave sufficient support to practising doctors and Catholic hospitals. There were many 'fine line' decisions.

The Mater had already established a leading position in dealing with some of the most difficult ethical issues. In November 1979, Sister Regis Mary Dunne, pioneer of genetic research in Queensland, left her laboratory and the cytogenetics counselling service she had

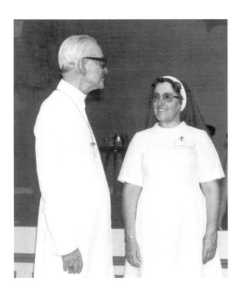

Archbishop Rush, who established the Queensland Bioethics Centre, with its first Director, Sister Regis Mary Dunne. MHHC

established with the paediatrician Dr Neville Anderson to study medical bioethics in the United States. Sister Regis Mary returned in 1981 to establish the Queensland Bioethics Centre to advise the Archdiocese and hospitals confronting medico-moral dilemmas.[63]

The difficult ethical dilemmas which preoccupied the Mater in the 1980s included the possibility of genetic 'engineering', which the chairman of the Mater Advisory Board, Kevin Cronin, described in 1981 as 'experimentation with the very core of life'. At the Mater Mothers' Hospital, Dr Edwin Esler was also concerned at the possibility of genetic manipulation arising out of the rapid developments in science which seemed to be penetrating to the very heart of the human genome.[64] The Mater's first large bioethics seminar in 1981 attracted 200 participants from places as far apart as Cairns and Tasmania.

As a response to dealing with a world in which ethical questions grew ever more complex, the Sisters of Mercy had enunciated their values and philosophy in a codified form in 1977. This kind of formalisation was part of a wider movement towards codifying policies in fields of endeavour in the corporate and government sectors, and in education. The Sisters' code took as its fundamental principle the inestimable value of each individual, which could not be measured by his or her usefulness or ability to contribute to a family or society. Every individual must, therefore, be treated with respect. The code demonstrated that ethical principles derived from theological underpinnings were, in fact, little different from the values recognised generally in the canon of medical ethics. Health care was to take precedence over all other tasks; clinical teaching or research could be undertaken only if the patient's well-being and comfort took precedence. In furthering this, the patient's spiritual needs had also to be satisfied, and, with the

SISTER REGIS MARY DUNNE was born in Toowoomba and educated at St Saviour's and All Hallows', before training as a teacher. Following her profession as a Sister of Mercy, Sister Regis Mary was appointed to the Mater laboratory to undertake newly established training in medical laboratory science qualifications. She qualified in 1954 and specialised in microbiology and became a senior scientist. She was awarded a Fellowship of the Institute of Medical Laboratory Scientists for her thesis on medical mycology and obtained her MASM for her published papers. In 1960, Sister Regis Mary pioneered cytogenetics in Queensland and for eight years provided Queensland's only diagnostic service. In 1961, Dr Neville Anderson and Sister Regis Mary established Australia's first genetic counselling service to assist clinicians, patients and families to deal with the complexities of genetic diagnosis. Sister Regis Mary studied at the University of St Louis, the Kennedy Centre in Georgetown and Loyola University in Chicago in preparation for establishing the Queensland Bioethics Centre in a house in Clarence Street, provided by the Mater. Her work included assembling a large library on all aspects of bioethical issues, which was made available for public use, and giving lectures and seminars all over Queensland.

Since 1981, Sister Regis Mary has sat on many federal and state policy committees, including the National Bioethics Committee, National Health and Medical Research Council committees, the Australian Ethics Committee and the Medical Research Committee, and the National Gene Therapy Research Advisory Panel. She has served on ethics committees for the Queensland Department of Health, several hospitals, three universities and the Queensland Institute of Medical Research. She has been made a Fellow of the Queensland Institute of Medical Research and been awarded outstanding service medals from Queensland Health and Griffith University and, from the Queensland University of Technology, an honorary Doctorate for 'Scholarship and contribution to medical science in Queensland'.

patient's consent, the next of kin were to be kept promptly, reliably and courteously informed; in every other circumstance, all information about the patient was to be kept secret.[65]

These principles were expanded in a series of guidelines on the most difficult medico-moral issues. Although the basic moral absolutes were regarded as immutable, it was always possible that particular applications could be modified as scientific investigation and theological developments opened up new problems or cast new light on old ones. Even though abortion was prohibited, drugs or other treatments could be allowed if they were essential to preserve the mother's life, even if fetal death resulted. Contraceptive measures, including hysterectomy, could be used in cases where they were necessary for the treatment of illness. There was no ban on organ donation and transplantation, provided the loss of organs did not deprive donors of their lives or the functional integrity of their bodies.

The care of the terminally ill was very important at the Mater, focusing as it did on increasing numbers of cancer patients and very ill premature babies. The Sisters stated that 'it is the function of the medical personnel to take every reasonable measure to sustain life, but to remain ever mindful of the best interests of the patient'.[66] The use of sedatives or analgesics to relieve suffering in the terminally ill was not considered to be euthanasia, even if life was shortened. Doctors could decide to cease active treatment in situations in which it was more merciful to let nature take its course. Care was to be holistic:

> The dying patient is to be given spiritual comfort and support at all times and after death the body is to be attended with care and dignity . . . the relatives of the dying patient are our special concern and are to be given every help.[67]

Courage was required, particularly as the public microscope was focusing ever more closely on all hospitals. Sister Angela Mary was quite sure that the Mater should discount any 'degree of scandal' which might arise in situations where the solid body of medical and moral opinion advocated a particular course of action as justifiable in a grave emergency.[68] After all, fear of criticism had never deterred the

Mater from difficult decisions in the past. However, it was necessary to ensure that the hospital staff were educated in ethics, and supported when difficult decisions had to be made.

Two important steps followed the Sisters' codification of ethical principles. The first was the appointment of the first hospital ethicist in Australia, Sister Deirdre Gardiner, a member of the Brisbane Congregation. Sister Deirdre was a science graduate who had worked in the Mater laboratory before studying at the Yarra Theological Union and graduating with special expertise in systematic and moral theology. She then studied in the United States at Georgetown University, Washington, where she graduated with a Master's degree in philosophy with a major in bioethics.[69] The second, the drafting of the Mater's first official ethics policy document by Professor Kevin Ryan, deputy chairman of the Advisory Board, was initiated in 1983. It began with the Mater's emphasis on total patient care – spiritual as well as physical – in which the dignity of each patient was pre-eminent. In recognising the need to adhere to the church's teaching in all decisions where morality or ethics were involved, the policy included recognition that no member of staff, or any patient, should be forced to act in a manner contrary to personal conscience, correctly formed. The right of all neonates to the same standard of care as older people was explicitly recognised. At the other end of life, every person was to be accorded the right to the best care available, but was entitled to refuse the application of extraordinary means to prolong life.[70]

The moral theologian Father Peter Gillam was available for consultation on emergency clinical decisions. All cases were very difficult; most were very sad. There was, for instance, a recommendation for tubal ligation for a patient in her early thirties who had been schizophrenic for many years and was quite unable to care for her five-month-old baby. As this was considered to be an instance of direct sterilisation, it could not take place at the Mater. On the other hand, the procedure was allowed for a patient with a severe heart condition because in this case the purpose for sterilisation was to prevent the patient's death. Saving a life was the reason for allowing a fetus to be removed from a woman in her twelfth pregnancy who showed signs of toxic shock from infection in her uterus due to premature rupture of the amniotic membranes. The baby would also have died if the infection had progressed, and was too premature to survive *ex utero*.[71]

Sister Deirdre discussed ethical issues with staff, conducted educational activities and worked with the ethics committees in each hospital on the Mater campus. A coordinating committee reviewed the issues arising in individual hospitals, supervised the ethics education program and examined research proposals for both their scientific value and their ethical standards.[72] Sister Catharine Courtney chaired the first Ethics Co-ordinating Committee and completed her term in 1989, with ethics committees running well in all four hospitals. Annual seminars included a program on 'Death and Dying – a Christian response' in October 1989. Educational work included programs for selected senior staff extending over a five-week period, with each session lasting one and a half hours; continuing education in ethics for the nursing staff; a seminar program to help staff appreciate their own contribution to the Mater's work, and another on health care and the law. Staff were supported when difficult decisions had to be made. The staff of the special-care nursery at the Mater Mothers' Hospital met monthly with Sister Deirdre and welcomed her with 'open arms'. Parents were always invited to attend discussions of ethical issues affecting their babies.[73]

The spiritual welfare of patients had always been emphasised at the Mater, indeed in all Catholic hospitals. These efforts were supported at a broader level by the Australian Catholic Health Care Association. In 1985, for instance, the Association's conference dealt with the ethical considerations involved in caring for the aged and the mentally ill. Pastoral care also occupied a large part of the program.[74] During the 1980s, formally organised pastoral care, both inside the hospital and after the patients left, became a means of fulfilling this part of the Sisters' mission, and helped to soften the harshness of modern technological medicine. Before that, however, many Sisters who had retired from nursing or administrative work spent years working in pastoral care: Mother Marcella McCormick, a former Superior-General, worked in this area, as did Sister Mary Madeleine, who had been in charge of the Mater Children's Hospital kitchen for many years, and Sister Mary St Edwin, formerly in charge of casualty at the Adult Hospital.

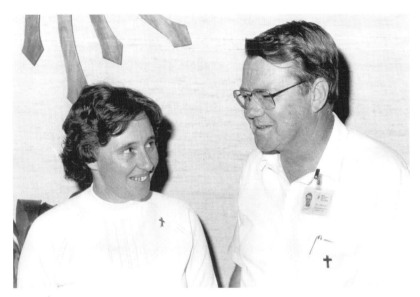

Sister Carmen Coffey and Father John Barlow of the Mater Pastoral Care
Department. MHHC

After faltering attempts in the late 1970s, the pastoral care department was established in August 1982, with Sister Carmen Coffey in
charge. The practice of pastoral care was no longer confined to a select
few. The Board believed that all staff should be encouraged to adopt
a pastoral approach to their work, and therefore the head of the new
department should be appropriately qualified with a position of high
status in the hospital.[75] The new department needed a large staff: two
priests, six religious Sisters, including a Dominican Sister and a Franciscan Missionary of Mary, a married layman and representatives of
all other faiths 'on call'. Pastoral care staff were available twenty-four
hours a day and, as well as direct care, conducted educational programs in various pastoral skills; in 1985, for instance, three seminars,
each of which attracted 100 people, were conducted on the theme
of mercy.

In these difficult areas, Sister Regis Mary Dunne, Sister Deirdre
Gardiner, Sister Carmen Coffey and Sister Brigid Hirschfeld demonstrated through their innovative work that there were many productive
new roles for Sisters of Mercy. These new directions revealed more
than the increasing complexity of work at the Mater hospitals. They

were also very important aspects of the Sisters' recognition that, ever since the second Vatican Council, their numbers had been declining and new strategies were needed to continue the Mercy mission.

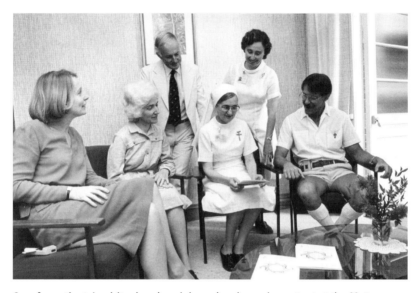

Care for patients' spiritual and social needs, always important at the Mater, was formalised in the 1970s and 1980s through the establishment of the Pastoral Care Department under Sister Carmen Coffey. Key people in pastoral care are shown here with Sister Carmen Coffey (standing at right): from left, Mrs Pat Neely, Director of Social Work, Sister Patricia McGinley, Dr John Waller, Medical Superintendent of the Mater Adult Hospital, Sister Mary Collette Anderson and Father John Chalmers. MHHC

PART THREE

MATURING

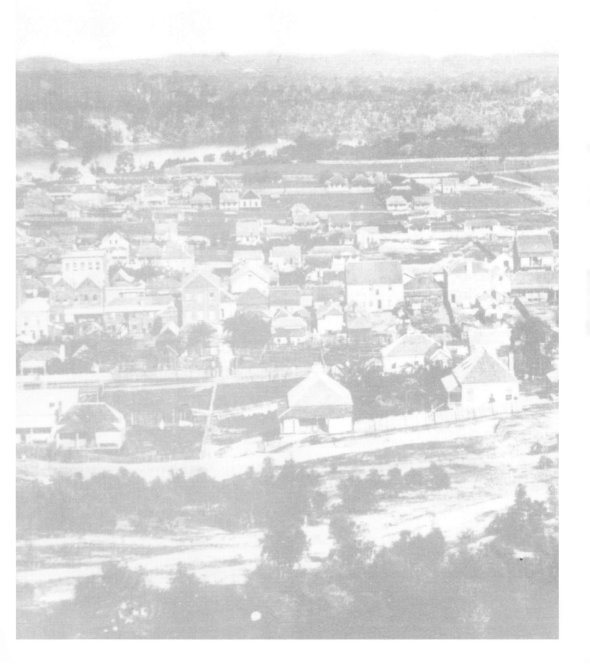

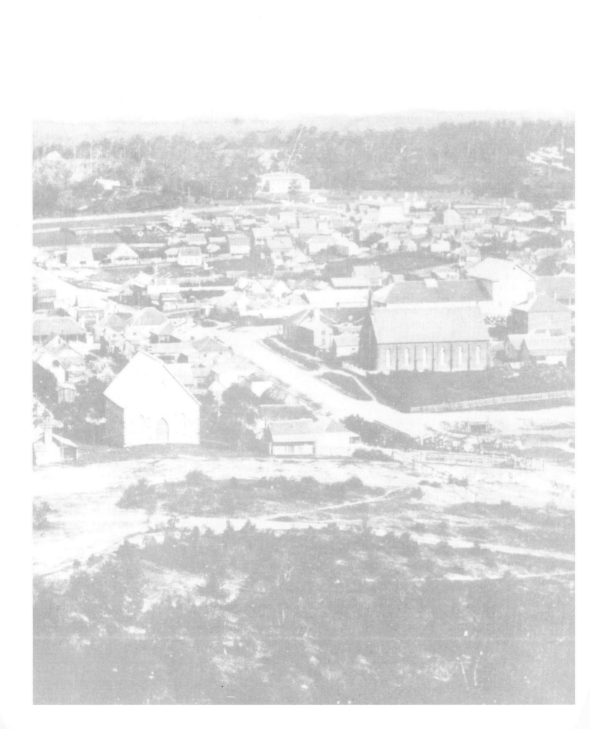

CHAPTER EIGHT

ADAPTING, RENEWING, GROWING

This hospital should be clearly distinguished by its
recognition of the dignity of the human person,
whatever the station in life of that person, by its attitude
to pain, suffering and death and by its compassionate,
caring concern for its staff. If in these and related areas
we are 'weighed in the balance and found wanting'
then we have failed in some way to leaven our hospital
life with the Christian principles we claim are our
inspiration and our motivating force.[1]

Dr Des O'Callaghan, Medical Superintendent, Mater public hospitals, 1962–1988

Determination, adaptation and innovation had proved durable strategies in meeting the opportunities and obstacles the Sisters of Mercy
encountered in developing their hospitals. In the 1980s, hard decisions had to be made about the ways in which a diminishing number
of Sisters could best pursue their mission. It became a question of how
to ensure that the hospitals continued to promote Mercy values and to
nourish the Mater spirit, while the Sisters prepared to relinquish the
reins of everyday control. There were no longer platoons of young,
fresh Sisters ready to take over and, in any case, governments dictated

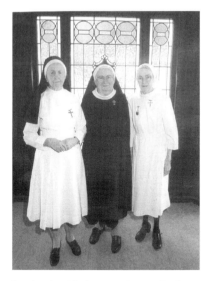

Lay leadership became increasingly emphasised at the Mater in the 1980s, and the Sisters' familiar white 'hospital' habits were gradually replaced by secular dress. Three of the Mater's most distinguished Sisters of Mercy show some of the habits: from left, Sister Mary St Rita Monahan, Sister Mercia Mary Higgins and Sister Gertrude Mary Lyons. MHHC

staffing levels. It was time to question, to define goals more clearly, to adapt, to innovate: clinging too hard to old ways could, after all, risk the longevity of the expression of the Mercy ideal in the Mater hospitals.

During the 1970s and 1980s, many Sisters felt real grief at ceding the charge of wards, departments and whole hospitals to lay leaders; others saw these sacrifices as a necessary part of the corporate ethic of ensuring the well-being of the Mater enterprise as a whole. Many Sisters had stayed at their posts for decades. In 1981, Sister Mercia Mary and Sister Mary St Rita retired after reigning over the pharmacy and laboratory for a total of fifty years, more than matched by Sister Stephanie Purtill who retired in 1983 after thirty-one years in charge of the radiographers.[2] Such dedication had been essential in the early days when the Mater struggled for survival with no financial assistance from government or the Church. In more ways than one, it had been a case of the poor helping the poor.

In the early 1980s, the Congregation made the difficult decision that the retiring age for Sisters should be no different from the custom prevailing in other workplaces. Sisters would retire at 65, and their positions would be advertised openly, a devastating development for those Sisters who had spent their working lives in the hospital. Adapting to changed conditions within the Sisters of Mercy and in society at large also meant another examination of the structure and operation of all the Mater hospitals, as well as a hard look at the Sisters' own Congregational structure and the ways in which their mission in hospitals, schools and social work could best be pursued. As always, much depended on the Congregational leadership.

In 1980, Sister Catharine Courtney ended her term as Superior-General. She had presided over a difficult era in which some of the most

challenging of the post Vatican II changes had
their full impact. When her term began in 1975,.
the lives of many Sisters had not changed much
'beyond shortening the habit and showing the
hair'[3] – big enough changes – but the next stage,
participation in Congregational governance, was
an enormous change from traditional unques-
tioning obedience to the Superior. Ironically, in
view of the Sisters' tussles with governments of
all complexions, their new Charter introduced
a system that worked in a way similar to many
political parties. All members of the Congregation elected a Chapter to develop policy, exercise
executive powers and choose the Congregational
Leader and her team of four or five councillors.
Between meetings of Chapter, the leadership
team, usually in office for six years, translated
Chapter's general aims into specific goals. The

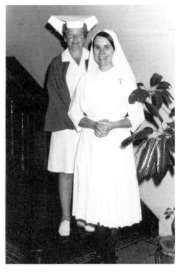

Sister Madonna Josey (in front)
was the last Sister of Mercy to
be Nursing Superintendent at
the Mater Adult Hospital. She
is photographed here with her
deputy, Miss Jill Marshall. MHHC

leadership team was responsible for the apostolic placement of the
Sisters, but in this era it rarely acted against individual wishes and career
aspirations.[4]

Sister Catharine Courtney was succeeded by Sister Kath Burke,
who preferred the title 'Congregational Leader' because she did not
feel superior and did not want to be a general.[5] When Sister Kath
became president of the Institute of Sisters of Mercy in Australia, she
was succeeded as Congregational Leader by Sister Madonna Josey,
formerly Nursing Superintendent at the Mater Adult Hospital. The
1980s were by no means easy years to carry the daunting responsibility of Congregational leadership. At a material level, the leadership
team was charged with protecting the property of the Congregation.
In both church and civil law, members of the leadership team were
trustees of the Sisters' assets. However, the leaders' primary focus had
to be the well-being of the whole Congregation, conserving its own
special traditions and, above all, promoting the authenticity of its
apostolic works.[6] In this context, the Mater hospitals were not just a
collection of health care institutions. The Mater was a corporate health

care ministry. The nuts and bolts of everyday administration, tussles with government over health policy and finance, even the promotion of clinical excellence, were only the tangible expression of the much broader concept of ministry, a sacred charge. The responsibilities were huge. Over and above aspiring to achieve excellent medical care, exercising a ministry meant attention to the spiritual needs of patients and staff, and stewardship of the Mater's corporate behaviour.

In the era after Vatican II, the church remodelled itself into the communion of the people, all of whom were charged with responsibility to exercise the church's apostolate. Nourishing the lay apostolate at the Mater, and developing the governance of the hospitals, became the subject of a process of 'future discernment'. All the signs in 1980s society indicated that it would be a difficult future to decipher. The economic shift from an industrial society to an information society was well underway, bringing with it rapid social change. Once-familiar jobs disappeared overnight in an increasingly complex economic system, infecting many people with a sense of powerlessness, and bringing to others real marginalisation and poverties of all kinds – economic loss, social deprivation, cultural confusion and religious disorientation. To some extent, the state's appropriation of the needs and problems of individuals through regulations and systems of many kinds only served to reinforce the sense that the individual was of little consequence in a mechanistic, globalising society, and had no influence on its dizzying pace.[7]

The dehumanising effect of an increasingly technological universe was accentuated by a new language – personnel officers became 'human resource managers'; services such as social welfare and health care became known as 'systems'; patients became 'consumers' or, even worse, 'clients'; hospital services became 'product lines'. The concept of stewardship was replaced in many organisations by devotion to the 'bottom line'. More than ever before, patients needed to know they mattered – really mattered. As Sister Angela Mary expressed it, 'medicine of the whole person' was not a technique, or a system, or a methodology – it was an attitude.[8]

All institutions, no matter how charitably inclined, faced the danger that mechanistic changes would become shaping forces, altering

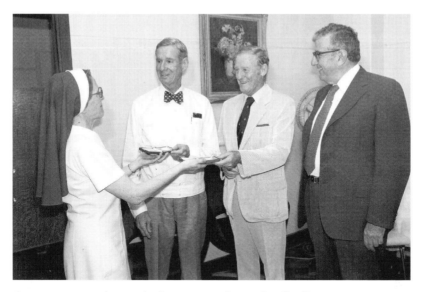

There were many changes in the 1980s, and some familiar figures were no longer seen so often at the Mater. Here, in 1980, Sister Angela Mary Doyle recognises the valued service of the orthopaedic surgeon Dr Michael Gallagher (next left) and the paediatrician Dr Stephen Clark Ryan (second from right), while Mr Kevin Cronin, Chairman of the Mater Advisory Board, looks on. MHHC

forever traditions and long-established cultures. In this climate, many younger Religious questioned the appropriateness of traditional ministries and searched for roles that seemed more likely to achieve social justice, particularly as falling numbers in religious orders brought an inevitable shift from hands-on service to management and governance, with many apostolic roles passed to the laity. Many women Religious found the search for their rightful place in the institutional church very difficult. Equally, it was often difficult for the Church, adjusting from the old hierarchical model to more participative structures, to recognise the value of articulate, educated, self-directed, professional women.

In this climate, it became even more important to see health care as a ministry with a goal – the just transformation of society – a human concept instead of a 'system' populated by 'health care professionals' and 'providers', in which medical procedures and practices were no longer evaluated only by their effectiveness in curing illness or relieving pain, but also, even predominantly, by their cost-effectiveness. Health care was rapidly being transformed from a human service to a commodity governed by the laws of economics. Other phenomena in the 1980s suggested, however, that society wanted a gentler and more intimate approach. Consumer questioning of medical practices, public pressure on governments to improve health care for Aboriginal people, and urgency in devising appropriate treatments for people affected by chemical dependency began to influence the medical model. It was clear that preventative medicine and health care delivery at community level would be emphasised increasingly, perhaps at the expense of the curative model. Resources would be stretched between hospitals and social welfare agencies as the impact of an aging population and many forms of social distress became more clearly manifest.[9]

These areas of emerging needs reached to the heart of the Sisters of Mercy: ever since the days of Catherine McAuley, meeting need in as practical a manner as possible had been their guiding principle. The Sisters had no wish to duplicate the Canadian experience, where a study on Catholic hospitals found that, although they differed noticeably from non-Catholic hospitals in their goals, they differed little in behaviour and performance, a chastening finding, given that the Church claimed compassionate work as its own mission and right, a stance reiterated by the Vatican II Decree on the Apostolate of the Laity.[10] But the Mater camel was well aware that rich governments were also looking for the eye of the needle. By 1983, the imminent advent of Medicare brought with it news of beds closed in public hospitals in other states by governments searching for value for the taxpayer dollar. This raised a fear which had haunted the Mater ever since it first successfully achieved government financial support: would governments continue to support the Sisters' hospital if they refused to provide some services for ethical reasons?[11]

In October 1984, the Mater Futures Task Force set about examining the shape the Mater should take to deal with a difficult and confusing present and an even more ominous future. More Sisters were moving into the background, increasing the danger that Mercy influence in the hospitals would be diluted at the very time pressures for cost-effectiveness and improved corporate performance were growing. The Mater Futures Discernment process, chaired by Sister Catharine Courtney, was a wide review, examining both overall governance and the direct, day-to-day administration of the hospital. Sister Catharine was well prepared for the task by her experience as Congregational Leader and her training in organisational theory and change management.[12] The Board examined the Mater's role, activities, procedures, and relationship to the Sisters' Hospital Council, and also looked at specialist questions such as Mercy philosophy, the possibility of incorporation, the indemnity of Board members, and relationships with the government. There were some pressing issues, not the least of which was the question of how to preserve the Mater ethos in a hospital owned by the Sisters of Mercy but which might not have Mercy sisters at key levels in future.

The Board was well aware that the Mater in Brisbane was not alone in struggling with these issues. A workshop convened by the Institute of Sisters of Mercy in Australia (ISMA) early in 1985 amply demonstrated that lay management would succeed the Sisters all over Australia. The Mercy private hospital in Melbourne was already under the management of a company limited by guarantee. In 1985, the national age profile of Australian Sisters of Mercy told its own tale. There were nine Sisters aged less than 30, 2,738 aged between 30 and 60 and 875 aged more than 60.[13]

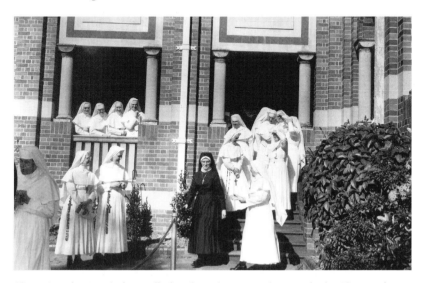

Sister Angela Mary is farewelled on her trip to Detroit to study the Sisters of Mercy health care system administered in Farmington Hills, Detroit, Michigan. The photograph was taken by Sister Mary Patrice Nally, pioneer of medical photography at the Mater. MHHC

The Futures Discernment workshops tackled a range of questions, such as the strengths and weaknesses of ownership and control by a religious congregation, the directions the congregation should take, and the type of congregation-owned institution which would best serve the hospitals' future needs and demands. As well as these large, philosophical questions, there were more practical issues to consider, such as the danger of lack of continuity in implementing policy when the congregational leadership changed every few years. This was important at a time when it was vital to maintain the individuality of the Mater, in view of both the Mercy mission, and the need to maintain distinctiveness as a marketing 'edge'. Unless Mercy values were translated from the words of mission statements into actions and practices, the Mater could become the same as any other hospital. A vision shared by staff in all divisions of the hospital needed to be instilled, maintained, reinforced and promoted.

Suggestions flew thick and fast: lay formation should be accelerated; health care and social welfare could, perhaps, be combined under one Sisters of Mercy umbrella; the Sisters' Hospital Council should be broadened to include both top and middle hospital management; the role of the Hospital Council should be publicised so that all Mater staff understood it; Mater management should develop a more collaborative model; the private hospital should be included in the Board structure; professional staff should be able to feel that they were adequately represented at Board level.[14]

Nationally, the Sisters of Mercy were looking at new forms of governance for their hospitals. The ISMA set up its own task force in 1984, with Sister Angela Mary as one of its members. She was convinced that the Australian Mercies could benefit from American experience. The Detroit Sisters had recommended that the Brisbane Sisters conduct a study to assess the feasibility of establishing a Sisters of Mercy Health System in Australia and invited Sister Angela Mary to spend a few months in Detroit getting to know their structure.[15] The Sisters of Mercy's health care corporation, based at Farmington Hills in Detroit, had been established in 1976. It was divided into sixteen divisions and managed a total of twenty-three hospitals with 5,560 beds and 18,500 employees. On this model, the Mater complex in Brisbane would form one division. An important advantage of the Detroit model was its ability to assist small or struggling private hospitals, a practice the Brisbane Sisters followed when Sister Michaeleen Mary went to Cairns to assist the Diocese to rebuild the Calvary Hospital. Integrated governance and management facilitated lay staff development and encouraged constituent institutions to share benefits with each other, maximising their strengths.[16]

The Detroit Sisters concentrated on ensuring that their values spread throughout all their hospitals and made creative efforts to contribute to the Church's social justice mission and medico-moral discussions. In August 1985, Sister Mary Concilia Moran, Sister Mary Maurita Sengelaub, John Quigley and E J Connors visited Australia from Detroit to advise on governance, developing the role of the laity and stimulating values permeation within the Sisters' ministries.[17] These issues formed the agenda for a major meeting at the Mater in October 1985. A large number of Mater people attended the session, among them Sister Jill Stringer, Sister Madonna Josey, Sister Eileen Pollard, Sister Deirdre Gardiner, Sister Josephine Crawford, Sister Anne Hetherington, Sister Angela Mary, and Assistant Administrator Mr Pat Maguire.

The Detroit team's recommendations pointed to a more integrated future. The Australian public–private pluralistic health system would continue, provided private hospitals were of high quality and relevant to modern needs. The viability and strength of the Catholic part of the private sector would eventually depend on significant reorganisation of the Catholic hospitals into a system of coordinated and interdependent institutions with strong values permeation throughout.[18] However, the independence of religious orders, once a strength, was deterring meaningful collaboration and stimulating competition between Catholic hospitals, a serious concern in the 1980s when government dominance of regulation and financing of hospitals could threaten the Catholic mission and philosophy. It was becoming increasingly difficult to retain the basic mission of caring for the poor. After much discussion, the Australian bishops agreed to write to the federal government communicating their strong theological, philosophical and sociological support for private hospitals. This and the bishops' advocacy of a Catholic Heath Care Association was a major break-through. As Sister Angela Mary reported, this was 'the first occasion on which the Bishops have indicated any concern for health care institutions or for the establishment of an Association to serve them'.[19]

The idea of an Australian Catholic Health Care Association (ACHCA) was not new. The health economist Paul Gross had advocated it in 1979, when health and hospital lobby groups were growing in number and strength, attempting to influence government policy and resource allocation. A national Catholic association would, it was hoped, show governments that Catholic hospitals could be proactive in the efficient, accountable use of resources and also demonstrate the church's responsiveness to the realities of social change.[20] The Mater strongly supported the move in 1982, donating $50,000 to fund the national secretariat, in addition to paying the levy of $5 per bed. The ACHCA set up a national council of state associations in 1983 with Sister Angela Mary as its Queensland representative. Sister Angela Mary became president of the Queensland Catholic Health Care Association, which met for the first time on 11 April 1985.

Discussions on the Sisters' future role in health care and participation on a wider stage were important milestones in succession planning. Stretching the lay management wings at the Mater was another. The foundation for the new era had been well laid in the 1970s with the inclusion of lay members on the Advisory Board. The next stage proceeded without J P Kelly, chairman of a succession of Mater advisory boards since 1938: he retired in 1980, after forty-two years of guiding the Sisters through a maze of changes in their hospitals. It was not a long retirement – J P Kelly died on 12 July 1984. The Sisters remembered him with admiration and enormous gratitude for his devotion to the Mater and perpetuated his name in the research foundation they established in 1982.

A Brisbane businessman, Kevin Cronin, succeeded J P Kelly. The new Advisory Board included a distinguished lawyer and future Supreme Court judge, Kevin Ryan; a management expert, J C Kable; a professor of civil engineering, Colin Apelt; an orthopaedic surgeon, Dr Anthony McSweeny; a physician, Dr Barry Smithurst; an obstetrician and gynaecologist, Dr Laurence Brunello; a solicitor, Margaret

Kelly; Sister Mary Etienne Flynn, Sister Mary St Margaret Kanowski, Sister Bernard Mary Crawford, Sister Geraldine Fitzgerald and, of course, Sister Angela Mary and her assistant, Pat Maguire.

The new Board established subcommittees to take advantage of this range of expertise – legislation and law under Professor Ryan, business management led by J C Kable, medical practice advances under Doctors McSweeny and Brunello, and Christian consciousness with Sisters Mary Etienne Flynn, Mary St Margaret Kanowski and Bernard Mary Crawford. These committees were asked to prepare a series of papers to present to the Board at two-monthly intervals. The papers commenced with a difficult subject which went to the heart of the Mater's mission. Professor Colin Apelt tackled the Mater's duty to the poor. He identified aged people, single-parent families, low-wage earners, disabled people, Aborigines, immigrants, refugees and single women as the most disadvantaged groups of Mater patients. Their access to hospitals was limited by excess demand on resources, a situation further complicated in the Medicare era by some people who could afford private insurance, and therefore private hospitals, opting not to be insured and using the free hospitals. There was also the difficult issue of providing adequate health care outside the hospital walls. In Professor Apelt's view, the Mater had an important opportunity to consider how services could be coordinated to suit the needs of Aboriginal people, who were often uncomfortable in hospital settings, the needs of recently arrived migrants and refugees with language problems – in fact services to all disadvantaged groups.[21] It was, he felt, time for governments and hospitals to throw away the too-hard basket.

Just how this could be done in a framework of increasingly rigid expectations of accountability and performance measurement was the question. The Mater Board and authorities in many other hospitals were preparing for the day anticipated by the health care economist Paul Gross in 1979. Gross predicted that in as short a period as ten years Catholic hospitals would be governed by boards accountable to the public and administered by lay managers. The Mater gathered all of its services under the new Board, including the Mater Private Hospital. This was a significant change. Until then, the Mater Private had been entirely separately administered. The Sister Administrator, Sister

Bernard Mary Crawford, was the first official Mater Private Hospital representative on the Board. The Board, while still not the decision-making body, continued to evolve to a structure similar to large commercial corporations, with committees on such topics as the public hospitals' budget, organisational design, and master plan development.[22] A temporary planning and research officer was appointed to assist with both short-term and long-term planning for the three public hospitals,[23] but a corporate strategic plan was not completed until 1993.

This was an era of sophisticated administration. The modern manager's briefcase was heavy with mission statements, policy formulations, strategic plans, organisational designs and budgetary models. These were necessary tools to deal with some stark realities. By 1985, uncertainties loomed. The Mater had become more dependent on government for both its operating costs and its capital expenditures, yet the government's expenditure on state hospitals was a vote catcher, while it was accorded little recognition for its contributions to the Mater. Therefore, in Sister Angela Mary's view, the Mater's future was assured only so long as it provided services the government could not supply.[24] Fortunately, the Mater was especially important in paediatrics and obstetrics, both essential in a rapidly growing city, but there was a cloud on the horizon. The new Queen Elizabeth II hospital at Mt Gravatt and the proposed hospital in Logan City south of Brisbane could dilute the demographic advantages that had always favoured the Mater. There was also concern that, although the Mater's ethical stance had never been publicly challenged, there was no guarantee that public opinion or government intervention would not put it in the position of either compromising its ethical stand or ceasing public hospital services, at least in part, a fate already suffered by some Canadian Catholic hospitals.[25]

Preparation for the future was punctuated by a year of public celebration of momentous past events. Nineteen eighty-six was the 125th anniversary of the arrival of the Sisters of Mercy in Queensland; the 75th anniversary of the Adult Hospital, the 25th anniversary of the Mater Mothers' and the 55th anniversary of the Mater Children's Hospital. Behind the scenes, revolutionary management changes were on the way. Sister Angela Mary returned from her study visit to Detroit

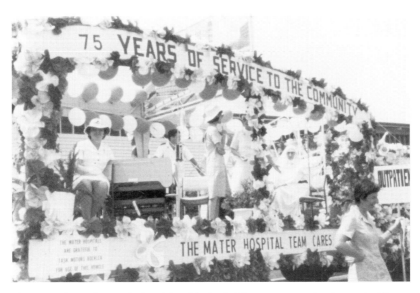

The Mater has a long relationship with the Brisbane community. In 1986, this Mater float in the city's Warana procession celebrated seventy-five years of care at Mater Hill. MHHC

armed with a report setting out the possibilities. From all the options she had considered, Sister Angela Mary recommended a structure for the Mater which would integrate more effectively all the Mater's services. The key would be the appointment of a chief executive officer to manage all the hospitals. The chief executive would be appointed by the Congregation and would be a voting member of the Board. The rigid separation between public and private hospitals would, she hoped, never re-emerge. This structure would be an important step to the ultimate goal of an incorporated board appointed by a Sisters of Mercy board of governance.[26]

It was not long before Sister Angela Mary's plan was realised. In 1987, the Mater Health Services Governing Board, empowered to develop policy and make decisions for the hospitals, replaced the Advisory Board. It was a significant stage in the long evolution from the Medical Advisory Board of the 1930s through the Advisory Boards of subsequent decades. The Sisters reserved some of their powers, particularly their canon law responsibility for property and their power to appoint the board and senior executives. There was continuity – Kevin Cronin remained as chairman, with the same deputy,

Professor Kevin Ryan. The new board included members with the skills required to cover all areas of decision-making likely to be necessary in a large hospital complex. The members included Charles McAnany, Queensland Manager of Bankers Trust Australia, a Supreme Court judge, Martin Moynihan, the professor of civil engineering at the University of Queensland, Colin Apelt, Shirley Gagen, a part-time nursing supervisor at the Adult Hospital and an active participant in community affairs, as well as Sister Kath Burke, Sister Mary Tinney, Sister Madonna Josey, Sister Angela Mary, the former principal of All Hallows' school, Sister Anne Hetherington, Dr Harry Barry, Dr John Burke and the assistant chief executive officer, Pat Maguire.[27]

The new Board's business was highly organised through a series of committees. An executive committee – Kevin Cronin, Sister Angela Mary, Dr John Burke and Pat Maguire – managed the day-to-day business of the hospital, finance committees scrutinised the hospitals' accounts, and a medical advisory committee recommended medical appointments. The Mater Private Hospital continued its medical and nursing practices committee and its management and planning committee. A member of the Board was assigned to take particular interest in one of the hospitals – Charles McAnany for the Adult Hospital, Sister Anne Hetherington for the Children's Hospital, Dr John Burke for the Mater Mothers' and Sister Mary Tinney for the Private Hospital.

As far as the Mater's everyday work was concerned, by far the greatest change was the end of Sister Angela Mary's long term as Sister Administrator. Her new position, Senior Director of Health Services for the Sisters of Mercy, reflected the wider interests of the Brisbane Congregation and provided her with the opportunity to rove more broadly than the Mater campus. Her brief included acting as a bridge between the Congregation and the chief executive officer, and liaison with the state government, the federal government and the universities in Queensland, as well as the national Catholic Health Care Association and the Sisters of Mercy health care corporation in Detroit.[28] At the same time, membership of the Sisters' Hospital Council was broadened, generally in line with the recommendations of the 'futures' task force, to include Professor Kevin Ryan as well as the chairman of the Board, Kevin Cronin.

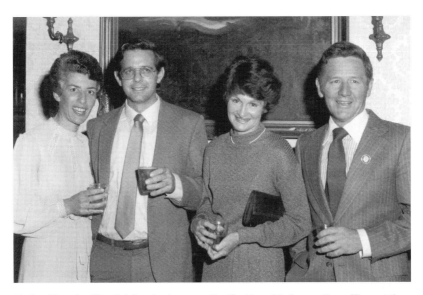

Mr Pat Maguire (far right), who became the first lay chief executive officer at the Mater in 1987, is pictured in 1981 with his wife, Anne, second from right, Mr Stan Walsh, who moved from the laboratory to the administration, and his wife, Christine. Stan Walsh became Pat Maguire's deputy in 1987. MHHC

Sister Angela Mary was succeeded at the Mater by its first lay chief executive officer, Pat Maguire, who had been carefully prepared for the position during his years as Sister Angela Mary's assistant. Almost immediately, Stan Walsh, a former laboratory technologist, who had successfully made the change to administration, was appointed to assist him.[29] Sister Angela Mary had no fear at all of lay leadership at the Mater. She had made her position quite clear in a major conference paper in 1985. It had, she said, taken twenty years for most religious orders to implement the Vatican II view that the laity should be partners of religious administrators, not their assistants, a reversal of the earlier view that Religious were on a plane above the laity. Acceptance of the lay apostolate came more easily when the numbers of Religious began to fall. In Queensland private hospitals in 1984, for instance, the proportion of Religious to lay staff was 2.8 per cent, in New South Wales it was 4.6 per cent and, in Victoria it was 3.3 per cent; proportions were even lower in the public hospitals – 2.3 per cent in New South Wales and Queensland and 0.9 per cent in Victoria.[30]

In this situation, Sister Angela Mary argued, sound management was essential to achieve harmony, cost-effectiveness and viability, while retaining a culture where shared values define fundamental character. Shared values should not, however, become an excuse for intransigence in changing direction when change was necessary. All religious orders continuing their health care missions must, therefore, specify their philosophy, their mission and their goals. Directing overall policy, enhancing material assets and appointing competent managers were also essential, particularly to assure quality of service. Sister Angela Mary also felt that a Catholic hospital should demonstrate cost-effectiveness in using public money; hospitals, she knew, could not expect the lion's share of the nation's health care resources.[31] Preventive health measures, including education, were necessary to reduce the number of patients who went home to the same conditions as those that had generated their illness. Boards and chief executive officers should share the view that Catholic hospitals must give priority to people over things, ethics over technology, and spirit over matter. Orientation and in-service training would become just as important for members of the Board as it was for the newest member of the Mater staff.[32]

With these ideals ringing in his ears, Pat Maguire started work as the Mater's first lay chief executive officer on St Patrick's Day, 1987. What faced him was the task of ensuring that the necessary efficiency in material development did not suppress the less tangible Mercy values on which the Mater was based. Maguire had recognised the creative tension implied by this dilemma in 1984 when he noted the variety of constraints which, if not handled well, could make the Mater very fragile. Externally, these factors included dealing with governments and complying with eighteen separate statutes, meeting the training requirements of the universities, and attending to the requirements of several separate workplace unions and professional associations. Internal constraints included walking the financial tightrope while providing medical care of a high clinical and ethical standard. Like all hospitals, the Mater faced the situation that Queensland ran on a cash accounting system, aggravated by historical budget processes, rather than a more forward-looking accrual basis. Next year's budget was always based on last year's, sometimes with escalation factors, sometimes without. The system provided no incentives to pursue efficiency

PAT MAGUIRE, CPA, FAIM, ABIA, was born in Brisbane in 1933 and educated by the Sisters of Mercy at Wooloowin and by the Christian Brothers at St Joseph's College, Gregory Terrace. He joined the staff of the Commonwealth Bank in 1951. Following transfers to Dalby, where he met his future wife, Anne, and to Nambour, he was promoted to executive cadet in the bank's administration in Brisbane in 1962. He resigned from the bank in 1966 to take up an appointment as accountant and first secretary at Mt Olivet Hospital. In 1969, he was appointed secretary to the Mater Hospitals Advisory Board. When Jack O'Brien retired in 1975, Pat Maguire was appointed Executive Director, Administration Services and served on the executive committee with Sister Angela Mary, Rex Ducat, Executive Director, Nursing Services, and Dr Des O'Callaghan, Director of Medical Services. He was appointed Assistant Administrator in 1980 and, on Sister Angela Mary's retirement as Sister Administrator, he became the first lay chief executive officer. His ready availability, affability and enthusiasm endeared him to all staff. Since his retirement in 1993, Pat Maguire has served on several Archdiocesan boards. Five of his six children and eleven of his grandchildren were born at the Mater Mothers'.

goals; it was built on negative sanctions and deficit financing. Special allocations rarely entirely satisfied needs, let alone ambitions for new services. Staff establishments were set rigidly by the government; new staff could not be employed without approval, even if the Sisters funded them in perpetuity.

Long-range planning in this situation was very difficult, if not impossible, particularly as annual survival from budget to budget was influenced by politicians' whims. This was even more serious in the mid-1980s, when it became clear that the proportion of gross domestic product spent on health care was declining. It had fallen from 8 per cent in 1977–78 to 7.5 per cent only three years later, and stalled at 8 per cent in 1989–90.[33] Costs, of course, had not fallen. This was the reality behind apparently impressive statistics. In 1967–68, $112 per person was spent on health care, rising to $505 by 1977–78. More than half the national health care budget was spent on hospitals in 1979.[34]

The phenomenon of the new Mater Adult Hospital had helped to consolidate an improved working relationship with the state. The Mater was represented on most important state health committees. Nevertheless, there were few rewards for efficient financial management; in Pat Maguire's opinion, the state looked for 'uniformity in the system and initiatives are to come from them'. He was philosophical:

> I adopt the attitude that if the Mater wishes to be a part of the public hospitals system in this state, we have to accept the vagaries that exist in the system – we are just as constrained as other public hospitals, although this does not imply that we just lie down and let the government walk over us.[35]

In Pat Maguire's view, some positive effects had flowed from wearying constraints – growth was orderly and measured, if not always exciting; and the Mater was more accountable, but retained the crucial elements of its autonomy. It had never been pressured into medico-moral compromise and the Sisters had complete liberty to establish the governing board they wanted.

The Mater's balancing act between compassionate care and cost-effective had been recognised during the 'Mater Futures' workshops in 1984. A decision that successful planning for change must be driven by the Mater's own distinctive culture was evident in future developments.[36] Emphasis on the Mercy spirit – compassionate care for patients, and recognition of them individually as valuable, whole human beings – was given voice more and more strongly in the closing years of the twentieth century and in the opening years of the twenty-first. Values and mission were given a prominent place in the executive management structure: Sister Anne Hetherington was appointed first director of mission effectiveness, responsible for the expression and application of Mercy values throughout the campus. Efficiency objectives were pursued by the Board just as strongly. After all, if the hospitals could not survive financially, the mission could not be expressed at all.

Staff changes had been in the wind throughout the late 1970s and 1980s. Visible manifestations of the movement towards lay leadership began in nursing. In 1977, Rex Ducat succeeded Sister Eileen Pollard as Director of Nursing for the Mater Public Hospitals, a position which became Executive Director, Nursing, in the new Mater structure. A former director of nursing for the Blue Nurses, a community nursing service, Rex Ducat was the first man to be appointed as a head of nursing in a major Queensland hospital.[37] Next, in 1986, came the appointments of the first two lay superintendents of nursing, the former principal nurse educator Karleen O'Reilly succeeding Sister Madonna Josey at the Adult Hospital and Rosalie Lewis succeeding Sister Mary Dorothea at the Children's. In the mid-1980s, two Sisters of Mercy remained in charge of Mater hospitals – Sister Jill Stringer at the Mater Mothers' and Sister Josephine Crawford at the Mater Private Hospital, where she was always known as Sister Bernard Mary.

One change caused real grief. Dr Des O'Callaghan, often known as 'EDoc', an acronym of his initials, died in January 1988, after twenty-six years in the demanding, frequently trying job of Director of Medical Services. He had presided over enormous development in the hospitals'

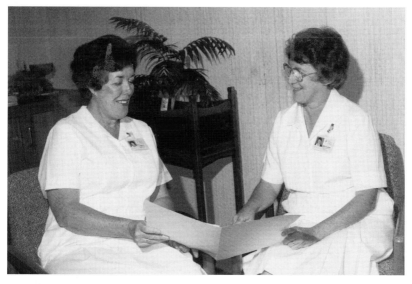

In 1986, Miss Karleen O'Reilly (at left) was appointed Director of the Mater Adult Hospital and Mrs Rosalie Lewis (at right) was appointed Director of Nursing at the Mater Children's Hospital. MHHC

clinical work, arbitrated disputes between doctors and departments, encouraged procedural reforms and worked his way through several administrative changes. Always conscientious, he was remembered fondly for his good humour in some awkward situations. As Dr John Herron put it, Des O'Callaghan 'always acted justly and he was scrupulous in seeking all possible advice before making a decision but having made it, he kept to it, even though on many occasions others disagreed'.[38] Dr O'Callaghan was succeeded by Dr James Griffin, and the position was renamed Executive Director, Clinical Services.

Even though daily bed costs in the Mater public hospitals remained the lowest of all public hospitals in the Brisbane area, increasing demand for services in all parts of the Mater ensured that finance remained a major worry throughout the 1980s. The hospitals were large and growing – public bed numbers were 481 in June 1970, 511 in June 1980 and 535 in 1990. Staff establishments had also grown.[39] The total staff grew from 1,130 in 1970, to 1,432 in 1980 and 1,737 in 1990. The numbers of permanent medical staff had shown the greatest growth; at least some of the visiting doctors' prejudice against staff specialists had, apparently, been overcome. The slow growth in the various therapies and social work demonstrated that, in a milieu of inter-disciplinary care, ancillary services were likely to be increasingly overloaded. The daily average cost of caring for a patient had, however, demonstrated the most remarkable growth between 1980 and 1984 – $122.29 to $206.85 at the Adult Hospital, $133.52 to $227.93 at the Mater Children's Hospital, and $108.72 to $177.25 at the Mater Mothers' Hospital. The introduction of the 38-hour week had had a huge impact, as had the decline in the number of Sisters of Mercy, who had always worked much longer hours, either free of charge or on low stipends.[40]

In an era of lean budgets, it was time to tighten up and supervise all the business enterprises at the Mater more closely.[41] Previously, the Congregation had owned the businesses – the art union, the Green Shop, the coffee shops, Reg Leonard House, the laundry and the Mater Private Hospital pharmacy. The Board and the Mater administration had not been involved in their financial management. Most were profitable, but the real profit leaders were the laundry, which helped to support the Private Hospital, and the first multistorey carpark, opened in May 1981, which consistently returned 20 per cent on the Sisters' investment.

The Mater Art Union had operated in splendid isolation from its own offices in Justice Chambers in Adelaide Street in the city, before moving to refurbished premises in Park Road, a few blocks from the Mater campus. Although ticket sales fell in the mid-1980s, when the development of similar art unions provided stiff competition, art unions nevertheless returned profits exceeding $1,000,000 annually. Even though the special administration committee remained, as required by legislation controlling art unions, the Congregation's Hospital Council supervised the art union more closely in the late 1980s. It had to respond when the Department of Justice chastised the art union for frequently exceeding the 35 per cent expenses limit and criticised its technique of mailing tickets to people who had not requested them, in the hope of expanding ticket sales.[42] The Sisters reviewed plans for all prize homes and kept a very close eye on operating expenses and sales' methods. The art unions had always had additional importance in raising the Mater's profile in the wider community. The government provided another valuable public relations opportunity when it chose the Mater as the official hospital for Expo 88, the world exposition held on the South Brisbane bank of the Brisbane River for six months during 1988.[43] Although the government regarded the accolade of caring for Expo patrons as a great honour for the Mater, it almost failed to eventuate. Late in 1987, the government had still not agreed to pay for the staff and the medications that the clinic on the Expo site would need.[44] This wrinkle was ironed out, and health teams from the Adult and the Children's Hospitals provided care for twelve hours each day for six months. The staff loved the experience, and the Mater name was put before visitors from all over the world.

The hospitals were not entirely reliant on external fundraising to supplement government subsidies. The Sisters continued to provide substantial material assistance. In the 1980s, the Sisters' projects included providing land for the Mater Children's Hospital school, reorganising the antenatal clinic and refurbishing bathrooms at the Mater Mothers', renovating old Ward 2 at the original Adult Hospital to provide a large meeting room, establishing a pastoral care centre in Ward 1, and, at the Mater Children's Hospital, converting the old babies ward to a permanent intensive care unit. The Sisters also paid the stipends of ten Sisters and two priests working full time in pastoral care at the hospital.

Staff salaries had become a major factor in escalating costs. In 1980, wages were 75.38 per cent of total costs. The Mater, like all businesses, had felt the impact of high inflation in the 1970s, one of the factors responsible for large award increases in nursing salaries. In the late 1970s, Sister Catharine Courtney had been very concerned that the Mater had still not faced the situation when religious sisters on low stipends would be replaced by lay staff on full salaries. At $3,300 annually in the late 1970s, stipends at the Mater were considerably lower than the $4,381 the schools paid their teaching Religious, and much lower than stipends paid in other states. In 1983, the Health Department, which controlled staff establishments, approved increased stipends for nineteen Sisters working in established positions at the Mater and agreed to annual reviews, an important step in facilitating realistic budgeting.[45]

There was also a serious anomaly affecting doctors, nurses and ancillary staff. The Mater had always been excluded from arrangements between state hospitals which allowed entitlements such as sick leave, recreation leave and superannuation benefits to be transferred if an employee left one hospital to work in another. There seemed no logical reason for the Mater's exclusion, because its public hospitals were working with staff establishments set by the Health Department on the same basis as other hospitals. It was particularly galling because the staff at St Vincent's public hospital in Sydney enjoyed reciprocity with the New South Wales state system, and this benefit was extended to Mater staff from Brisbane who moved interstate to work in public hospitals.[46] Rectifying this situation was also in the Mater's interests because it was deterring capable staff from applying for Mater jobs, and frustrating existing staff hoping for job experience elsewhere.

Retaining competent nursing staff was a particular worry in most hospitals in the 1980s. The wastage rate of nurse trainees at the Mater, 5.6 per cent in the early 1980s, was much lower than the state average

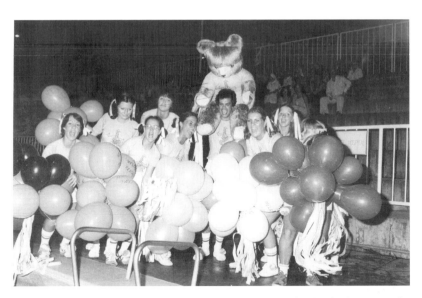

The annual swimming carnival in 1970 brought out an enthusiastic cheer squad, including, from left, Leanne McKnoulty, Jennifer Moran, July Clark, Susan Cleary, Louise Shields, Graham Wemyss with the Mater Bear, Margaret Briggs, Karen Milano and Julietta Valks. MHHC

of 16.4 per cent, but was quite bad enough. The 1970s and 1980s were years of rapid change in nursing and nurse education. Many nurses felt inadequately prepared for the duties they were expected to perform in an increasingly technological medical milieu. Many trainees did not complete their courses and registered nurses began to leave the profession.[47] Even worse, many Queensland registered nurses found it very difficult to gain employment in interstate hospitals because their educational standard was inferior. Behind the scenes, the development of a tertiary program for nurses was proceeding, infuriatingly slowly in Queensland and more rapidly in the southern states. In the mid-1970s, Sister Eileen Pollard was one of two Queenslanders the Royal Australian Nursing Federation appointed to a national working party on goals in nurse education which prepared a submission to the federal government on funding the transfer of nurse education into the tertiary education sector. In Queensland, the Sisters of Mercy's McAuley College, which had begun as their teacher training college, seemed the most appropriate place to develop tertiary nurse training for the Mater hospitals. As well as being asked to help plan this move,

Sister Eileen Pollard acted as a consultant to the Catholic teachers' college at Ascot Vale in Melbourne.

The 840-hour curriculum had been the first stage in changes which began to move the old-fashioned nurse education curriculum in Queensland to a more rigorous academic standard. This old disease-oriented, hospital-based curriculum was replaced with a much broader concept, a systematic approach to the patient's total needs, including health promotion. By the 1980s, task-oriented nursing had been replaced by a patient-centred approach which emphasised the preparation and implementation of patient care plans. Sister Eileen Pollard was very close to the action in nurse education and urged it on at every opportunity. Her study tour of hospitals in the United States, the United Kingdom, Europe and Asia in 1973 had filled her with ideas on preparing Queensland nurse education for the transition from apprenticeship training to the tertiary education sector. Sister Eileen was asked to join the Board of Nursing Studies' task force on developing a new, broader curriculum, a vital stepping stone to a nursing course at tertiary education level. The slightly expanded 1,200-hour curriculum, introduced in 1982, was the next advance. The training school had also changed when men had been admitted to the general nursing school in the mid-1970s, a path first trodden by John Collins, when he started nursing aide training in 1971. By the late 1970s, men had been admitted to midwifery training at the Mater Mothers'.[48]

At last, in 1975, the Commonwealth government announced that nursing education would be moved to tertiary institutions by 1990. The Commonwealth government insisted that, to qualify for funding, all Colleges of Advanced Education be interdenominational, multipurpose institutions: Sister Eileen Pollard was quite happy that McAuley College would not remain a 'uni-function, unisex college for nuns'.[49] In 1978, she was devastated that the Queensland government had decided not to fund the move to McAuley. Nurse education was, therefore, established in tertiary institutions in other Australian states years before Queensland, where the Queensland University of Technology and the Australian Catholic University inaugurated nursing degree programs in the 1980s. The end of the Mater nurse training school came in August 1989, when the last intake of trainees began the hospital-based curriculum. It was the first Brisbane hospital to phase out hospital-based training. By the time the final group graduated in 1992, the Mater had educated 4,000 nurses and the nursing staff establishment had grown to 900.[50]

The nursing division at the Mater was large and complex. In the 1980s, a nursing management advisory committee was established as a discussion forum for Rex Ducat, Executive Director, Nursing Services, the nursing superintendents of the three public hospitals and the principal nurse educator to develop major policies. By the mid-1980s, the nursing structure had been expanded to include a nursing process committee. Sister Judy Chalker's section was vigorously helping the Private Hospital to achieve accreditation, working on projects ranging from an evaluation of the standard of documentation of nurses' notes in patients' records to Sister Eileen Pollard's idea of replacing medication trollies with locked cupboards at each patient's bedside. This innovation, first applied in the Mater Private Hospital, streamlined ward paperwork. Some doctors, anchored in the old attitude that patients should have information, as well as medication, dispensed in frugally measured doses, resisted the accompanying innovation of charts at the end of patients' beds, because patients would know more about their medication regime. In 1986, the Mater and the Queensland Nurses Union were awarded a federal grant of $80,000 for a three-year research project to implement and evaluate a program to prevent nurses' back injuries. This was a real feather in the Mater nursing research cap – it was the only nursing project chosen from 114 applications to the National Occupational Health and Safety Commission.[51]

Mater nurses also suffered from the pressure on hospitals to reduce costs, which meant that fewer staff were somehow expected to maintain the same level of care. The Mater adult intensive care and coronary care units, for instance, were staffed at a level appropriate to seven beds, but were operating with ten beds during 1984.[52] By the end of the 1980s, nurses in the general wards were coping with a huge range of sophisticated devices – electronic thermometers, blood-glucose-measuring devices, patient-controlled analgesia machines, automatic apparatus for monitoring vital signs and syringe drivers for drug delivery – in addition

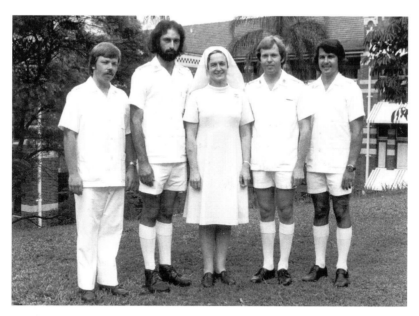

Men became very important in nursing in the 1970s and 1980s. Here, Sister Jill Stringer is photographed with the first male midwifery students, from left, Mr A Gordon, Mr P Rankin, Mr K Josey and Mr J Green. MHHC

to increased responsibility for quality-assurance and infection-control programs.[53] In this era of increasing technology, the Mater conference in September 1988 with the theme 'caring in the age of technology' was very welcome. Inservice training was also essential because ward equipment was becoming more and more sophisticated. The education process was by no means one-way. Mater nurses were also involved in education programs for a range of conditions. At the Mater Children's Hospital, for instance, nurses worked with patients and their families in areas such as diabetes, neonatal lung disease, asthma and spina bifida, as well as with cystic fibrosis patients who were growing up and moving to care at the Adult Hospital.

Although hospital-based nurse education had been very limited in extent and academic rigour, it did have the advantage of providing student nurses with broad practical training. The opportunity for practical work in university programs was more restricted and it was more difficult for newly graduated nurses to adapt to ward nursing conditions. The Mater developed a preceptor program – an experienced nurse working with each new clinical nurse – to integrate graduates into clinical situations with a practical understanding of their role and responsibilities. This form of mentoring was also very important in assisting nurses returning to the profession, many of whom had been away for years. These initiatives were, to some extent, self-interested. Nursing shortages were beginning to be felt in hospitals in many parts of the world, and these programs were seen as helping the Mater to be a 'magnet' for nurses.[54] Lunchtime seminars enabling nurses to hear about papers given at conferences also helped to develop professionalism. Supportive work in the Nursing Personnel department included attendance at job fairs and addresses to university students, as well as information campaigns aimed at overseas and interstate nurses to maintain nursing staff levels.

Medical staff training was also a critical issue in the 1970s and 1980s. The various specialist colleges retained their monopoly of training for the medical specialties, and from the 1960s onwards hospital-based training programs had largely replaced the older 'apprenticeship' model. The colleges, therefore, set standards which hospitals had to meet in order to be accredited for training in the various specialties.[55] Hospitals that were not fully accredited had difficulty retaining those resident medical officers who hoped to progress to appointment to a registrar training position for a particular specialty. The need to establish and maintain training programs was a major factor in the formalisation of medical departments in the various hospitals. The Mater noted in 1975, for instance, that the establishment of the department of surgery had helped to maintain both staff levels and training accreditation. On the other hand, the Australian College of Paediatrics accredited the hospital for only one year of postgraduate training in 1975 because the Children's Hospital was small and, in the College's opinion, operated too few sub-specialties for advanced paediatric training. Within ten years, however, the position had been rectified and by the mid-1980s the Mater Children's Hospital was part of a great increase in postgraduate medical education at the Mater. More registrars were passing their examinations, joint training sessions were being held with the Royal Children's Hospital and registrars were encouraged to undertake research projects. Indeed, as early as 1982 the Mater could report that it had a high reputation as a training hospital for medical students and that more medical students applied for positions as resident medical officers at the Mater than at any other hospital.[56] The improvement in Mater training programs did not entirely solve the shortage of staff specialists or trainees. The hospital was still recruiting from the United Kingdom in 1990, a practice begun in the mid-1970s.[57]

By the end of the 1980s, the most urgent improvements in the Mater public hospital system had been achieved. The first board with decision-making powers had been established, lay leaders were working in senior positions in the administration and in the hospitals, and the old apprenticeship training systems for nurses and specialist doctors had been replaced with modern programs. At the same time, the 'grand dame' of the Mater family, the Mater Private Hospital, had been re-positioning itself to take its place in the Mater's future.

CHAPTER NINE

KEEPING THE FAMILY TOGETHER

A private hospital today must operate on a reasonable
level of profitability or convert to another use.
The current Federal Government cannot afford to
allow the private health insurance schemes to collapse,
but in the short term the future for any private hospital
is far from bright.[1]

Sister Catharine Courtney, 1979

Rationalisation of health services, a concept generated by the growing
push to economy and efficiency in spending the health care dollar,
was demonstrated graphically at the Mater in the 1980s by events
at two of the hospitals, the Mater Private and the Mater Children's.
The movement towards integration of all the Mater hospitals appeared
threatened, first by the difficult question of the future of the Private
Hospital, and second by a proposal to move the Children's Hospital.

The management changes at the Mater in the mid-1980s had integrated all parts of the Mater complex under a single administrative
structure. Until then, the Mater Private Hospital had been very much
a world of its own. It was the senior hospital, the first to be opened
on Mater Hill, yet rarely was it featured in external public relations
material, or in internal reports. Sometimes its staff felt overlooked,

even unimportant to the Mater as a whole. In reality, the reverse was true. Although administratively separate until the 1980s, the Mater Private Hospital had always been extremely important to the Mater hospitals. In the days before the Sisters working in the public hospitals were paid stipends, the Private Hospital had supported them and their convent. Whenever possible, it had channelled its profits to the public hospitals.

The Private Hospital had also been vital in maintaining a healthy complement of honorary medical specialists for the public Adult Hospital. Before 1976, when visiting medical officers were paid for the first time, the opportunity to be admitting doctors to the Private Hospital was an honorary doctor's sole pecuniary reward for work in the Mater public hospitals. The Mater Private continued to be regarded highly among Brisbane's private hospitals; the right to admit patients remained prized, even though competition among private hospitals increased during the 1970s and 1980s. The Uniting Church had opened its large Wesley hospital at Auchenflower, while the Presbyterian Church's St Andrews' hospital and the Catholic Holy Spirit hospital were greatly enlarged. In contrast, the old flagship of the Mater fleet was floundering. Its fabric was deteriorating, and its finances were shaky.

In 1977, the Sisters investigated future possibilities for the Mater

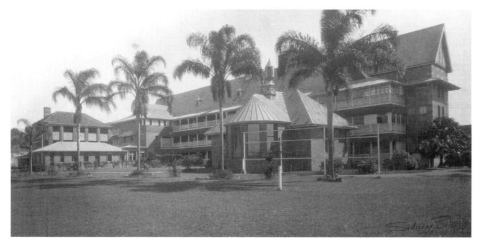

The original Mater Private Hospital was a gracious, beautiful building, even from the rear. This photograph, taken in 1940 before the side wing was built, shows the original operating theatres in the right foreground. MHHC

Private, specifically to identify the types of services it might offer one
or two decades ahead, and the alterations the building would require.[2]
There were numerous imponderables. The fortunes of all private hospitals fluctuated. They had had a precarious existence under the original
national health insurance scheme, Medibank, which reintroduced free
public hospital care in the early 1970s, but most were flourishing only
a few years later, when the Commonwealth paid private hospitals a
subsidy of $16 per occupied bed per day for providing medical care,
regardless of who they treated or how efficiently they were treated.
To succeed, private hospitals had to have their beds as fully used as
possible.[3] These changes, ostensibly to relieve overcrowding in public hospitals, were due in no small part to the lobbying of doctors'
organisations determined to protect private medicine in all its manifestations.[4] The strength of the private medical lobby seemed to grow
in direct proportion to the increase in government involvement in the
medical insurance industry. The Australian Medical Association clung
hard to the old private fee-for-service model.

The 1977 investigation identified surgery as a strength the Mater
Private could develop, but substantial capital expenditure was needed
to ensure its position in the surgical front rank. Patients and doctors
were only too aware that the facilities and equipment in the newer
private hospitals were more up-to-date. Even though they were costly
and became obsolete quickly, the latest in accommodation and technology had to be supplied. In 1976, work commenced on a new
operating theatre block to contain four new theatres, adjacent to new
intensive care and coronary care units, with a recovery ward, facilities
for the blood bank and a central sterilising department on the top
floor, ten single rooms, five with ensuite bathrooms, on the second
floor, and streamlined administration offices on the ground floor.[5] The
new block, always known as 'St Gabriel's', was the brainchild of the
Sister Administrator of the Private Hospital, Sister Mary St Gabriel
Corbett. Sister Mary St Gabriel knew all corners of the Mater complex.
She had been Sister Administrator of the public hospitals between
1954 and 1966, and Superior of the convent before becoming Sister
Administrator of the Mater Private in 1974. She was not alone in
her enthusiasm to improve the hospital. The Mater Private had loyal

supporters among the business community. A senior public servant, Sir David Longland, architect Robin Gibson, shoe-store entrepreneur Sir Robert Mathers and Dr Ian Ferguson had organised nearly 100 people to donate $111,000 to help fund the new intensive care unit.[6]

There was a downside to this progress. Some rooms had to be closed to accommodate the new facilities and running costs rose. Pat Maguire, assistant administrator of the Mater, was concerned that, if the intensive care unit cost as much to run as the Holy Spirit's unit, it would be difficult for the Private Hospital to operate profitably.[7] The new work cost almost $2,500,000; the Private Hospital would need a large loan. It was time for a searching examination of the hospital's finances and methods of operation. The Mater Private, the Mater Mothers' private and the intermediate section of the Adult Hospital had not been exempt from the scrutiny of the management consultants whose recommendations in the 1970s had formed the basis of the modernisation of the Mater administration. Several major changes in the time-honoured system had been implemented. Firm targets and cost objectives were set, depreciation charges on buildings and equipment were established, and the cost of operating the convent was separated from the operating costs of the private hospital, but at the end of the 1970s much remained to be done.[8]

In 1979, Pat Maguire investigated the financial operations of the Mater Private Hospital.[9] He was not happy with the situation he found. Monthly cost controls, through measurement against an authorised budget, could not be implemented because statements of receipts and payments were still used instead of profit and loss statements. The hospital had traditionally shown a small surplus, but this was a mirage. The full costs of operating the laundry, a major source of income, had not been shown. It appeared, therefore, that the hospital itself had not actually made a profit for twenty years. The problem was serious, and structural. An enormous proportion of the Private Hospital's expenditure, 81.48 per cent, was spent on salaries and wages, an unfavourable comparison with other private hospitals which contained labour costs at 70 per cent. If this level of spending continued, the position would deteriorate even more when more Sisters of Mercy were replaced by lay nurses.

High labour costs could not be excused on the grounds that the hospital was inordinately busy; its bed-occupancy figures fluctuated between 69.6 per cent and 75.5 per cent, when 80 per cent was recognised as a viable occupancy figure for a private hospital.[10] The Mater Private was under-used. In contrast with the hospital's glory days in the early 1960s, when 119 patients was the daily average, by 1979 the daily average had decreased to about 80 patients. The position had to be rectified quickly. Fading finances could not be tolerated. Through discussions at the hospital during his investigation, Pat Maguire had decided that nursing care had to be organised around one team for each nursing unit, and inefficient practices in the catering department had to be curtailed.

Fortunately, there would be no need to retrench staff, because the enlarged operating theatres and specialised new units would need nurses. Another important economy could be achieved by combining the convent and hospital kitchens. A central plating system in the ground floor pantry serving the other floors would reduce inefficiency. Other necessary economies removed some of the touches that had made the Mater Private special. Sterling silver cutlery and utensils would be replaced with stainless steel; the fine bone china crockery was shelved in favour of utilitarian pieces able to survive industrial dishwashing machines. Catering and cleaning staff were organised on a strict shift system; the former practice of staff working the hours which suited them was abandoned.[11] The old system provided valuable employment to people who badly needed it, but the hospital's position decreed that savings through reorganisation – some $185,000 in a single year – were too important to sacrifice. In a climate of changing government health-insurance policies, private hospitals had to be profitable. In acknowledging this reality, church-run private hospitals, which ploughed their profits

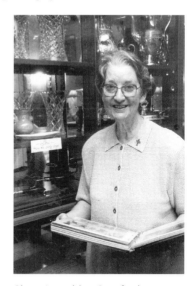

Sister Josephine Crawford, known as Sister Bernard Mary during her many years at the Mater Private Hospital, became Sister Administrator in 1981. On her retirement in 1987, Sister Josephine became the Mater archivist. MHHC

back into their hospitals, ran the risk of being confused with a growing phenomenon on the Australian hospital scene – private hospitals owned and managed by private companies which sought profits for their shareholders.

In 1980, jubilation at the opening of the Mater Private's new extensions masked these underlying financial worries. Sister Josephine Crawford succeeded Sister Mary St Gabriel as Sister Administrator in 1979. She was already very well known to the patients, nursing staff and doctors, having worked at both the Private Hospital and the Mater Mothers', and also had training through the Australian Institute of Management in her management arsenal. Reorganising the Mater Private and increasing its efficiency and cost-effectiveness were her first tasks as Sister Administrator. It was not easy. Many of the nursing staff resisted the changes, but Sister Josephine accepted this philosophically: 'I couldn't be worried about that because it was the hospital that was the big issue'.[12] The operating theatres were new and shiny, and bristling with the latest equipment, but other parts of the 1910 building were aging, and lagging behind the standards Sister Josephine wished to establish, and which many doctors demanded. Taking the hospital's quality to new levels and ensuring it never lapsed were her goals.

The first step was the appointment of a core group of advisors – Pat Maguire, Sister Angela Mary Johnson, a member of the congregational leadership team, and Margaret Ryan, the Congregation's bursar; an accountant, Brian Grace, was appointed administration officer. A management consultant recommended appropriate systems and processes. Work on a master plan for the hospital began in 1981. The advisory group concentrated on finance; a project control committee coordinated all aspects of the private hospital's rejuvenation.[13] Eliminating over-staffing and reorganising the hospital into six twenty-bed nursing units was an essential step. Lay registered nurses were appointed as charge sisters in each of the six nursing units. Much of the Mater Private's distinctive flavour and popularity with patients came from the high number of Sisters of Mercy on its staff. In lean times, with fewer Sisters available, this precious resource had to be stretched as far as possible. A Sister of Mercy was appointed to liaise with patients in each nursing unit. During 1981, the Mater Private's financial situation began to recover, but it still had to recognise competition from other private hospitals. A business-like attitude was essential.

The Mater Private pharmacy, established in the 1930s as a private retail service, was an important wing of the business. The pharmacy's profits were directed to congregational revenue; most were reinvested in the hospital. Because Queensland law required pharmacies to be owned by pharmacists, the private hospital pharmacy had been registered in the secular name of Sister Mercia Mary Higgins, at that time the Sisters' only qualified pharmacist. She was, therefore, the legal owner of the pharmacy, managed for many years by a local lay pharmacist. However, at the age of 81, Sister Mercia Mary was on the verge of retirement. Fortunately, by 1981 there were six pharmacists in the Congregation.[14] The pharmacy was established as an independent legal, financial, professional entity, owned and administered by the Sisters of Mercy.[15] The laundry was next to be examined. It was a very profitable enterprise. In the 1982–83 financial year, for example, the laundry's profit stood at $160,732.[16] Efficient systems introduced by a new manager, Brian Fennelly, and new machinery, such as a $350,000 batch control washer, reaped rewards – the laundry's income was $1,054,236 in the 1983–84 financial year and it had contracts to wash the linen for the Mater public hospitals, the Mater Private Hospital and the Holy Spirit Hospital.[17]

The development of new businesses was essential in modernising the Mater Private. The ever-increasing range of new medical technologies provided a valuable opportunity to catch up with Brisbane's more modern private hospitals. In August 1982, the Mater Private was the only Brisbane private hospital without an angiography unit, a matter emphasised by the radiologists, Doctors Robert Morgan and James Bolger, in their submission to install such a unit, and a CAT scanner, at the Private Hospital.[18] The nurses' dining room and Wards 1 and 2 on the ground floor provided appropriate space, but losing beds also meant losing income in tight financial times. However, the risk seemed worthwhile. More patients would be admitted because the new service was available as an intrinsic part of the hospital.[19] Space was leased to the radiologists, and the new service began in 1983.

Leasing valuable ward space to the radiology practice ended a service the Mater Private offered in the early 1980s. At that stage, the private section of the Mater Mothers' was overwhelmed with patients. The front wing on the third floor of the Mater Private was made available to private obstetric patients and their babies, a boost for both hospitals which used to advantage their co-location on the one site. The patients loved the large rooms, the verandahs, the views and the breezes, and the staff loved having mothers and babies in their midst. However, this space was needed for patients displaced by the construction of the radiology rooms. The experiment of housing overflow private patients from the Mater Mothers' at the Mater Private finished at the end of 1985.[20]

More business-like practices helped the Mater Private Hospital to turn the financial corner remarkably quickly. After years of trading losses, the hospital reached the break-even point at the end of the 1980–81 financial year, despite a substantial loss in the first half of that financial year.[21] The hospital was then able to budget for a daily average of eighty patients. However, even in 1982, the salary bill remained stubbornly high, and the new operating theatres were far from paying their way, losing $300,000 in a single year.[22] Overall, however, the position continued to improve. By 1983, a surplus of $308,568 was predicted which, with reserves, would provide a total surplus of $726,880. The Mater Private was back on track and, by 1985, bed-occupancy figures were generally ahead of budget estimates and it was at last free of debt.[23] The Mater Private had survived, when other private hospitals had closed.

In the mid-1980s, private hospitals comprised 21 per cent of Australia's health market. The Commonwealth's bed subsidy had risen from its original $16 to $40 in 1984–85, some 22 per cent of patient accommodation fees at the Mater Private. However, both the Commonwealth government and the state government scrutinised private hospitals very closely. Value for the taxpayer dollar was the keynote. The state government regulated private hospitals through the issue of licences and approving building works, and private hospital earnings were controlled through a Commonwealth categorisation process.

No one could relax in this highly regulated climate. Continual work was necessary to keep the old Mater Private building in working order. In 1982, the roof was leaking, more en suite bathrooms were badly needed, and the hospital still did not have an adequate isolation area. The roof alone cost almost $70,000; the total price for all the urgent renovations was $375,000.[24] With fifteen private hospitals in the Brisbane metropolitan area, competition was stiff and margins were always tight. Increases in nurses' salaries in 1982 were an added pressure, but the Mater Private was able to contain its fees at levels lower than Brisbane's other major private hospitals. In October 1983, the daily fee for a bed in a shared room was $118 at the Mater Private, between $120 and $130 at St Andrew's, $130 at the Wesley and between $130 and $140 at the Holy Spirit; fees for private rooms began at $135 at the Mater Private, whereas the lowest private room fee at St Andrew's was $150, at the Wesley, $155, and at the Holy Spirit, $160.

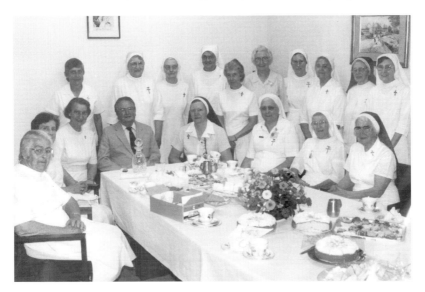

Dr Tony McSweeny was a highly valued visiting orthopaedic specialist at the Mater Private Hospital and was also a key member of its clinical and nursing practices committee. Dr McSweeny is pictured at his farewell on 4 December 1985 with, seated from left, Sister Mary Mechtilde Slattery, Mrs Anne McSweeny, Sister Bernard Mary Crawford, Sister Marie Therese Rosenberg, Sister Pascaline Mackey, Sister Gertrude Mary Lyons, Sister Alphonsus Mary Kennedy, and, standing from left, Sister Eileen Pollard, Sister Mary John Patch, Sister Ignace McLoughlin, Sister Mary St Maurice O'Brien, Sister Mary Michele Quinlan, Sister Mary St Gabriel Corbett, Sister Mary Emilia Crowe, Sister Mary Lorenzo Conroy, Sister Denise Lannigan and Sister Francesco O'Brien. MHHC

Even so, fees at the Mater Private had increased considerably since the 1981–82 financial year when ward bed fees were $96 and those for private rooms, $126.[25]

Quality assurance through formal accreditation was one means of ensuring that the Mater Private would remain in the top echelon of Brisbane's private hospitals. Many private hospitals were investigating formal accreditation, primarily to secure the highest classification in the Commonwealth's emerging system which paid a range of patient benefits according to a hospital's grading.[26] The movement towards hospital accreditation had a long history in Australia, promoted since the 1950s by the medical profession's enthusiasm for a system of accreditation for public acute-care general hospitals. While the Commonwealth adopted accreditation in the 1970s,[27] Queensland's public hospitals remained outside the accreditation process even in the 1980s – the government was determined that no outside body or interest group would look at its institutions. Queensland private hospitals generally trod the accreditation path before the public hospitals did so.[28]

The Mater Private Hospital took its first steps towards accreditation with the appointment of Sister Eileen Pollard to coordinate the complex process. Every nook and cranny of the hospital was meticulously scrutinised. An array of committees investigated and evaluated all aspects of patient care, the pharmacy, medical and nursing practices, medical records – essential to ensure good data and to prepare standards, policies and procedures – and operating theatre services. Surgery was a critical area and spawned several subcommittees covering such areas as infection control, environmental services, and safety and fire prevention. A register of visiting medical officers was established, and a committee comprising Doctors Tony McSweeny, Laurie Brunello, Harry Barry, Gavin Carroll and John McCaffery reviewed all applications for visiting rights. The nursing development task force offered active education programs in areas ranging from nursing management to the correct procedure for treatment of cardiac arrest. The administrative structure was clarified. The nursing superintendent, Sister Mary Michele Quinlan, and the Director of Administration, Brian Grace's successor, Gerry Wyvill, reported to the Sister Administrator who liaised with the visiting medical staff and reported to the Mater Board and thence to the Congregation's Hospital Council. At last all was ready for the accreditation team's visit in November 1983.[29] The Mater Private Hospital passed its critical test, with suggestions that it modernise the accounts system, and became one of only seven accredited private hospitals in Queensland. It had been a full team effort; every department from the nursing to the gardening had participated.[30]

Accreditation came just in time for the commencement of the new national insurance scheme, Medicare, on 1 February 1984. Medicare continued free hospital care, but aimed to shift a greater proportion of health resources from the private to the public sector. Private insurance membership started to fall during 1983 and 1984, in anticipation of Medicare's introduction. Nationally, the number of people with private hospital cover fell by 14.3 per cent between June 1983 and December 1986 and the proportion of private bed days fell by 13.4 per cent.[31] The Mater Private was placed in the highly sought-after Category 1, which received the highest subsidy. In return, the hospital was expected to maintain at least four intensive care beds, and to ensure that a doctor was in the hospital twenty-four hours a day. The Mater Private at least had the advantage of access to the Code Blue team from the Adult Hospital when cardiac emergencies occurred. Dire predictions that some private hospitals would not survive sent shudders through all private hospital administrations; all hospitals looked to their laurels.[32] On top of these pressures, the Mater Private knew that its accreditation review, due in 1986, would expect to find that services and accommodation had continued to be upgraded.

In 1984, the Mater Private again reviewed its facilities. Patient days were lower than predicted, reflecting a fall in the numbers of people subscribing to private health insurance, and expenditure per patient per day was higher, $244.97, compared with the budgeted figure, $180.33.[33] After a brief financial reprieve the hospital made a $69,895.84 loss in 1984, which not even the laundry's profits could make up. It was clear that the new private radiology practice had been a boon, but it now needed to expand. Discriminating patients were also tiring of four-bed wards, and the hospital looked for ways to create more single and two-bed rooms with en suite bathrooms.[34]

In mid-1984, the Mater Private was registered for 130 beds, but 150 beds would be an optimal number.[35] Other private hospitals were rapidly developing new specialist units and there was always the fear that, if the Mater Private did not continue to demonstrate an innovative approach, it risked its precious Category 1 classification.[36] An examination of the hospital's potential indicated five possibilities – vascular surgery, neurology and neurosurgery, radiology, day care for minor surgery, and cancer treatment.[37] There were some factors which could give the Mater Private an advantage. Cancer treatment could tap the benefit of co-location with public hospitals on a large campus, an advantage which no other private hospital in Brisbane possessed. The Mater's Queensland Radium Institute sub-centre was to be redeveloped with three new linear accelerators. Vascular surgery, which could share one investigative laboratory with neurosurgery, would benefit from significant demographic changes. Elderly people have the greatest need for vascular surgery and the older proportion of Australia's population was growing rapidly.

Neurosurgery, a strength at the Mater Private since the days of Dr Geoffrey Toakley, had not developed as a particular specialty at any other private hospital. The treatment of neurological conditions had benefited greatly from developments in scientific and technological medicine. The neurosurgeon Dr Michael Redmond thought that huge advances in brain tumour treatment had been largely unexplored in Australia, providing an important opportunity for the Mater to develop its care for patients with very serious and distressing illnesses.[38] Neurosurgery developed rapidly at the Mater Private: there were, for instance, thirty-eight neurosurgical operations in the first six months of 1985, compared with forty-four for the whole of 1984.[39]

Gastroenterology was another possibility because the Holy Spirit endoscopy unit was operating at peak capacity. Eye surgery was another. The unit at St Andrew's private hospital was operating at full stretch, and there was the opportunity to benefit from synergy with the progressive Mater Adult Hospital ophthalmology department. A more enlightened attitude at Queensland Health also helped the planning for future growth. In 1985, the Director-General, Dr Peter Livingstone, suggested that the private firm providing radiology services to the Mater Private could also develop radiology at the public Adult and Children's Hospitals. The Mater received this suggestion warmly, both for its convenience and as a way of further strengthening ties between the private hospital and the three public hospitals. Dr Livingstone also indicated that the restrictions on doctors maintaining consulting rooms in private hospitals would be modified to allow specialists this right.[40] Many Mater specialists already maintained consulting rooms in the privately owned Taylor Centre in Annerley Road opposite the Mater Children's Hospital, but the opportunity for consulting rooms in the centre of the Mater campus was obviously attractive to the specialists, and to the hospital. This type of development was particularly appropriate to the diagnostic specialties but, through the availability of specialists based at the hospital, was also likely to enhance neuro-surgery and vascular surgery. The Queensland government's adoption of the idea of co-locating private and public hospitals on a single campus, as was developing in New South Wales in the mid-1980s, was less exciting to the Mater, which had successfully maintained co-located hospitals for three-quarters of a century.

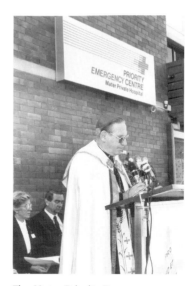

On the medical front, these possibilities were exciting, but a nagging doubt remained – could the existing private hospital support further development? Its design, size, and aging structure were considerable obstacles. An engineering report in 1984 revealed that, although the structure of the old building was still sound, the walls between the rooms, which provided crossways stabilisation of the structure, did not conform to current Brisbane City Council regulations. Care would also need to be taken to ensure that any proposed extension did not overload the foundations.[41] Closer examination of the existing hospital revealed more and more problems. The bathrooms were too small to allow nurses to use lifting aids; there was no piped oxygen or

The Mater Priority Emergency Centre was an important innovation at the original Private Hospital in the late 1980s. In this photograph the Centre is blessed by Bishop John Gerry in 1988 with Sister Michaeleen Mary Ahern, Administrator of the Mater Private Hospital, and the Premier of Queensland, the Hon. Mike Ahern, seated behind the Bishop. MHHC

suction in the ward areas; many doorways were too narrow to move beds directly to the operating theatres in accordance with modern surgical practice. There were some options for extending the building.

A new southern wing could be constructed to extend the hospital towards the public Adult and Children's Hospitals, but this would mean removing Loyola, the chaplain's residence, and this site had already been earmarked for the Children's Hospital. Another option, a northern extension, could mean replacing the complex of workshops which formed the engineer's department. This would be expensive and would also mean finding a suitably convenient site for a department which was always critically important to the hospital's operations. Dr Harry Barry suggested that the new Mater Private could be built on the site of the old Adult Hospital.[42] However, the old Adult Hospital building had already been earmarked for administrative functions.[43]

Several of the hospital's honorary medical staff took an adventurous view, favouring an entirely new hospital to be built where the convent stood joined to the hospital at all three levels. Building on the convent site would allow additional facilities for day care for patients after minor surgical procedures. This scheme could also allow the old Mater Private to become an aged care centre and a central support area for home care services. This convent option, was, perhaps, the most convenient but was likely to be the most difficult to achieve. The convent was the home of the Mater Sisters who had already had to face a diminished role in medical and administrative work at the Mater.

Proposals were further refined through meetings of all visiting medical specialists and investigations by Charles M Campbell and Associates, architects and health planners.[44] The Campbell report differed from the doctors' views, favouring a phased redevelopment of the hospital's existing site. This would take advantage of the treasured views and breezes, avoid the enormous cost of demolition and rebuilding, and conserve the Sisters' capital investment in the existing building. However, even this modified scheme included the construction of a new block to replace the kitchen and expansion into the convent.[45] A review of the Campbell studies suggested another option to avoid the problem of placing a new wing to face due west – never a desirable aspect in Brisbane – and, even worse, to look directly into the convent.[46] This review recommended a new block between the north-west section of the hospital and the northern wing of the convent to avoid significant difficulties in the existing hospital – the 1980 extension had cut off air flow to the rear of the 1910 building and had closed the rear verandahs, forcing all traffic through the central corridors. The existing ground floor could provide expanded diagnostic services east of the main entrance, a redeveloped west end would include a new kitchen, a staff canteen, stores, pharmacy, medical records and administration offices, with day surgery at the western end of the second floor, and general renovation and refurbishment throughout. Redevelopment was necessary to meet expected accreditation requirements for accommodation and services, but even this conservative solution would cost between $9,000,000 and $10,000,000, and would require some intrusion into the convent to provide essential additional beds.[47]

Although a new convent could be built on the hill below St Laurence's College, the original convent building was a very precious home to the Mater Sisters. It had direct access to the chapel, a convenience which might not be available if the convent were to be moved further to the west. Broaching the suggestion to the Sisters who lived at the convent was extremely difficult. As Sister Kath Burke, the Congregational Leader, remembered, 'the Sisters at the Convent were extremely nervous, it was an awful period for them – they feared that they might be chased out'. That was a terrible prospect for a very strong, close community who shared decades of dedication: many had given forty, fifty and sixty years of their lives to the Mater.[48] The position was made even more tense for Sister Kath and her assistant in the negotiations, Sister Madonna Josey, because there seemed no alternative to use at least part of the convent site. The congregational representatives held meetings at the convent where they were faced with implacable resistance. The planners, not the Sisters, were disappointed. The decision not to interfere with the convent could have come at huge cost. Sister Madonna even felt that 'it was almost a death note sounded for the Private Hospital'.[49]

The next possibility was a wing adjoining the new public Adult Hospital. The existing library was already scheduled for demolition.

This option would retain the open space in front of the original Private Hospital and allow better sharing of facilities with the Adult Hospital, repairing to some extent the physical separation between the hospitals, a phenomenon which some regarded as 'piecemeal development', made worse by a clutter of small, low-rise buildings.[50] A way out of the dilemma suddenly presented itself. Ridgewood Developments, a company which had provided land for Mater prize homes at Algester, told Pat Maguire it owned three blocks of land in Vulture Street on a hill facing the Mater, only a stone's throw away. Sister Angela Mary and Pat Maguire, convinced that an entirely new hospital was the only solution, immediately offered to buy the land.[51] Costs remained an issue. Developing an entirely new private hospital while the original one was still operating guaranteed an income stream, but there would be no government subsidy for capital works at the private hospital. The Sisters would need to use their own funds, and inevitably raise a large loan.[52]

Negotiations and reassessments of the position dragged on during 1987, the year Sister Josephine Crawford retired. The new Sister Administrator, Sister Michaeleen Mary Ahern, had no doubt that an entirely new hospital was necessary. Quite apart from structural and design problems at the old hospital, changes in health funding and insurance were expected to require private hospitals to provide a day surgery unit, and accident and emergency facilities available twenty-four hours a day.[53] Doctors also continued to press for consulting rooms close to the hospital, a real possibility if the Mater secured sufficient new land between the Vulture Street site and Stanley Street, opposite the main gate of the Mater campus.[54] Sister Michaeleen Mary, the Director of Nursing, Sister Mary Michele Quinlan, Pat Maguire and John McAuliffe, a member of the Board who advised the Sisters on property acquisitions, toured the potential site and negotiated many times with its owners and the Congregation.

Nineteen eighty-seven was a difficult year to contemplate such a large and risky new venture. Australia's health insurance system was still in a state of flux. The Commonwealth government withdrew its bed day subsidy paid to private patients from 1 October 1986. The focus was again on the private insurers. The private health insurance funds increased benefits under the 'basic table' to $184 for patients in a Category 1 hospital, $154 for a Category 2 hospital and $124 for a Category 3 hospital.[55] Retaining Category 1 status was clearly very important, particularly as there were substantial cost pressures from increases in nursing salaries. Although salaries were still far from luxurious, nursing staffs had long ceased to be the badly under-paid resource on which hospitals relied to keep their financial heads above water. A salary increase of 12.8 per cent in August 1987 forced increases in private hospital fees, no comfort at all to patients still leery about repeated changes in national health insurance.[56] Patient numbers at the Mater Private dropped dramatically in April and May 1987. Changes to the national Health Insurance Act in March 1987 generated fear, exacerbated by media publicity emphasising that private patients would have to meet an increased gap between hospital fees and insurance rebates. There was some strength in numbers. The Queensland Private Hospitals Association, which the Mater Private supported, negotiated with the private health funds to increase the benefits paid to patients.[57] The Mater Private adjusted its fees so that the gap between the hospital fee and the health fund rebate was between $15 and $25 per day.[58]

Long-term viability and ways of financing a large debt on a new hospital were key issues.[59] The Mater Private redevelopment committee, chaired by Kevin Cronin, chairman of the Mater Health Services Governing Board, met regularly during 1987 to consider submissions on the proposed new hospital. There were many of them. Doctors Clem Marrinan, Harry Barry and John Herron presented a detailed medical brief for a hospital of 200 beds, larger than the existing hospital's 130-bed capacity. Flexibility was to be the keynote, so that any reorganisation required by future medical innovations could be accomplished without undue disturbance. As well as the accepted emphasis on oncology, neurosurgery, vascular surgery, day surgery and diagnostic facilities, more general medical beds would be needed to care for an aging population. First-rate intensive care and coronary care units and a proper post-surgical recovery ward were also high priorities.

Plastic surgery, eye surgery, sports medicine and a women's health centre were also on the agenda. Because a separate unit for adolescent patients would require facilities to cope with infectious diseases and the psychiatric needs of drug-dependent patients, the doctors' submission recommended against adolescent medicine at the new private hospital.[60] An accident and emergency centre, which the orthopaedic surgeon Dr Robert Cooke was keen to establish, was a real possibility. This centre, he thought, could include an out-of-hours roster of general practitioners, an innovation already established at the Sunnybank Private Hospital. Other suggestions included private hospital accommodation for children, and a facility for AIDS patients. The emphasis would be on shorter stays in hospital. It was clear that the new health insurance system would not favour caring for long-term patients in a private hospital.[61]

For the Sisters, the decision to build a new hospital involved much more than planning its services and raising sufficient finance. These were the easy issues. Reconciling the provision of a splendid new hospital for the affluent with the Sisters of Mercy mission to the poor and needy was far more difficult. The position in 1987 was entirely different from the situation faced by the Sisters at the beginning of the century. In the 1980s, operating costs and most of the capital costs for the public Adult, Children's and Mothers' hospitals were supplied by the government. A private hospital to support a public hospital was no longer needed. Much of the burden of this decision lay with Sister Kath Burke, the Congregational Leader. At the end of 1987, she went to New Zealand to spend a month in isolation. There, she prayed and thought deeply. It was a long, tough, anguished tussle. Then, realisation came: 'this decision about whether we redevelop the Mater [Private] or not is peanuts compared with decisions that people had to make in the beginning when they had absolutely nothing' and, what was more, had to find supporters in a sectarian climate.[62] Many of the Sisters also recognised that poverty and need are not only matters of financial resources. Illness brings fear, grief, loneliness and many other deprivations which only the richest in spirit can withstand. On 21 January 1988, the Sisters took the momentous decision to build a new hospital in Vulture Street.[63]

The implications were huge. The land alone had cost $1,300,000, provided from fundraising profits. Hospital construction would cost

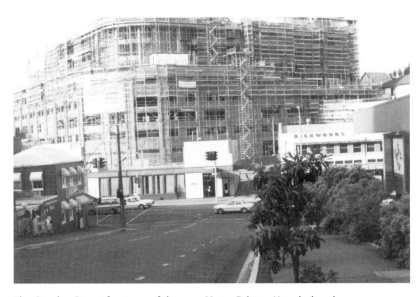

The Stanley Street frontage of the new Mater Private Hospital under construction. The little blue building at left was a favourite corner shop for Mater staff. MHHC

$35,000,000, a cost exceeding $250,000 per bed for a hospital of 130 beds. The faithful ANZ bank and the Archdiocesan Development Fund would both advance $10,000,000, but the Sisters would have to find the rest, and cope with interest on the loan at 12 per cent, the rate prevailing in 1988. This meant annual repayments of somewhere between $1,070,000 and $1,090,000 each year, making the position very tight – the existing operating surplus generated by the Private Hospital was $1,080,000. There were also other considerations. The Sisters were committed to new nurseries and other facilities at the Mater Mothers' at a cost of some $9,000,000, expenditure which was unavoidable to reverse the decline in private patients at the Mothers'.[64] It was essential, therefore, that the new Mater Private be a viable proposition. The management consultants Graham Wright and Associates recommended an emphasis on surgery – five operating theatres for a 130-bed hospital, with two additional theatres for day surgery. Fourteen private rooms in each thirty-bed ward were recommended to accommodate the trend in all private hospitals to single-bed rooms.

On top of these worries, some of the Sisters were far from happy with the decision and questioned the large amount of money to be spent on those who were not the most needy, at the expense of low-cost housing which would have to be demolished in order to make way for the new hospital. This was a pertinent issue. Old working-class suburbs in inner Brisbane were becoming 'gentrified' as wealthier people began to seek the convenience of residence close to the city, as they were in cities all over the world. Poorer people were finding it increasingly difficult to remain in their familiar neighbourhoods, and the Sisters could spend their surplus funds on more low-cost housing. There was also lingering concern that most pressure for the new hospital had come from doctors, who wanted 'the latest, the biggest and the best', a matter more of professional status than of patient care.[65]

In the late 1980s, however, medical specialists were in a position of considerable strength. Several private hospitals competed for eminent specialists, particularly those practising in the newer specialties.[66] Private hospital costs were also rising faster than the inflation rate and, in a declining private insurance market, health insurers were not at all keen to increase benefits to match costs. A financial feasibility study in 1988 revealed the gloomy news that the best the Sisters could expect would be a return on their investment of somewhere between 2.5 per cent and 8.7 per cent, depending on utilisation of the hospital and final costs. The whole project would have to be managed very carefully. Fortunately, the Sister Administrator of the private hospital, Sister Michaeleen Mary, soon revealed her talent for planning and project management. She was well aware that, if the new hospital stumbled, every one of the Sisters' works could be set back considerably.

The budget for the new hospital was $38,500,000.[67] The successful tender for construction, at $28,888,000, left some leeway for the construction of rooms for specialists, even after the cost of the land had been included. The medical centre with its forty suites was timed to open at the same time as the new hospital, to entice a wide cross-section of health practitioners to have a close association with a major private hospital. Senior nursing and design staff formed committees to plan the nursing units to ensure two major benefits – quality and efficiency. All patients were to have either city or mountain views, individual medicine cabinets, and bedside phones to communicate with the nursing staff. Nothing had been left to chance. The senior architect, Glynne Fletcher of the firm Peddle Thorp, had designed the Mater Adult Hospital as well as hospitals in the United Kingdom and the Middle East. He knew the language of clinical staff, and another architect, Tony Giammichele, was a registered nurse who had studied nursing to experience first-hand how a well-designed hospital really functioned, or should function. Regular newsletters kept the hospital community and its neighbours informed of progress. The building, constructed by Baulderstone Hornibrook, proceeded very quickly, and was 'topped out' in October 1991. Internal construction was completed in August 1992, and the hospital was handed over in that month, eight weeks ahead of schedule. It had been completed in seventy-eight weeks. The total cost had risen to $50,000,000, which included the cost of the medical suites and new carpark.

No matter how splendid the new building, its success would depend on the reputation of the existing Mater Private. Quality assurance programs continued; the Mater Private Hospital secured its third successive accreditation certificate in 1989. Bed-occupancy figures at about 66 per cent were reasonable, if not wonderful, in a climate of continuing uncertainty about private health insurance. Patient figures were actually better than they looked, because increased use of day surgery meant that many patients were not in the hospital at midnight, when governments insisted the day's figures were calculated. Admissions rose in the early 1990s, but more of the patients were acutely ill, requiring intensive, expensive nursing supervision. However, the

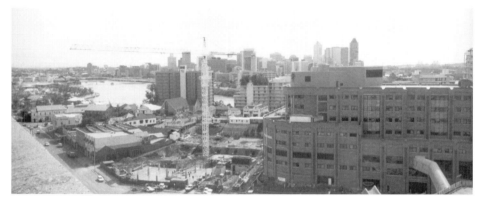

The site works for the new Mater specialist centre (on left) and rear of the new Mater Private Hospital (on right), with the Brisbane River in the background. MHHC

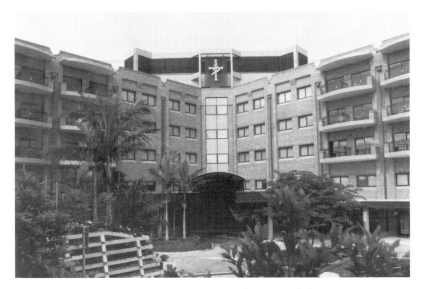

The Vulture Street entrance to the new Mater Private Hospital. MATER PUBLIC RELATIONS
AND MARKETING

busy hospital was finding it difficult to retain registered nurses, even
with its program of providing clinical experience to students from the
Australian Catholic University who, it was hoped, would choose the
Mater Private when they graduated. Nursing shortages were well and
truly affecting private, as well as public, hospitals.[68]

In this climate, new initiatives were very important in distinguishing one hospital from another. During the years the new building
was rising above Vulture Street, new services kept the hospital competitive. The Mater Private Priority Emergency Centre – the first in
any Queensland private hospital – opened on 15 September 1989.
The centre filled a growing gap in medical services. Fewer and fewer
general practitioners provided after-hours or weekend care; public
hospital emergency centres were overloaded.[69] The centre was also
an additional gateway to admission to the Mater Private. However,
the centre attracted many critics. The Consumers Association worried
that people could be taken to the centre in an unconscious state and
wake to find a big bill. The Brisbane Locum Service, an organisation
which provided an after-hours general practitioner service, sought a
Supreme Court injunction to prevent public advertisement of the centre on the grounds that the Medical Board of Queensland did not allow

doctors to advertise. Dr Robert Cooke, whose company managed the centre, was prosecuted by the Medical Board and found guilty of seven charges – four regarding advertising a medical practice and three of canvassing for patients.[70] The Medical Assessment Tribunal dismissed all charges, but the Medical Board appealed to the Supreme Court, where Dr Cooke's lawyers argued that the prosecution was unreasonable, in view of the Wesley Hospital openly advertising its breast clinic and St Andrew's its cardiology clinic. The Supreme Court found in favour of Dr Cooke.[71] This worrying incident was not the end of the troubles for the Mater Private's emergency centre. Dr Cooke's group moved the clinic to St Andrew's which was closer to the centre of the city and already had a large cardiac centre and nuclear medicine centres, as well as accommodation for 250 patients and a private children's ward.[72] The Mater Private did not give up and operated its emergency centre itself.

Laser surgery, in a special centre opened by the premier, Mike Ahern, on 15 March 1988 was another significant innovation.[73] Lasers were suited to delicate cutting as they reduced the blood loss, allowing more procedures to be conducted on a day surgery or outpatient basis. This was a coup for the Mater Private; doctors from all over Australia came to demonstrations of the new technology in ophthalmology, gynaecology, neurology and dermatology, as well as ear, nose and throat procedures. These were important years for the Mater Private to spread its wings. Allowing visiting orthopaedic surgeons to bring their students to examine patients in the Mater Private helped to include the private hospital in training schemes, assisting the Mater to maintain its place as a multiple hospital system.

Continuity between the original and new private hospitals was important. In fitting out the new building during 1992, this principle was kept in mind, so that while the latest in technology, such as a laminar flow operating theatre with Queensland's first Howarth Exflow unit, was installed, the ambience of the original Mater Private was recalled in the timber on the walls and in the furniture. Continuity in mission retained its primacy but, as the Congregational Leader, Sister Madonna Josey, said, articulating the Catholic hospital mission and maintaining this identity with confidence was a greater

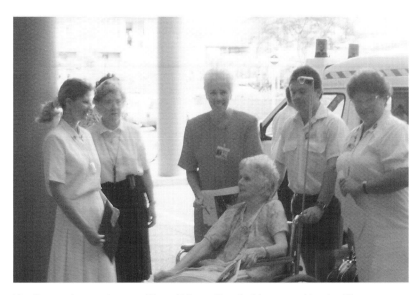

The first patient at the new Mater Private Hospital is greeted by the Sister Administrator, Sister Michaeleen Mary Ahern, second from left. MHHC

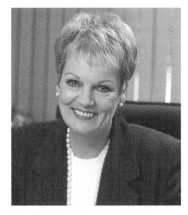

Mrs Pat Snowden, appointed Director of Nursing at the Mater Private Hospital in 1996. MATER PUBLIC RELATIONS AND MARKETING

challenge in a highly competitive society.[74] The spectacular 'Mater bronze', sculpted by Sister Gail O'Leary, was installed in the foyer of the new hospital to convey a simple message: 'This then is what Yahweh asks of you, to act justly, to love tenderly, and to walk humbly with your God'.[75] The new Mater Private was opened on 7 February 1993 and patients were transferred from the old hospital on 10 February. It was a spectacular achievement; at a time of economic recession, it was the largest building completed in Brisbane.

As far as the Mater public hospitals were concerned, the early 1990s reflected further changes in government hospital policy. After more than thirty years, government had passed from the conservative coalition to a Labor government with very firm ideas about the development of health services. New legislation, the *Health Services Act 1991*, introduced hospital regions to replace the 1920s concept of hospital districts. Regionalisation of many government services was a major early initiative of the

Goss Labor government which took office in December 1989. The Mater was placed in Brisbane South, one of thirteen health regions in Queensland. On the surface, things seemed little different. The government agreed that Mater staff would continue to be employed by the Sisters of Mercy and that the Mater's own standards and values could continue to be applied. Further, the Mater was the only public hospital in Queensland to retain its own board. However, the line of accountability changed. The Mater was to be accountable to its regional director for planning and finance, making direct access to senior levels in Queensland Health more difficult.

The effects of regionalisation and rationalisation were felt first at the Mater Children's Hospital. The Mater Board had already received the support of the Queensland Paediatric Society for its plans to redevelop the Children's Hospital. Changes to relieve pressure in key areas could be nothing more than temporary relief. A submission to the government for urgent funding for a brand new children's hospital, sweetened by the Sisters' offer to fund fifty-five new beds themselves, was under consideration when the government changed.[76] Regionalisation affected these plans as much as the change of government. The Paediatric Society was wary about the possible effects of the organisational changes on health services in Brisbane South. It preferred coordination of services by a central agency, rather than diffusion by *de facto* local health authorities. It was also concerned that absorption of the separate board of the Royal Children's Hospital into a regional authority would compromise that hospital's ability to provide the range of services planned for the future. At that stage, the Society felt that the Mater, with its separate board, had a better chance of retaining its ability to plan and deliver services to rapidly growing areas south of Brisbane.[77]

A bombshell in 1992 put all plans on hold. Sister Angela Mary had secured a place on the board of the Brisbane South Region which then horrified her by strongly recommending that the Mater consider moving the Mater Children's Hospital to the Queen Elizabeth II hospital seven kilometres away at Mt Gravatt, which had been under-used since the government opened a new public hospital slightly further south in Logan City. The Logan hospital was expected to develop into a major teaching hospital with 450 beds by 1993, incidentally putting pressure on the Mater Adult Hospital to clarify its role and the specialties it proposed to develop. If the Mater were to move to QEII, as the Queen Elizabeth II hospital was popularly known, the government could move the dental teaching hospital from Turbot Street in the city to the Mater. This proposition should not have come as a complete surprise. Ten years earlier, the then Health Minister, Mr Brian Austin, had suggested that the growing number of hospitals on the southside – the Mater, the Princess Alexandra, the QEII, and the Greenslopes Repatriation Hospital, which the Commonwealth was considering selling to the private sector – would duplicate services. He went further and asked, 'Should Brisbane have two Children's Hospitals or would it be better to have one with improved facilities?'.[78]

In May 1992, the Mater Board considered how best to deal with an unwelcome proposal without antagonising the government. It examined all options, beginning with the most basic question – did the Sisters want to continue in health care, or reallocate resources from health to another field?[79] Quite apart from financial uncertainties and the stress of dealing with governments and health funds, there were other risks, such as dealing with the public in an increasingly litigious climate. If the Sisters remained in health care, specifically child health, a site closer to population growth areas in the extreme south of the city might be the most convenient for patients and doctors. On the other hand, paediatric services on the existing campus could share facilities with the other hospitals. There was also the option of withdrawing from paediatrics to concentrate on adult health. However, the Mater Children's was a central part of the Mater's mission. Moving would split the Mater family and affect other Mater services, particularly the convenient link with the Mothers' hospital.

There were some advantages in the government proposal. The QEII hospital building was larger than the Mater Children's and fifty years younger. It had six operating theatres, modern accident and emergency and intensive care departments, a day surgery unit and excellent radiology facilities. A QEII paediatric centre could become a tertiary-level paediatric hospital providing highly specialised care to patients from all over the state and a major paediatric training centre, as well as providing primary and secondary services to its local community.

There was no doubt, however, that the government wanted to rationalise health care services in the Brisbane south region, bringing inpatient care as close as possible to where people lived. The possibility of replacing the Mater Children's with the dental hospital fitted the government's policy to shift resources from acute hospitals to community care. Rather than make an instinctive choice, the Mater Board agreed on a feasibility study of four options – redevelop at South Brisbane, move the Children's Hospital to QEII, build a stand-alone children's hospital next to the new Logan public hospital, or build a new hospital on a new site, yet to be determined.[80]

The study began in May 1992.[81] A steering committee formed for the study was chaired by Ross Dunning, deputy chairman of the Brisbane South Regional Health Authority. It was weighted in favour of the government, and included Peter Read, executive director of policy and planning in Queensland Health, and Dr John Golledge, regional director of the Brisbane South region. Grace Grace and John Van Leent represented the affected unions. Sister Angela Mary and Pat Maguire were the Mater's only representatives. The parameters of the study defined a southside children's hospital catchment area as south from the Brisbane River to the New South Wales border, west from Moreton Bay to the western border of the Darling Downs Health Region. In addition, a tertiary-care paediatric hospital would also serve patients from remote Queensland, the Northern Territory and northern New South Wales. This was a young area. In 1992, 41 per cent of all children in Queensland lived in the catchment area; growth to 44 per cent by 2001 was predicted. The child population, 276,983 in 1991, was expected to grow by 19 per cent to 329,595. The greatest increase was expected in former rural areas rapidly becoming Brisbane's dormitory suburbs – the Redland Shire, Logan City, Albert Shire and Moreton Shire. The expansion to the south-western area between Brisbane and Ipswich was expected to accelerate between 2001 and 2006. Large new suburbs such as Springfield and Forest Lake were emerging, and more were planned.

The majority of families with children, therefore, lived in suburbs between fifteen and forty kilometres from the inner urban area, where both Brisbane's children's hospitals were located. The Royal Children's Hospital was in a similar position relative to Brisbane's spreading northern suburbs. The first option, maintaining the existing Mater Children's Hospital site, would maintain economies of scale, but would be less convenient for people further to the south, and marginally less convenient to growing south-western areas. The QEII was some seven kilometres closer to the young population and could be a convenient location for community health services, but these advantages might not compensate for the need to relocate QEII's existing adult services to other hospitals, or address the possibility that visiting medical officers and the existing Mater Children's staff could resist the additional travel. Developing an entirely new hospital at the Logan hospital site, or on another site, would involve huge capital costs, and further dislocate paediatric and neonatal services. The cost equations were revealing. Redevelopment on the Mater site was estimated to cost $35,100,000 in capital expenditure, with an estimated operational cost of $40,400,000. The QEII option was estimated at $48,800,000 in capital costs and $43,200,000 in operational costs. Although at first glance, redevelopment on the existing site had financial advantages, a net present value analysis ranked the QEII option first, largely through questionable recurrent savings due to redeployment of staff.

The feasibility study defined the QEII option as a hospital with 125 beds for primary-, secondary- and tertiary-level care with outreach to the Logan and Redlands areas and to 25 secondary- level beds at the Mater site. The New Life Centre at the Mater Mothers' would remain the tertiary referral centre for neonatal patients, including neonatal surgery. The existing Mater Children's Hospital was a tertiary paediatric hospital with 139 beds in wards ranging from an original Nightingale ward to a new medical ward designed for contemporary treatment modes. However, outpatient consulting rooms were inadequate, space for multidisciplinary clinics was exhausted, and research funding was in short supply. Nevertheless, the Mater Children's staff included world authorities in areas such as sleep studies, growth and development and child protection. The Mater Children's had demonstrated its commitment to community paediatrics for years, and had appointed Australia's first Director of Ambulatory Paediatrics. It had pioneered day surgery for children in Australia and, in the early 1990s, more than 50 per cent of surgical patients were day admissions. These successes, however, only highlighted the existing hospital's inadequate space for outpatient clinics and multidisciplinary services. There was a huge and growing need for outpatient services all over the Brisbane south region, highlighting the need for coordinated regional services, particularly in mental health and child protection.

Wider consultation produced some interesting results: paediatricians and the ambulance service preferred redevelopment on the existing site; the unions feared that QEII staff would lose their jobs; people in the vicinity of the QEII hospital were concerned about the loss of convenient acute adult medical and surgical services. There was a trace of anachronistic bigotry in some responses from people who construed the possibility of the 'Mater Mt Gravatt' as a Catholic 'takeover' of a state hospital, an ironic reversal of the source of the proposal.[82] The Mater was not unaware of either the advantages of moving the hospital or the risks of insisting on retaining the Children's Hospital at South Brisbane. The risks of intransigence were many. First, the drift of young populations to the outer suburbs could threaten both the Mater Children's and the Mater Mothers' and, second, the regional health authority could develop a paediatric retrieval hospital at Mt Gravatt independently of the Mater, accompanied by strenuous efforts to make the Royal Children's Hospital the major paediatric hospital for the city, with the likely consequence that the Mater Children's would wither. If this possibility eventuated, it would be necessary to protect the Mater Mothers' New Life Centre as the desired neonatal surgical and referral centre for the region and beyond.[83] Clearly, if the Children's Hospital remained at Mater Hill, it would need new doctors in emerging sub-specialties who were also trained in research in order to reach the standard of Australia's leading children's hospitals.[84]

As part of the investigations, architect Glynne Fletcher was asked to estimate the cost of building a 150-bed children's hospital at Mater Hill. This study demonstrated that there would be significant savings in sharing equipment through retaining all the hospitals on the Mater site.[85] A study of paediatric services in south-east Queensland considered three options. Both children's hospitals could be consolidated into one; the two hospitals could be retained with the Mater Children's upgraded to 150 beds, with minimal development of paediatric services in outlying areas and beds; or there could be one tertiary-level hospital, the Royal Children's, with the Mater continuing as a secondary hospital servicing the Brisbane South region. By September 1992, the Mater's options had been reduced to two – relocation to QEII or redeveloping the Children's Hospital somewhere on the Mater site.[86] Finally, in February 1993, all the studies were complete, including Pat Maguire's concern that the costs of duplicating expensive services such as pathology and the therapies at QEII had been underestimated.[87] His concern was justified: quite apart from major repairs, the QEII needed complete rewiring.

Throughout the feasibility study process, relations between the Mater and the regional health authority had been strained. The Mater's curiosity about the genesis of the proposal, and its urgency, was not satisfied until years after the issue had been laid to rest. The Mater discovered that the government had insisted that the Region reduce its adult beds by 200, the number at QEII, without affecting the Mater Adult Hospital. The unions' concern made it clear that the proposal had been presented to them as emanating from the Mater. However, to the annoyance of the Region, Sister Angela Mary stated in no uncertain terms that the Mater had no desire to move the Children's Hospital, and that the proposal had arisen in the Region. Further, she said, the Mater Children's catered for low- and middle-income families who needed to use public transport, easily available to South Brisbane but almost unobtainable to QEII; and real economies from sharing central services with the other Mater public hospitals would be sacrificed by moving the Children's Hospital.

For a while there was silence from the government. Then in March 1993, Sister Angela Mary and Pat Maguire were invited to see the Minister, Ken Hayward, only to find that senior officers from Queensland Health and the Region were also present. The Minister asked when they would be ready to move the Mater Children's to QEII. Sister Angela Mary and Pat Maguire were astounded. Fortunately, the Board relied on the judgment of its representatives who immediately responded that the Mater Children's would not move.[88] A letter from the Minister arrived on 16 March which gave the Mater just two days to respond formally to the proposal that the Mater Children's be moved to QEII. The Board and the Sisters of Mercy responded immediately: the Mater Children's Hospital would stay at South Brisbane and, further, the state should support its redevelopment. The Mater family would remain intact and open its arms more broadly to the wider world.

CHAPTER TEN

INTEGRATING CARE

The strength of the Mater hospital remains in its special
ethos based on the care and dedication of staff in all
categories. This ethos will be a major strength in the
current atmosphere of change and economic stringency.

Dr James Griffin, 1991

Since the opening of the first Mater hospital in 1906, the Mater based
its distinctive ethos on the Sisters of Mercy's mission, values and philosophy of care. For at least seven decades, the Sisters' presence in
wards, departments and offices was a visible expression of the Mercy
mission in action. Mercy values were communicated implicitly in
interactions with staff and patients, and explicitly in ways as diverse
as nurse education programs and negotiations with governments. The
expression of Mercy values was essential not only in giving real meaning to the Sisters of Mercy's enormous investment in time, money and
property at the Mater but also in maintaining distinctiveness in an era
when developments in health policy could have integrated services
to the point where the Mater hospitals were indistinguishable from
any other.

The concept of 'integration' was expressed in several ways at the
Mater from the 1980s into the twenty-first century. The old notion of

the Mater hospitals as a family united by a distinctive culture had been affirmed with the inclusion of the Private Hospital in the administrative structure; the Mater had been integrated more closely with the state health system through increasing reliance on government, both voluntarily in accepting grants for capital works and operating expenses and involuntarily through the imposition of government funding and health policy regulation. Constant efforts were made throughout the 1990s and in the early years of the new century to emphasise the Mater's ethos and to strengthen its distinctiveness. Values and ethics were integrated in staff education, consciously re-stated in annual reports, and expressed in approaches to patient care.[1]

'Integration' had a slightly different meaning in Australian health policy. Since the 1970s, when particular specialties were assigned to certain general hospitals and not to others, health services were said to be 'integrated', rather than rationed. Many expensive scientific and technological services were 'integrated' in tertiary-care hospitals, serviced by feeder hospitals offering less complex primary or secondary care. Integration was an active influence inside hospitals, too. Care of individual patients was 'integrated' through the efforts of multidisciplinary teams; inpatient care became steadily more 'integrated' with care in the community. On the face of it, the idea that patients could be cared for in the comfort of their homes, surrounded by their familiar communities, seemed kinder than long spells in the colder, more routine-bound surroundings of hospital wards. Thus, while integration in this guise appeared positive, it could not hide the fact that more responsibility for their own recovery was thrust upon the patients as the health care dollar was spread more and more thinly. The move to reduce inpatient care and to expand day care and outpatient services was largely driven by government funding requirements. Nevertheless, integrating hospital and community care provided a golden opportunity for the Mater to reinforce its distinctiveness and to nurture its own ethos, while expanding its array of activities and penetrating more deeply into the Brisbane and south-east Queensland communities.

The development of cancer treatment at the Mater in the 1990s demonstrated the range of linkages which could be involved in an integrated health care service. With the incidence of cancer grow-ing rapidly in the Australian population, care of cancer patients was an obvious area for the Mater to develop. It had taken a leading role in the treatment of cancer since 1928, when it became Queensland's first cobalt treatment centre. The first deep X-ray machine did sterling service for almost twenty years.[2] The Queensland Radium Institute centre at the Mater attracted some remarkable staff who stayed for many years. Dr Eileen Harrison, for instance, was a radiotherapist for almost thirty years between 1949 and 1977. Until his retirement in 1994, Dr Robert 'Nobby' Bourne worked with the Queensland Radium Institute for thirty-seven years, twenty-eight of them at the Mater, where he had trained as a medical student in the 1950s. Dr Bourne was also a very active presence in the College of Radiologists. He served a term as chief examiner, was Rouse Fellow in 1979 and federal president in 1992–93. Nobby Bourne spread his wings over-seas as a consultant for the World Health Organisation in New Guinea in 1993. He was actively engaged in research, publishing numer-ous papers, and was appointed a University of Queensland clinical professor in 1992.[3] The Queensland Radium Institute expanded its centre at the Mater from two to four linear accelerators in 1993. It employed six full-time radiation oncologists and was able to broaden its services with, for example, a multidisciplinary breast clinic.[4] The integration movement had reached the Mater Radium Institute cen-tre and it was jointly administered with the Royal Brisbane Hospital centre.

The Mater's cancer services developed on several other fronts in the 1990s. Dr John Mackintosh was appointed the Mater's first full-time oncologist in 1991. Surgery and inpatient care remained important, but day care services, palliative care and research were increasingly emphasised. Day care and palliative care fitted well with the growing movement towards integrating inpatient services with care outside the hospital. Modern chemotherapy could be administered as a day care service. In 1991, the Queensland Cancer Fund contributed $225,000 towards funding a day care oncology centre for radiation therapy and chemotherapy.[5] The unit opened in the old Adult Hospital building in 1992. Cancer care at the Mater was coordinated by the collaborative cancer group. By 1995, the Mater was the only hospital system in Australia providing cancer services to adults and children as both public and private patients. The day care oncology service grew five-fold in its first four years.[6]

Supporting patients who could no longer be helped by active treatments was a very important aspect of compassionate comprehensive care. In 1991, the Commonwealth government allocated $1,500,000 over five years for the development of a pilot palliative care program at the Mater. As part of the National Demonstration Hospitals Project, which had continuity between hospital and community care as its focus, palliative care became an important dimension of the Mater's expanding hospital and community linkages. Special-purpose grants were always important in establishing new services, but securing permanent funding to continue them was a persistent strain. Only a funding reprieve in 1995 allowed palliative care to continue. Art and poetry projects were introduced as creative therapies to help patients through the emotional swings of cancer diagnosis and treatment.

Research was a very strong focus. The opening of the Francis Munnich laboratory at the Queensland Radium Institute in 1995 made bone marrow transplants, a very important treatment for intransigent leukaemia, possible at the Mater.[7] The Queensland cord blood bank, the third in Australia, was established in 1996 to build on the Mater's strength in cancer research and treatment. Once again, the co-location of hospitals on the Mater site added to efficiency – the close proximity of the Mater Mothers' assisted in the harvesting of cord blood, and simplified its transfer to the laboratory at the Adult Hospital where the vital stem cells were separated and stored. The cord blood bank was supported by Lions service clubs and Ronald McDonald House charities, a further development in the Mater's relationships with community organisations.[8] Collaborative projects between the Queensland Radium Institute and the Mater's haematologists developed in the mid-1990s.[9] Dr Robyn Rodwell and Dr Kerry Taylor published many important papers in haematology. By 2003, they were managing clinical trials of Glivec, which targets the molecular abnormality in chronic myeloid leukaemia cells, and in 2004 they were supervising bone marrow transplants as a day care service.[10] These developments also allowed Mater cancer care to reach outwards. Regular visiting services in oncology and haematology spread to Rockhampton in central Queensland. A ceremony in 1999 honoured the Sisters' service in developing cancer care with the blessing of a Celtic cross, inspired by a sixth-century cross in Cardonagh, Donegal, carved by Dr Bruce Kynaston, a former director of the Queensland Radium Institute.[11]

The multifaceted approach to treatment developed for the care of cancer patients was applied even more broadly to another disease becoming increasingly prevalent in modern Australia – diabetes. In the mid-1990s, the disease affected about one in twenty Australians, and in 1998, when Her Excellency Mary McAleese, President of Ireland, opened the Queensland Diabetes Centre at the Mater, the grim prognosis was a likelihood that this proportion would double by 2010.[12] About half the patients at Queensland's first multidisciplinary endocrinology investigation unit at the Mater Children's, which opened in December 1996, were diabetic.[13] The diabetic centre started work in 1997, with Dr David McIntyre as director. It was deliberately structured to care for adults, pregnant women and children and was the only diabetic unit in the state integrating the care of all three patient groups. In addition to medical services, the centre developed educational services, including a kitchen to help patients plan appropriate meals, and a variety of outreach programs, including a twenty-four hour telephone advice service which would, it was hoped, decrease patients' need to be admitted to hospital. Response was immediate; the centre treated 2,000 patients in its first six months. Particular needs were included, such as a special clinic for adolescent patients, and an eye clinic to identify and treat the eye conditions which frequently affect people with diabetes. The clinic coordinated its care with the patients' general practitioners, and developed training programs in endocrinology, as well as outreach programs in regional and country Queensland.[14]

The introduction of day care services across a number of areas helped to reduce average lengths of hospital stays from 7.5 days in 1970 to 4.2 days in 1993.[15] Day care was a significant weapon in the fight against escalating costs. In 1991, for instance, an inpatient cost $350 per day, in contrast to a day patient at $150 per day. The ability to treat more patients for the same total cost put considerable strain on essential areas. In 1981, when the new Adult Hospital opened, the pathology department put decades of cramming into small spaces behind it and moved into the almost unimaginable luxury of occupying the entire sixth floor. By 1991, only ten years later, the department was again feeling very crowded.[16] In the spirit of integrating health services, it was responsible for processing specimens for the QEII and Logan hospitals, as well as neuropathology for the whole of Queensland.

Automation helped to some extent in the final years of the century. The Lamson pneumatic delivery system brought samples automatically from the wards to the department; the addition of the Queensland-made Pathfinder machine enabled samples to be divided without human handling, and forwarded to different sections of the laboratories for testing.[17] Specimens also began to arrive by car from collection points in southern Brisbane suburbs when Mater Pathology opened its private practice in 1986. By the year 2000, pathology was a vastly different department from the one Dr John Bell had joined in 1969. As well as being director of pathology at the Mater, John Bell became a director of the Red Cross Blood Transfusion Service, a member of the executive of the Red Cross in Queensland, and a member of the state Council for Maternal and Neonatal Morbidity and Mortality and belonged to the state branch of the College of Pathologists. In recognition of his own research and the work he fostered, Dr Bell became a professor at the University of Queensland in 1994.

The rapid increase in day surgery produced an enormous histology workload for the pathologists and a great deal of diagnostic work for the radiologists. As well as studies of numerous parts of the human body by X-ray, ultrasound, CAT scanning, mammography and echocardiography, the modern radiology department also conducts treatments such as correction of mechanical disorders of fallopian tubes. Dr John Masel, director of radiology for almost twenty years until his retirement in 1996, oversaw the department's move to a central position in the new Adult Hospital close to the accident and emergency section, the outpatient department and the operating theatres. However, like Pathology, it soon found this space, which seemed huge in comparison with its old quarters, too small. In some respects, the integration concept was reversed when paediatric radiology separated from the main department in 1996.[18]

The pharmacy was becoming increasingly busy but still operating on its traditionally frugal lines when Bob Marshall became chief pharmacist in 1993. Many changes were necessary to prepare the department for the twenty-first century. Drug therapies of many kinds, and new drug delivery systems, became even more important in innovative modern treatment. The Mater was a challenging environment for professional pharmacists. Most drugs were mass-produced only in adult dosages, so Mater pharmacists needed to produce medications in dosages suitable for tiny babies and children. Sister Marie Therese Rosenberg and Joy Bostock introduced ward pharmacists in the 1960s, an important Mater innovation; by the 1990s, pharmacists were core members of interdisciplinary teams in the wards where patient-controlled analgesia delivery systems were introduced, even in the Mater Children's.[19] Linking inpatient care to care in the community became a significant area of the pharmacy's work. Reviews of patient medication were conducted in patients' own homes when general practitioners requested them, and, with funding from the

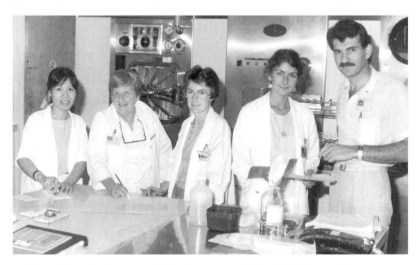

Staff members of the Mater Public pharmacy with the chief pharmacist Joy Bostock (second from left): from left, Phuoc Pham, Karen Bristowe, Smaranda Clintoc and Chris Stephens. Joy Bostock was an enthusiastic supporter of fundraising to improve staff amenities and swam 1,000 lengths of the swimming pool in aid of the funds. MHHC

Commonwealth government, the Mater pharmacy's practice grew to include medication reviews in nursing homes. In 1995, the pharmacy launched the Queensland Medication Helpline. Managed by Geraldine Moses, it was Australia's first public 'call-in' centre to answer public queries about medications. The Helpline grew to include a national service for the public, as well as a service for the health professions to report adverse drug reactions.[20]

The development of specialties at the Adult Hospital was reflected in the hospital's structure in the 1990s. Oncology became a separate division, and was one of three divisions alongside the more traditional divisions of medicine and surgery. Surgery, particularly, felt the pinch of government funding policies predicated on the expectation that hospitals could somehow deliver more services with fewer resources. Throughout the 1980s and 1990s, waiting lists in public hospitals, particularly for elective surgery, were a continuing cause of irritation in the community, and a source of anxiety for hospital administrators. The Mater's efforts to reduce waiting lists were considerably assisted by the day surgery program which began in 1988, freeing inpatient beds for new surgical patients. Development of new day surgery orthopaedic and gynaecological procedures also helped to ensure that 50 per cent of all surgery was performed as day surgery by 1996, a factor which also helped to bring the Mater's surgical infection rates below the national average.[21] Even so, tight budgets lengthened waiting lists for more complicated elective surgery. Shortages of nurses and specialists, particularly anaesthetists, added to the frustration. The medical superintendent of the Adult Hospital, Dr John Waller, told the Board in 1995 that patients brought to the hospital by ambulance were sometimes moved to other hospitals after assessment, a situation deeply offensive to the Mater's emphasis on comprehensive care for every patient presenting to the hospitals.[22]

Patients who once would have spent several days as inpatients were considered ready for discharge in much shorter times. However, most needed support when they returned to their homes. Discharge planning became an important wing of modern acute hospital care. In 1995, the Commonwealth appointed the Mater as a lead hospital for discharge planning, to assist five other Australian hospitals perfecting their systems.[23] The Mater model was underpinned by a continuum of care philosophy which ensured that patients were monitored after discharge, and was also a vehicle to demonstrate Mercy values in action. By the mid-1990s, the national centre for care management had been established at the Mater and the hospital was involved in international collaboration on discharge planning. The Domiciliary Allied Acute Care and Rehabilitation Team (DAART) became a mainstream district service linked to the Mater. The era of increased integration between hospital and community care put increasing emphasis on the role of general practitioners and primary health care, a necessary step in the development of health promotion strategies aimed at reducing the incidence of serious illness. In 1993, the Sisters of Mercy subsidised a general practice and primary health care division, with equal funding from the Commonwealth, and by 1994 the Brisbane South general practitioner clinic had opened at the Mater.[24]

The multidisciplinary clinics that developed at the Mater Children's Hospital in the 1970s and 1980s had already established a path for integrating inpatient services with various forms of community

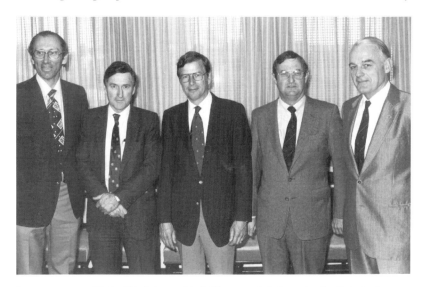

For many years, Mater Week brought visiting specialists and scientists to the Mater for lectures, seminars and discussions. This photograph shows Mater surgeons, from left, Dr C Elmes, Dr Mervyn Neely, Professor Keith Kelly, 1985 Visiting Professor to the University of Queensland, Dr Michael O'Rourke, and Dr J Herron. MHHC

care. However, it was clear that neither of Brisbane's aging children's hospitals could hope to accommodate all the new specialties within paediatrics. Greater coordination with the Royal Children's Hospital was inevitable in the 1990s.[25] Specialist clinics helped to reduce the need to keep children in hospital as inpatients. The ambulatory services building, named for Mother Patrick Potter, became a focus of developments in the 1990s. Day care services of all kinds expanded rapidly from their introduction in 1992; more than 1,000 children were treated as day patients in the first year alone.[26] In 1994, the babies' ward moved into a new area in the Potter building which also provided rooming-in space for parents. The former babies' ward in the main building was made available for an expansion of paediatric respiratory medicine, an area which benefited greatly from large grants – $500,000 to each children's hospital annually for five years – from that mainstay of Queensland's public hospitals, the Golden Casket lottery.[27] Professor Brian Hills' respiratory medicine laboratory, which also included the study of sudden infant death syndrome, was renamed the Golden Casket laboratory. Professor Hills, a physiologist who had graduated in chemistry and engineering before studying physiology, was a world authority on surfactant, or 'surface active agent', which helped to improve lung function, particularly in babies born with immature lungs.

By the mid-1990s, respiratory medicine, nephrology, psychology and paediatric endocrinology were significant specialist areas. In 1999, Dr John Burke established the Queensland centre for paediatric renal transplants; the establishment of the cord blood bank and the introduction of bone marrow transplants put the spotlight on the treatment of leukaemia and other childhood malignancies. Dr Ram Suppiah was the first full-time oncologist in a unit which emphasised family care. He hoped to increase the proportion of patients who could be treated at home by a multidisciplinary team. Community partnerships were essential in pursuing this goal. In 1999, the Home Care Program for children with cancer was introduced, with funding from the Leukaemia Foundation, Kids with Cancer and the telecommunications company One.Tel. Coordinated cancer care ensured that each young patient had a case manager.[28] Families of children who did not survive serious illnesses and accidents were not forgotten. The University of Queensland Child Health Department at the Mater developed 'An ache in their hearts', the world's first comprehensive intervention program for parental grief.

The Mater Children's Hospital's role as a tertiary referral hospital put great pressure on all its services. Many cases treated in the emergency department, the busiest paediatric emergency service in Queensland, were the result of accidents. The Queensland Injury Surveillance Unit started work in 1987 and within a few years was collecting data from many hospitals outside Brisbane. Falls, road accidents and drownings headed the list of child accidents studied in the unit under the direction of Dr Rob Pitt.[29] The unit's successful advocacy for compulsory fencing around swimming pools was a major factor in halving the tragic incidence of child drownings.

Psychological services were also increasingly needed. Waiting lists lengthened for appointments with the psychologists when resources in the community became more limited.[30] Increases in the number of psychology positions during the 1990s were made possible by grants from various agencies, enabling the hospital to treat young people up to the age of 18 and, in 1999, to establish a project to manage withdrawal from dependence on alcohol in a special five-bed unit.

A Commonwealth Medicare Incentive Package provided funding to continue the rehabilitation and neuromuscular diseases clinic.[31] Cochlear implants, which revolutionised life for deaf people, available at the Adult Hospital since 1988, were introduced at the Children's Hospital in 1994, and expanded into an outreach program to rural Queensland in 2003. Developmental paediatrics, still with Dr Michael O'Callaghan at the helm, became an increasingly important area with a larger staff. An Autistic Spectrum Disorders Clinic, the first in Queensland, was opened in 1996. Cranio-facial surgery was a different form of multidisciplinary care. Several different surgical specialties could be involved in any one operation, which could last for more than twelve hours. Many operations were life-saving; all saved children from the risk that their disfigurement could cause others to reject them. In 1989, one of the earliest patients, Robert Hoge, by then a Year 12 student and a prefect at his school, visited the Mater where, as a four-year-old in 1977, he had undergone complex surgery to repair his face after a large congenital tumour was removed.[32]

For children treated as inpatients, the hospital was livelier and more cheerful than ever before. Young people from the Church of Jesus Christ of Latterday Saints brightened the foyer with colourful paintings, and entertainment was brought into the modern era. The children became active participants in entertainment programs in 1990, when the radio industry funded a Radio Lollipop studio. Radio Lollipop began in the Queen Mary's Children's hospital in Britain and by 1990 there were five studios in the United Kingdom, and one other Australian station in Perth. The Mater's redoubtable maintenance staff constructed the station, and the staff interviewed 200 applicants to find the eighty volunteers needed to run it. By the end of the 1990s, the Mater's Radio Lollipop station was managing a satellite station at the Logan Hospital. In 1999, the Mater Children's scored another first when Dr Wendy Moody, then the only Australian to hold a doctorate in human and animal relationships, introduced the Pet Assisted Therapy Scheme, PATS, with Honey, a friendly German Shepherd, brought to the hospital by her owner, Jean Cowley.[33]

These were by no means the only innovations in paediatric care. The idea of a Mater Children's private hospital, first mooted in 1977, became a reality in 1998 when the Mater opened the first dedicated private children's hospital in Australia.[34] A feasibility study had found that a private children's hospital, managed on the same lines as the Mater Mothers' private, was likely to recoup the initial investment within three years, even though there was considerable concern in the mid-1990s that fewer people were subscribing to private health insurance.[35] The establishment of the new private hospital was an appropriate use of level 4, the remaining floor in the Mother Patrick Potter building.[36] Only three floors of the six-storey building had been opened in 1986, accommodating adults' and childrens' ear, nose and throat clinics and the ophthalmology outpatient department. A medical ward was relocated to the fifth level in 1991, and the babies' ward to level 6 in 1998. The new 25-bed hospital, the third Mater private hospital, was bright and cheerful, based on a seaside theme, complete with playrooms. Each patient's room had its own computer with

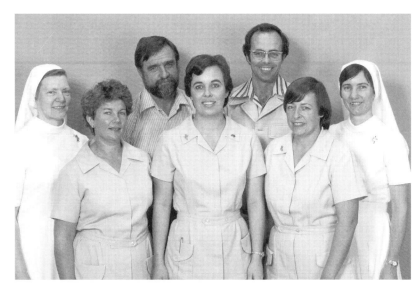

Mater volunteers who worked with the Red Cross in Kampuchea from November 1979 to March 1980: from left, Sister Marie Therese Rosenberg (chief pharmacist), Ms D O'Neill (paediatric nurse), Mr J O'Brien (radiographer), Miss M McCarthy (paediatric nurse), Dr David Wood (paediatrician), Mrs V Devine (Nursing Supervisor) and Sister Patricia Kirchner (Principal Nurse Educator).
MATER PUBLIC RELATIONS AND MARKETING

internet access. Parents were included, with their own advisory panel, a lounge, and double beds for overnight stays near their children.[37]

Outreach programs were a natural extension of the Mater Children's growing integration of inpatient and community care. As well as local programs as diverse as the investigation of the possibility of a Chair in Community Paediatrics, a positive parenting column in Quest community newspapers and continued involvement in Camp Quality for cancer patients and camps for diabetic patients, the Children's Hospital spread its wings overseas. Between 1969 and 1979, volunteers from the Children's and the other Mater hospitals served with the International Red Cross in Kampuchea, and, in 1989, Mater Children's nurses celebrated the third exchange with Toronto Hospital for Sick Children.[38] The sister-hospital relationship with Zhejiang cancer hospital in China continued, and plastic surgeon Dr Richard Lewandowski established the Operation Smile partnership for third-world children with facial deformities, with surgeons giving their services as volunteers.

The cranio-facial clinic, one of only two in Australia during the 1990s, demonstrated growing interdependence between local and overseas programs and between the hospital and community organisations. Lion's clubs and Rotary clubs assisted in bringing children to the Mater.[39] The unit developed its own group of fundraising friends, led by Mrs Alayne McDougall, Mrs Geraldine Anderson and Mrs Jan Seymour. The Wu family from Taiwan were very generous supporters in bringing children from the Philippines and New Guinea for treatment. All the children suffered from distressing conditions; some operations were Australian firsts. In 1997, a little girl underwent the first operation of its kind in Australia for agenia, a condition where her teeth were piled on top of each other preventing her from opening her mouth fully.[40] Planning an expedition to India early in 2005 involved organising treatment for 150 children and developing training programs for local doctors and nurses.[41] In 1993, Project Nadezha, meaning 'hope' in Russian, began when Alina Chuhhynova was brought from Russia to the Mater Children's for treatment for her progressive neuromuscular condition. Vera Derestov from Brisbane's Russian community sponsored her. This initiative developed into a program funded by the Russian community for Russian doctors and therapists to come to the Mater for training and for Mater doctors to treat patients in Russia. In 1998, the project was formalised by a signed agreement with the Russian Health Ministry.

Integrated services and outreach programs were also developed at the Mater Mothers' where economic stringency in the 1990s was felt particularly acutely. By the early 1990s, 145,000 babies had been born at the Mater Mothers', a tertiary referral hospital like the Mater Children's. In the early 1990s, almost 14 per cent of babies were admitted to the neonatal intensive care unit.[42] The special-care nurseries were always crowded. Under these conditions, Queensland Health's reluctance to fund an adequate nursing establishment added to the stress. In 1990, senior staff, including the Director of Nursing, Sister Jill Stringer, RSM, made presentations to the Board, convincing it to explain to the Health Minister that the Mothers' Hospital might not be able to continue to provide appropriate and safe care if its staff establishment was not increased. Headlines in the *Sunday Sun* publicised the difficulties. The government agreed to increase the nursing establishment, but there was a sting in the tail – if, in future, the Mothers' could not cope safely with demand on its resources, serious consideration would have to be given to the transfer of patients to the Royal Women's.[43] The government insisted that the Mothers' develop a plan to reduce admissions. However, even with a fruitful relationship with the Royal Women's Hospital, overcrowding persisted.[44]

A major extension offered some relief, and allowed the Mothers' to modernise its services. The New Life Centre, opened on 14 April 1991, provided new operating theatres, labour wards, a birthing centre where patients could be attended by midwives, and new special-care nurseries. The government provided $5,000,000 for the new wing. Mater fundraising covered the remaining costs, including a new chapel where people who had played an important part in the development of the Mater Mothers' were commemorated. The Stations of the Cross, for instance, were a memorial to John Ohlrich, who supervised fundraising to pay for the hospital.[45]

The number of Mater births continued to rise in the early 1990s and included sets of quintuplets in 1991 and 1992 and ten sets of triplets and 114 sets of twins in 1993. The resilience of tiny babies continued to amaze the staff. A set of twins born at twenty-four weeks gestation survived; Matthew Bird, born at twenty-three weeks, spent 113 days in the intensive care nursery. The challenge was not only to ensure that the latest developments in neonatal medicine were incorporated into the Mater regime – it was the only Australian unit accredited for the full three years of specialist training – but also to try to identify babies at risk as early as possible. In 1995, the appointment of Dr Fung Yee Chan, Queensland's first registered specialist in maternal fetal medicine, was a major step.[46] The Mater Trust was an essential supporter of fetal medicine and by 1996 was providing $500,000 each year to develop the service; this included a telemedicine connection to Kirwan Women's Hospital in Townsville in 1998.

Community services, carefully integrated with the Mater Mothers' overall philosophy of care, became an increasingly significant area in the 1990s. The Commonwealth's Alternative Birthing Services Program funded a community midwifery care pilot scheme to provide antenatal care in a woman's own home. This program relied on the Mater's staff midwives and the patient's general practitioner. The community midwifery scheme was cost-effective and also helped ease the load on the hospital. However, a trial to allow a private midwifery practice to use the hospital had to be abandoned in 1993, a victim of the growing problem of medical indemnity insurance which particularly bedevilled obstetrics during the 1990s.[47] It was not long before the Mater Mothers' became the first Queensland maternity hospital with an early-discharge program, necessary to address the persistently high demand for beds.[48] The budget crisis reached its height in 1995, when the hospital was in danger of recording a $4.7 million budget deficit. Sixteen beds were closed.[49] However, lean budgets did not prevent the development of a more comprehensive women's health centre based at the Mater Mothers' Hospital, integrated with a related 32-bed gynaecological ward in the Adult Hospital.[50]

Jenny Skinner, with degrees in nursing administration and public sector health management, was appointed executive director to manage the demands of the growing hospital and the range of new services which supported its patients.[51] A young parents group and a playgroup for former premature baby patients were established, and there was a special project to help mothers of very low-birthweight infants to breastfeed. Outreach services were very important. Midwives visited a clinic in nearby Peel Street to help drug-dependent mothers, and in 1999 Mater Mothers' staff were part of an exchange scheme with Di Kariadi Hospital at Semerang, Indonesia, and supplied fetal heart monitors to Bougainville.

Some very familiar figures left the Mater Mothers' in the mid-1990s. Sister Jill Stringer, RSM, retired after twenty hectic years as Director of Nursing, and Sister Margaret Kanowski, RSM, a member of the original 1961 staff, retired after forty-five years. To everyone's regret, Dr Aldo Vacca resigned as director of obstetrics. He had been the only staff obstetrician for several years in the 1980s, when demand for his services grew rapidly; he had been on call at all hours of the day and night. In 1995, Dr James King, who had established many important services, including maternal fetal medicine, resigned as medical superintendent to establish Queensland's first perinatal epidemiology

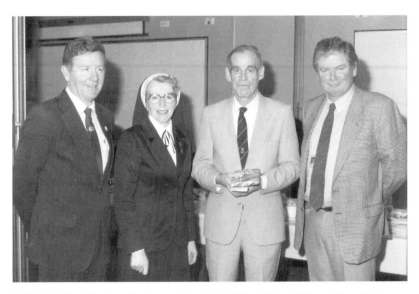

Dr Edwin Esler, first medical superintendent of the Mater Mothers' Hospital, second from right, on his retirement in 1986 with Mr Pat Maguire, Sister Angela Mary Doyle and Dr Esler's successor, Dr James King. MHHC

centre and to manage the secretariat for the Queensland Council of Obstetric and Paediatric Morbidity and Mortality.

All the developments in the rapidly changing 1990s – burgeoning specialist clinics, care for patients in the era of early discharges, closer relationships with community services – required close attention to administration and support services. However, continuing shortages in nursing and medical staff were a serious challenge to the modern Mater. The need to rely more and more on nurses supplied by agencies to supplement its own staff went against the grain at the Mater with its emphasis on its own value systems and philosophy of care. Agency nurses were expensive and needed a great deal of support, particularly when they first started work.[52] Nurses in all Queensland hospitals were well aware that the growing emphasis on hospital management had increased career opportunities for nurses in the administrative stream, while nurses who remained at the bedside reached a ceiling at the level of ward charge nurse.

In 1991, a new career structure was introduced in Queensland to address this situation and, hopefully, to halt the steady march of experienced registered nurses out of the hospitals. 'Job redesign' opened career paths in four streams: clinical nursing, nurse educa-tion, research and management. The new structure created a five-level hierarchy from Director of Nursing at level 5 to registered nurse at level 1, completely changing nursing services. New positions, clinical nurse consultants, managers and clinical nurses at levels 4 to 2 were advertised. In-service education was very important in easing the new structure into the hospitals. Assistant Directors for Nursing for edu-cation were appointed to each of the Mater public hospitals – Sister Patricia Kirchner, RSM, Irene Howgego and Marina Noud. In 1993, nursing at the Mater reverted to its earlier decentralised model; each hospital was free to employ its own nurses to match its needs.[53]

A new 'stream', nursing research, was the only centralised service, supported to some extent by external funding. Grace Croft, with a doctorate in nursing and wide experience in nursing and nurse educa-tion in the United States, was appointed to the position of Assistant Director of Nursing – Research, and a nurse researcher was appointed to each of the Mater public hospitals. The Nursing Research Cen-tre, established in the casualty section at the original Adult Hospital, supported staff undertaking research and further study and, more importantly, involved nurses in projects addressing clinical practice issues in each of the hospitals. In 1997, the Mater's Nursing Research Centre became the Queensland centre for the Joanna Briggs Insti-tute, which advocated research-based knowledge to inform nursing practice, a model established in medicine some years earlier. Mater nurses participated with nurses from other hospitals and staff from the universities in evaluating research to inform nursing care, and were acknowledged in publications of the Joanna Briggs Institute. Using research evidence to improve outcomes for patients became embed-ded at the Mater, as it was internationally.[54]

The introduction of the new career structure coincided with extremely busy times in all the hospitals and was made even more difficult in the prevailing climate of stalled hospital funding by Queens-land Health's requirement that the Mater reduce its nursing staff. This requirement, and the introduction of a 38-hour week for the nursing staff, made the whole process of job re-design and restructuring partic-ularly traumatic. By the end of the 1990s, when the new structure had overcome the worst of its teething problems, Karleen O'Reilly retired as Director of Nursing at the Adult Hospital, a position she had held since 1986.[55] She had overseen many changes since being appointed Principal Nurse Educator in 1977. The new Director of Nursing, Irene Lake, came from Victoria where she had commissioned the new Northern Hospital and worked as chief nursing officer and director of specialist medical services.[56]

The multitude of services put an enormous emphasis on education in all areas across the Mater campus, from clinical pastoral education, which ran its first eleven-week course at the Mater in 1989, to education for hospital administrators, to postgraduate medical and nursing courses. The University of Queensland maintained departments of Child Health, Medicine, Obstetrics and Gynaecology, Radiology and Surgery at the Mater. The university introduced a new system in 1990, requiring all medical students to complete all units of their clinical training at the same hospital. Most hospitals welcomed this development, hoping it would encourage young graduates to stay for postgraduate training. In the early 1990s, the Mater was still relying on overseas recruitment to fill its medical staff establishment, and in 1995 ran a pilot program to find ways of attracting young specialists to make their careers in hospital service, rather than leave to enter private practice.[57] Dr John Cope, director of postgraduate medical education at the Adult Hospital, had established a centralised continuing medical education centre in May 1990, which helped to increase the number of registrars who passed their specialist examinations. Education and the development of specialties were boosted by the introduction of joint appointments with the University of Queensland. Several senior doctors, such as Dr Bell in Pathology, Dr Bourne at the Queensland Radium Institute, Dr Vacca in obstetrics, Dr Tudehope in neonatology and Dr Fung Yee Chan in maternal fetal medicine became clinical professors. Medical education also had an outreach dimension; the paediatric registrar rotation program, for example, was extended to Toowoomba in 1992.

Education was extremely important in ensuring that staff in all clinical areas, ancillary medicine departments and administration had access to appropriate professional development. Management and leadership courses were developed, and in 1994 the Sister Angela Mary Doyle Scholarship Fund was established to enable Mater staff to study spirituality or philosophy. Education at the Mater was growing so rapidly that it needed to be properly coordinated. In 1998, the Mater Education Centre was established to foster an integrated multidisciplinary approach, with the educator Dr Neil Carrington as its first director. This, it was hoped, would create an educational environment supportive of staff development, inservice training and initiatives in continuing education, as well as a productive environment for research.[58] By 2004, the Education Centre had held national conferences on leadership in health education, and on leadership to generate high performance.[59]

Educational initiatives were more than a means of encouraging skilled staff to stay at the Mater; they also demonstrated that Mater care extended to staff as well as patients. The Mater's staff could have populated a small town. In 1996, 3,800 staff were required to run the Mater hospitals, caring for the multitudinous needs of 60,000 inpatients and 350,000 outpatients. In the 1990s, a series of awards was designed to show the Mater's appreciation of the staff. In 1991, for instance, 500 people, almost 20 per cent of the staff, were awarded badges recognising ten years' service. The long-service awards, originally the idea of a wardsman, Richard Bucknall, revealed that many Mater staff had stayed a great deal longer than ten years. In 1994, Helen O'Brien was recognised for her forty-four years at the Mater. Ms O'Brien started work as a cadet in the laboratory and did not retire from the Pathology Department until 1997. Clinical and research staff were frequently recognised internally and externally for excellence in their fields, but in the 1990s such recognition spread more broadly. Lyndell Cotton of the palliative care unit was the Queensland Cancer Fund nurse of the year in 1994, Dr Jenny Brown, director of obstetrics and director of planning, was the Queensland Business Woman of the Year in 1995, and in 1999 the Women's Network Australia named Dr Fung Yee Chan its executive woman of the year in science and medicine.[60]

Staff retirements also highlighted decades of experience at the Mater. Pat Maguire retired as chief executive officer in 1993, after almost twenty-five years at the Mater; Dr Laurie Parker retired in 1991 after thirty-eight years as an ear, nose and throat, visiting medical officer; Dr Bill Everingham retired after twenty-seven years as a visiting plastic surgeon; Dr Elsie Harwood, the neuropsychologist who had developed the Children's Hospital's work in trauma care, retired after twenty-eight years; Mrs Pat Neely retired after twenty-one years in social work; the former general practitioner Dr Paul FitzGerald resigned after supervising the emergency department for eighteen years; and in 1996 Rex Ducat retired as Executive Director, Nursing Services after twenty years at the Mater. Dr John Waller, AM, medical director of the Adult Hospital when the new hospital opened in 1981, retired in 1997 after nineteen years in that challenging post. He had also been state president of the Royal Australian College of Medical Administrators and president of the Queensland branch of the Australian Medical Association, as well as holding a senior rank in the Australian Army Medical Corps. His ability and personality were recognised as vital in maintaining a cohesive spirit in the hospital.[61]

'Retirement' could, however, mean a new career at the Mater. Sister

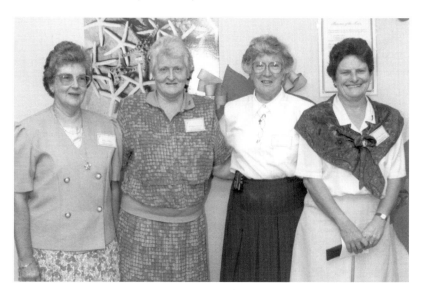

Helen O'Brien (far left), a member of staff in the Pathology Department for forty-four years, with, from left, Sister Margaret Kanowski, who worked at the Mater Mothers' Hospital for forty-five years, Sister Michaeleen Mary Ahern, a former Administrator of the Mater Private Hospital who became a member of the Redevelopment Planning team for the new Children's and Mothers' hospitals, and Sister Deirdre Gardiner, the first Mater ethicist. MHHC

Angela Mary's remark that Mater hospitals 'show many beginnings and many endings' in her final report as the Sisters of Mercy's Senior Director of Health Services was prophetic. Sister Angela Mary became executive director of the Mater Trust – her fourth separate career at the Mater. Mrs Betty Kennedy, a Mater nurse trainee in the Second World War era, retired after almost fifty years' association with the Mater. She left the hospital when she married in 1950, but responded to a desperate call from Sister Gertrude Mary in 1962 to help out for one day – she stayed as a triage nurse until she retired in 1994. This was not the end of Betty Kennedy's association with the Mater: she continued to run the Past Nurses Association and to produce its newsletter. Owen McGuiness retired after many years' work managing staff establishments, reorganising the superannuation scheme and negotiating with the unions, but returned to continue in industrial relations on a part-time basis until 2004.[62]

Retaining staff for decades was a strong element in Mater tradition. Forging and maintaining close links with the wider community was another. The focus on relationships with the community in modern health care suited the Sisters of Mercy approach. They had, after all, begun as 'walking nuns' seeking and addressing needs in the communities where they lived and worked. Some of the Mater Sisters' work in the final decades of the twentieth century further demonstrated nonjudgmental, practical compassionate care and also reflected a growing closeness in the relationship between medical care and social work. In the 1980s, for instance, the Mater Sisters supplied furniture for an emergency accommodation centre at nearby West End. Developing outreach services meant recognising needs – the Mater's and the wider community's. Language guides were introduced to help in diagnosis and treatment for people who do not speak English, a very important service in the Mater catchment with its increasingly diverse multicultural community.[63]

The Sisters sponsored AIDS research, including a study on how best to meet the needs of AIDS patients, a project that became known as the AIDS Needs Assessment Study.[64] Their work with sufferers and their families, which began very soon after the disease first appeared in the 1980s, was important in helping to dispel the fear, hurt and increasing alienation which AIDS patients and their families frequently felt; even in 1987, the international year of the homeless, many AIDS sufferers were turned out of their accommodation. By the end of the 1980s, the Sisters of Mercy had provided houses for AIDS sufferers in Brisbane, Rockhampton and Cairns and were planning more. Sadly, the addresses of all the houses had to be kept secret to avoid community hostility. Sister Angela Mary was an active presence in activities to highlight the needs of AIDS patients. She was appointed to the national AIDS advisory council, addressed large audiences on World AIDS days, and organised candlelight vigils in King George Square in the centre of the city.[65] High visibility in the community was essential: it soon became clear that the battle to control the spread of AIDS would be more effectively fought through education in workplaces and classrooms, supported by new treatments and scientific work in hospitals and laboratories. Associate Professor Joe McCormack's work in infectious diseases was important to AIDS treatment at the Mater.[66]

Supporting families and community carers was a key to enhancing the effectiveness of treatment regimes across a wide range of clinical areas. Partnerships with business and community service organisations produced the most effective services. In 1996, the Reg Leonard units, built with assistance from Queensland Newspapers to accommodate parents from remote areas whose children were patients, were refurbished, but they could not supply the demands of the 1990s. Licensees of the fast-food chain McDonald's sponsored the construction of Queensland's first Ronald McDonald House to provide accommodation for country children and their families during courses of treatment at the Children's Hospital. The original concept had come from an American football star, Fred Hill, whose daughter was seriously ill, and the idea spread to other countries where the golden arches dotted the landscape. The Variety Club, the entertainment industry's charitable organisation, provided $150,000 and the Sisters of Mercy, $50,000. At least 250 firms in the building industry donated materials and services and McDonald's licensees outfitted the house with furniture and electrical appliances, part of the $750,000 they raised for the project. Ronald McDonald House was opened in nearby Allen Street in May 1990, and was extended in 2005.[67]

The Mater's diverse neighbourhood included one of Brisbane's largest Aboriginal communities. Many Aboriginal people had lived in the Brisbane area for countless generations, but some came more recently from much further afield. Unfortunately, as well as all the usual health needs, the incidence of serious diseases such as diabetes is higher among Aboriginal people than it is among people of European descent. Part of the problem arises from the unavailability of many nutritious traditional foods. Western diets higher in fats and refined carbohydrates, supplemented by alcohol, take their toll on European people but have much more serious consequences for Aboriginal people. The Mater's Aboriginal and Torres Strait Islander liaison service was established in 1997 to build on earlier initiatives, such as Sister Mary Dorothea's special immunisation clinics at the Children's Hospital in the 1980s. Glenda Brown was the first liaison officer, and was succeeded by Sharon Lam Sam. The liaison officers visited people in their homes, and various outreach programs were developed, including adolescent health services and parenting programs for Indigenous men. Mater medical staff visited Indigenous health service clinics to develop outreach services in essential areas such as respiratory medicine and obstetrics. The respiratory medicine outreach service was extended to far north Queensland.[68] In 1998, the aim of improving health partnerships with Indigenous people was captured in the 1998 Mercy Week theme, 'Many peoples; one community'.

World Expo 88, which ran for six months on the banks of the Brisbane River at South Brisbane in 1988, provided a different kind of neighbourhood experience. The government chose the Mater

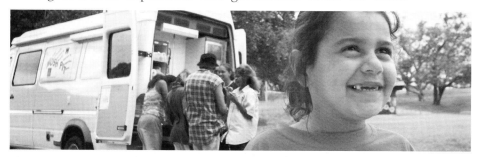

The Mater's relationship with its local community and services to its neighbours have become increasingly important. Here, the MOSH PIT van visits Musgrave Park at South Brisbane. MATER PUBLIC RELATIONS AND MARKETING

as the official hospital for Expo, an opportunity to raise the Mater's profile.[69]

The integrated services developed at the Mater during the 1990s were a response to trends in overall health policy and the expectations of patients. Some patients, however, did not enjoy their experience at the Mater. Sister Madonna Josey was appointed as the patients' representative to be an advocate for all patients. Although some patients felt that basic care was being overlooked in the modern highly technological hospitals, she found that most complaints stemmed from inadequate communication. Some patients felt that no one really listened to them or, if they did, failed to respond appropriately to their concerns, or did not explain either the diagnosis or the treatment options comprehensively in plain English. These lapses in communication were enough to send some patients scurrying to the newspapers or, more ominously, to their solicitors.[70] The late twentieth-century emphasis on consumer rights brought a wide range of new requirements as governments responded to community demands.

The kaleidoscope of inpatient, outpatient and outreach services developed at the Mater in the 1980s and 1990s changed the Mater's clinical profile substantially. The purpose of the Mercy Mission – delivering the best possible health care to all who need it – had always required continual innovation. Nurturing links between the hospitals and the wider community, creating outreach services, as well as developing clinical services, formed the core business of the modern Mater hospitals. Keeping the core business alive, active and distinctive and enabling it to grow was the task of the Mater's management: it was a particularly difficult challenge in the 1990s.

CHAPTER ELEVEN

MANAGING PARTNERSHIPS

The Mater is grateful for the enormous support given
by a wide spectrum of partners, who work closely
with us to deliver and develop our health care services
that include the Queensland government, Queensland
Health, health insurance providers, universities and of
course our dedicated staff and volunteers.

Mater Annual Report, 1999

Partnerships had always played a significant part in the Mater's development. In the hospital's earliest days, the Sisters of Mercy developed
partnerships with doctors and the community to realise their health
care vision. Over the years, partnerships between the Mater and volunteer workers and fundraisers produced facilities and equipment,
and partnerships between the individual Mater hospitals nurtured
the development of multidisciplinary services. The partnership with
the government, necessary to provide funding for the Mater's public
health services and capital injections for new buildings, was always
the most troubled partnership. In the 1990s, the level of government
funding for the Mater's public health services strained the relationship
severely.

All public hospitals were under considerable strain in the late twentieth century. New technologies and startling scientific discoveries were widely publicised, stimulating clamour for the latest treatments to be widely available. Demand was one thing, supply was quite another. Access, equity and efficiency were critical questions on both sides of the turn of the century. Health services were thrust into the public mind through wide-ranging publicity focusing on long waiting lists for elective surgery and specialist appointments in the nation's acute care general hospitals. The Commonwealth had failed to address the causes of falling subscriptions to private health insurance, and waiting lists in the public hospitals lengthened. The old constitutional divide in Australian health policy remained: the Commonwealth provided most of the funding, but the states were responsible for deciding where, and on which services, the money would be spent. Rather than producing a coherent system, Australian health policy remained little more than a series of policies about who paid for medical or hospital treatment, and how the money was distributed.[1]

Health expenditure, at about 9.3 per cent of the national gross domestic product in the early 1990s, had not greatly increased its share of national resources for decades, despite the higher costs of scientific and technological services. The real difficulty for hospitals was the decreasing proportion of the health budget spent on them: 46 per cent in 1975–76, in the early days of national health insurance, had fallen to 35 per cent by 2001–02.[2] The shift away from inpatient care was a challenge to the most adaptable clinician; the strain on costly services, and the necessity to accommodate financial pressures, was a nightmare for hospital administrators. All public hospitals were under-funded.[3] In the tense 1990s, the harsh realities of tight funding and high patient expectations meant that hospitals needed continually to refine their services, while improving both their standard and variety.

Demographic changes increased demand. Aged people, who generally need higher levels of health care, became a larger proportion of the population. The Australian population at the 2001 census was just under 19 million, double the population in 1947; in the same period, the population over 65 had trebled.[4] Demographic factors were an interesting mix of influences on the Mater in the 1990s. The growth in the aged population certainly influenced the Mater patient profile, but the Mater catchment showed some interesting variations. The rapidly growing outer suburbs still contained a high proportion of young families. However, areas nearer the coast, in, for instance, the Redland Shire, had attracted 'sea-changers' – elderly people, retirees and younger families seeking to escape the city – a growing Australian phenomenon. On the other hand, areas close to the Mater – South Brisbane, West End, Woolloongabba – were caught up in the growing inner-city 'gentrification' movement and the rapid development of apartments in areas close to the centres of cities. Many younger people came to live in the Mater's immediate suburban environs in the final two decades of the twentieth century.

Pressures for economy in a climate of rising demand led, almost inevitably, to both levels of government attempting to increase their control over the whole health system, public and private. Increased government control over the system, in the interests of keeping costs down, eroded the autonomy of hospital administrations and challenged staff at the clinical coalface.[7] Controlling patients and their expectations was, however, much more difficult. Universal health insurance increased public expectations of more and better services, although both the increasingly highly qualified staff necessary to deliver the services, and the technologies thought likely to achieve better results, were costly.[6] Hospitals were somehow expected to flourish in a discordant atmosphere generated by rising expectations clashing with falling funding. The Mater, with its mixture of public and private hospitals, adult, paediatric and obstetric care, inpatient services and community care, had to juggle more balls in the air than any other part of the Queensland hospital system.

Pat Maguire retired as chief executive officer in 1993 after almost twenty-five years at the Mater. He had negotiated substantial land purchases which allowed the Mater to expand to the other side of Stanley Street, and had directed major capital developments, such as the new Mater Private Hospital and the Mater's own complex of suites for specialist doctors. Pat Maguire's successor, Mark Avery, was charged with the task of managing a growing organisation through difficult financial times.

MARK AVERY arrived at the Mater in November 1993. Unlike Sister Angela Mary Doyle and Pat Maguire, the chief executive officers who preceded him, Mark Avery was new to the Mater. His experience in health service administration had been acquired outside Queensland. Before he took up duty at the Mater in 1993, he had eighteen years' experience in the administration of hospitals, community health organisations and aged care. He had spent ten of these years in Catholic hospitals in New South Wales and the Australian Capital Territory, coming to the Mater from Calvary Hospital in Canberra, where he had been chief executive. In an era of growing coordination within the Catholic health care sector, he had a broad perspective on developments outside Queensland. In his first few years at the Mater, Mark Avery appointed several executives from interstate, a move not entirely welcomed. During his term as the Mater chief executive, he changed the Mater's organisational structure, oversaw the development of Mater Redlands and the Mater Medical Research Institute, and managed a complex master planning process which guided the redevelopment of the Mater Children's Hospital. Mark Avery left the Mater for private consultancy shortly before the inauguration of the incorporated Mater Misericordiae Health Services Ltd.

The Mater had lived its whole history in a climate of economic stringency; some financial pinches had been acute, others were a persistent ache. Managing change – medical developments, administrative growing pains and the vagaries of government policies – had also been a persistent motif on Mater Hill. All hospitals were being forced increasingly to compete for scarce government resources and for private-sector partnerships. To be effective competitors, hospitals relied very heavily on their clinical reputations, which, in turn, relied on attracting and retaining highly skilled nursing staff and the most able doctors. This was a troubled area. Professional nurses chafed at the almost impossible requirement of providing high levels of patient care with fewer staff, and many doctors felt exploited by unrealistic expectations of the services they could provide within the constraints of a highly regulated system. Staff doctors, whether resident medical officers, registrars training to enter specialties, or staff specialists, were under similar pressures, and were just as stressed.

On top of this pressure, growing competition between hospitals for health care resources meant that public hospitals had to prove their value. As early as 1984, with the Mater Private Hospital already accredited, the Mater Board was aware that accreditation of its public hospitals could soon become a condition of Commonwealth funding.[7] However, a decade passed before accreditation of public hospitals in Queensland was required. The Mater public hospitals were surveyed by the Australian Council on Healthcare Standards (ACHS) for the first time in July 1995. Apart from a requirement to improve isolation facilities at the Children's Hospital, the Mater passed its assessment with flying colours and became the first public and private hospital system in Australia to be accredited as a whole.[8] Gaining accreditation for three large public hospitals at the first attempt was a remarkable achievement; every department in each of the hospitals had met the exacting ACHS standards for both current performance and planning to meet future goals. Generally, the Mater was praised by the ACHS for its clinical pathways, provision of workshop training in clinical path analysis and documentation review. Accreditation surveys became a regular triennial feature until 2000, when the Private Hospital became one of the first Australian hospitals to be accredited for four years.

Persistence in ensuring that Mercy values permeated the entire ethos of the Mater hospitals was a factor in this success. The ACHS surveyors noted that the reputation of the hospitals within the community was very high; this, they believed, was largely due to the dynamism of the organisation and the sensitive, caring manner in which services were delivered.[9] Clearly, the Mater spirit was more than a motivating force. It was a significant asset to be protected. All assets were under pressure in the state government's lean funding regime during the 1990s. The government had an enticing motive for financial toughness. In all states, the Medicare funding agreements with the Commonwealth provided state governments with some latitude to conserve some of the funding the Commonwealth allocated for hospitals. The regime of split responsibilities placed on the states the onus for the full marginal cost of any increase in hospital budgets during the term of the Medicare agreements. However, this strict Commonwealth line came with a carrot: the states could keep any surpluses. This was a strong incentive for the states to keep the budgetary screws wound tightly, but ineffective in achieving the Commonwealth objective of forcing the states to match Commonwealth funding growth.[10] All hospitals' expenditures had increased sharply. At the Mater, for instance, the operating budget in 1993, $2 million weekly, was more than a fifty-fold increase from $2 million annually twenty-five years earlier.[11]

In the mid-1990s, the financial tightrope became even more insecure, when the implications of new funding methodologies really hit home. This was the era of 'casemix' funding, based on a concept of 'diagnosis related groups', or DRGs. The two terms, 'casemix' and 'DRGs', sent shudders through the administrative offices of all large hospitals, particularly tertiary referral hospitals, where the high proportion of seriously ill people, requiring long courses of expensive treatment, could distort funding formulae to a tertiary hospital's disadvantage. There was one bright spot in the new system: casemix enabled better recognition of the work of specialist nurses in day care services, including the Mater's diverse range of specialist clinics, but, overall, the Mater feared that it could lose $1.4 million in funding in the single year 1995–96.[12]

There was worse to come. In 1999, the Mater Adult Hospital was reduced from the highest funding category, Category 1 Group 1, to Group 2, which further reduced the weightings allowed for certain DRGs. To achieve the same funding, the Adult Hospital would have to treat 15 per cent more patients.[13] Even worse, this demotion implied that the Mater Adult Hospital was not a tertiary-level hospital. Staffing in the intensive care and emergency units was the source of the problem in 1999 when these areas were given additional weight in deciding categorisation. In each unit, one full-time specialist was supported by four junior doctors. The problem was rectified by increasing specialist staffing to four in intensive care and three in the emergency department; both units had a full complement of accredited training positions. Despite this substantial investment and repeated applications,

Group 1 status was not restored.[14] Effectively, the Mater was subsidising free public hospital services. This anomaly was but one component of an effective state 'debt' to the Mater which grew over the ensuing years and was magnified by scant government funding for any of the outpatient clinics.

A structural sleight of hand had contributed to the problem at the Mater. The Commonwealth required trials of casemix funding, but allowed the states to select the hospitals where casemix benchmarks would be established, leading the states into the temptation of choosing hospitals with fewer complicated, expensive services. In the Mater's view, if the Commonwealth imposed the system, it should measure the benchmarks and then, perhaps, recognise both the strain on tertiary hospitals and the inequities in hospital categorisation. The Queensland Hospital Benchmarking Prices Model did not reflect either the costs of medical and surgical supplies, including pharmaceuticals, or the rapidly rising costs of public risk insurance premiums, met by the state for government hospitals but not for the Mater.[15]

The old issue of how a patient should be compensated when a medical error is made, or alleged, became more prominent in all hospitals in the 1980s and 1990s. The inadequacy of the social welfare system to provide adequate long-term care for disabled people exacerbated the problem. Medical indemnity and hospital insurance cover seemed to many to be the best means of accessing the large sums needed for long-term care if injury resulted from medical mistakes. The notion that 'insurance' paid was a comforting shibboleth – in reality, the whole community paid through higher medical and hospital costs necessary to meet sharply rising insurance premiums.[16] The Mater and its staff did not escape from the increasingly litigious climate across the nation. In 1992, solicitors expert in insurance law briefed the Board about the medical litigation process, using as their example a particularly tragic instance that occurred at the Mater in the 1980s. In this case, the Court found that two staff doctors had been negligent, but also highlighted evidence that Mater systems, particularly the advice available to inexperienced staff at night, could have contributed. As the lawyers explained, hospital administrations are usually sued as well as individual staff members, because litigants see a large organisation as more likely to be able to fund damages than any one person, however well insured. In any case, if staff members of any organisation are found to have breached a duty of care, the law ascribes a vicarious liability for the staff to the employer. In these instances, trials become battles between the hospital's insurer and the staff member's insurer, rather than between patient and doctor or between doctor and hospital. In some instances, damages were increased by out-of-court settlements, preferred by hospitals which always want to avoid adverse publicity.

After this case was concluded, the Mater Board indemnified its doctors, apart from instances of criminal conduct, conduct under the influence of alcohol, or serious, wilful misconduct.[17] Nevertheless, risk management became increasingly important. Informing patients of the possibility of risks from any procedure was an obvious aspect. However, because negligence can also arise from inaction, unnecessary medical treatment also became an issue, with the feeling that some tests and procedures were generated unnecessarily from the age-old medical fear of having 'missed something'. Such medical intervention-ism could add to patient pain and distress, and also to hospital costs. Risk management in this situation became increasingly difficult as the available technological options increased.[18] The Mater's unusual rela-tionship with government added to the complexity. The government's legal advisers took the view that because the Mater accepted funding to carry out public health services and used its assets for this purpose, it bore the liability for carrying out those services. The government's 'long pocket' was not to be available to the Mater when litigation arose.[19] In the Mater's view, the substantial cost of public risk insurance premiums – $1,387,936 in 1999 for the public hospitals alone – was another component in the state's growing debt to the Mater.[20]

Wage pressures added to the financial strain. Changes to indus-trial awards limited resident medical officers to forty hours' work a week, and nurses to thirty-eight hours, considerably increasing salary costs. The Sisters considered funding some critical new positions, but this solution could have pushed mercy and charity to the limit. After all, the Sisters had already provided land free of charge for substan-tial public health services.[21] The government was also wary of such strategies, fearing that the Sisters' funding for new positions could be withdrawn, leaving the government in the position of either funding the positions or risking the odium of forcing retrenchments.[22] The Queensland government exacerbated the problem when it changed from a cash accounting system to accrual accounting in 2001. There was no compensation to the Mater for the substantial accrued liabilities for public hospital staff recreation leave and long service leave entitlements, which appeared on the books when the new system was introduced, adding a further $28,787,646 to the state's effective debt to the Mater.[23]

In this tough funding regime, the Mater drew on its own resources to subsidise its public hospital services, as indeed it had many times in the past. The Mater's private means included the enormous contribution of the Sisters of Mercy in providing land, buildings, equipment, research funding and countless grants of one kind or another, profits from the Mater's businesses from the laundry to the carparks, surpluses when possible from the private hospitals, the income from the art unions and the work of armies of volunteer fundraisers. By the turn of the twenty-first century, the net current value of 'donations', apart from land and buildings, amounted to a vast sum – almost half a billion dollars.[24] However, the base of social capital developed since 1906 was just as formidable a resource: a rich stock of active connections among people both inside and outside the Mater, a wide network based on trust, mutual understanding, shared values and dedication to a common goal.[25] This network was more than a large 'support group' for the Mater; it also amounted to a substantial electorate in political terms.

Building relationships and raising funds was ground the volunteer auxiliaries had been fertilising for decades. The volunteers had raised hundreds of thousands of dollars over the years. In the single year 1992, for instance, the Adult Hospital auxiliary raised $220,000 for badly needed equipment.[26] The auxiliaries had attracted remarkable women who dedicated years of their lives to the Mater and had developed their own strong and loyal following. Mrs Joy Shields started with the Mothers' auxiliary in the 1960s, and was still guiding it thirty years later; Mrs Felix Dittmer spent years leading the Children's Hospital auxiliary, and Mrs Cath Schmidt was secretary of the Adult

Hospital auxiliary for more than thirty years. Her husband, Harry, a sports journalist with the *Brisbane Telegraph*, spent many hours doing the auxiliary's typing. By the 1990s, the Children's Hospital had an additional auxiliary, the Friends of the Cranio-facial Unit, led by Mrs Alayne McDougall, Mrs Geraldine Anderson and Mrs Jan Seymour.

The level of activity maintained by the voluntary auxiliaries into the twenty-first century was all the more remarkable because a great deal of the work relied on women. Fewer women were available for voluntary activity in the final decades of the twentieth century. With many more women in the paid workforce, the community was beginning to recognise the real value to the economy of the voluntary work of generations of volunteers, particularly in social services and health care. In the 1990s, the Mater's army of volunteers were busy across the campus helping in patient care as well as fundraising. Volunteers supported the work of the child abuse team; 'cuddlemas' and 'cuddlepas' helped to nurture frail premature babies when their parents were not able to be at the hospital; others propelled heavy trolleys of magazines and other comforts up and down the wards, or dispensed thousands of cups of tea and coffee, with their listening ears ever ready to support the families of very ill patients. By 1993, 170 volunteers contributed 24,000 hours of service annually, which had more than doubled by 1996. In 1992, Sister Pamela Barker of the Franciscan Missionaries of Mary was appointed to organise and coordinate volunteer services, which were still growing when Vicki Franklin took over in 1997.[27] By the end of the century, 450 volunteers were working in ninety different areas across the campus, and had broadened their services to include, for example, a transport service to bring patients to the hospital for appointments, support for patients in the oncology unit, play activities at the Children's, and an arts and craft service to help combat boredom, always a problem for long-term antenatal patients. Outside the hospital, many women busily knitted brightly coloured woollen caps for tiny babies in the special-care nurseries.

In addition to the work of the voluntary auxiliaries and occasional large donations and bequests the Mater had developed several successful forms of fundraising.[28] Of these, the art unions and the *Courier-Mail* Children's Hospitals' Appeal, shared with the Royal Children's Hospital,

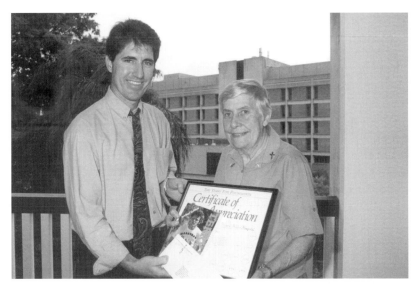

Sister Eileen Pollard, enthusiastic fundraiser for the Queensland Cancer Fund, is shown here with Mr Richard Langton from the Queensland Cancer Fund receiving the Fund's Certificate of Appreciation, awarded to the Mater as the most successful corporate fundraiser for the Terry Fox Fun Run. MHHC

were the most widely known. Imitation can be the sincerest form of flattery, and a plethora of art unions, offering houses, boats, cars and overseas holidays as prizes had appeared once it was obvious that the Mater Prize Home art union was highly profitable. Nevertheless, the Mater art unions, buffeted by competition, remained a valuable wing of fundraising, particularly for the Children's Hospital, and a significant means of reaching a wide section of the community who might otherwise not contribute to the Mater. Mater people did not raise money solely for the Mater. Sister Eileen Pollard's enthusiastic participation in the Terry Fox Fun Runs to raise funds for all kinds of cancer research helped the Mater to achieve the accolade as the Run's highest corporate fundraiser for several years.[29]

During the 1980s and 1990s, the Children's Hospital won valuable support from a remarkable Brisbane identity, the antique dealer Cecilia McNally. Often dubbed the 'Duchess of Spring Hill', Miss McNally was a passionate advocate for this historic inner-Brisbane suburb, where her fairs celebrating the area's history and sense of community drew thousands of people from all over the city. During the

1980s, Miss McNally donated the proceeds of the fairs – in some years more than $50,000 – to various Mater causes, such as instruments for microsurgery and a portable ventilator for the neonatal emergency retrieval service, and ran special events such as a dinner dance to help the parent aide unit.[30] Cecilia McNally died in 1996, leaving the proceeds of an auction of her house and its valuable collection of antique furniture to the Mater Children's, a bequest worth $1.3 million.[31]

All voluntary work was personalised public relations. Public relations became extremely important in this competitive era. Hospitals advertising their services and publicising their 'firsts' and 'onlys' became an increasingly evident phenomenon. In the late 1980s, state hospitals embarked on aggressive marketing and public relations campaigns, attracting substantial media attention, with a noticeable impact on morale at the Mater. Some Mater staff were worried that their hospitals might be perceived in the general community as being in decline.[32] It was an annoying situation – all the Mater hospitals were full of wonderful human interest stories. Attracting the media was, however, only one part of the task. A much broader strategy was needed, including reviving the annual reports as a vehicle for strong and clear messages, a valuable technique J P Kelly had used to the Mater's advantage in the 1950s and 1960s, and enclosing the corporate message in every piece of art union promotion. However, it was obvious that it would be counter-productive to tie all publicity to fundraising – it was first necessary to win the public's interest.[33] There was nothing like having people in the grounds to raise awareness of the things the Mater hospitals actually do: the Mater's first Open Day in 1993 attracted 3,000 people.[34]

The key to the Mater's public image was its distinctly different personality. The Mercy mission and values formed the foundation of the Mater's character and the face it presented to the world, a factor recognised by the strategic planners in the 1990s in developing a mission statement. Often derided as empty 'corporate speak', mission statements can crystallise objectives. The mission statement written to help 'position' the Mater in the health care future, both inside the hospitals and in the community, was simple and direct:

> In the spirit of the Sisters of Mercy, the Mater Hospitals offer compassionate
> service to the sick and needy, promote an holistic approach to health care
> in response to changing community needs, and foster high standards in
> health-related education and research. Following the example of Christ
> the Healer, we commit ourselves to offering these services to all without
> discrimination.[35]

The Sisters continued to drive a strong corporate culture, believing that the Mater's strength lay in the quality of its people and that, in order to be a healthy institution, the Mater must be willing to be shaped and reshaped. A great deal of effort in the 1990s was invested in staff selection and formation, essential to keep Mater values alive.[36] Each annual report in the late 1980s and 1990s included prominent statements of the Mater's mission, values and philosophy. One hundred members of the staff contributed to the identification and statement of the Mater's values: mercy, care, dignity, commitment, quality.[37] The Mater Private joined in, and produced 'Philosophy in Action' to inform its staff and integrate the hospital's mission in all of its activities.[38]

To be effective, mission statements must be supported by management strategies. The Mater, in common with government departments and commercial organisations of all kinds, adopted the latest offerings from the growing discipline of professional management. This was an era of experimentation with systems and structures. Management was no longer an arcane art practised by remote figures in hospital administration; all executive directors of individual Mater hospitals and ancillary services were to be responsible for their own budgets, a certain recipe for stress in times of high pressure to improve patient services within 'existing budgets', always a euphemism for smaller budgets in real money terms.

Each hospital developed its own operational plan to fulfil a new corporate plan, introduced in 1994 to guide development for the final five years of the twentieth century. Similar new management structures and management systems were introduced at other hospitals and were *de rigeur* in the state system with its plethora of executive directors and district managers. Different forms of management for the individual hospitals were tried. In 1995, for example, two-year appointments were offered to Dr Peter Steer, as executive director of the Children's Hospital, and to Dr John Waller, as executive director of the Adult Hospital, as a means of exploring the appropriate clinical direction for both hospitals. Dr Jenny Brown, executive director of the Mater Mothers' Hospital, was appointed director of planning.[39]

The traditional role of director of medical services was disappearing in the evolving realm of hospital management. There had only ever been two such appointments at the Mater – Dr Des O'Callaghan in 1962 and Dr James Griffin in 1988. Jim Griffin had been part of the team which established the QEII hospital, and was its first medical superintendent after many years working in Queensland government hospitals all over the state. Moving to the Mater, Jim Griffin developed the program to recruit doctors from overseas and greatly improved the Mater's relationship with the University of Queensland. He forged the Mater's relationships with overseas hospitals, particularly with the Zhejiang cancer hospital in China. Dr Griffin improved strategic planning and initiated the development of 'Code Brown' disaster management software, the first in Australia.[40] Dr Griffin resigned in July 1999 to enter private practice.

In the late 1990s, a number of new and altered executive positions reflected the elevation of planning and strategy in the new Mater structure. Dr Jenny Brown was responsible for strategies aimed at enhancing relationships with the universities; Jenny Skinner succeeded David Kelly as chief operations officer; and Dr John Gilmour, as acting director of mission and ethics in Sister Deirdre Gardiner's absence overseas, was responsible for developing closer partnerships between the Sisters and the Mater's lay staff.

Despite managerial restructures and the vigour of voluntary work, needs could always be expected to outstrip resources. The Mater Children's pleaded its need for increased resources in 1986, when the Medical Superintendent, Dr John McNee, estimated that capital expenditure of $30 million would be needed within a decade if the hospital was to have any chance of keeping up with demand for its services. His belief was based on the knowledge that more than 65 per cent of Brisbane's child population lived south of the river. Sister Mary Dorothea Sheehan even feared that, if no assistance was forthcoming, the only Catholic children's hospital in Australia could be lost. The medical staff thought that donations had been lost in the past because the Children's Hospital had no infrastructure to accept large sums of money.[41] The only available mechanism for large donations was the J P Kelly Foundation, established in 1982 to support medical research. However, the Children's Hospital's needs were much broader, and its advocates recommended a foundation which would fund buildings as well as research.

Secure funding for specialist units had also been a persistent worry. Specific-purpose donations and allocations from grant bodies helped to develop the Mater's specialist services, but a considerable level of discretionary capital was urgently needed.[42] Other hospitals – the Royal Brisbane Hospital, the Royal Children's Hospital and the Royal Women's Hospital – were pertinent examples close at hand of the foundation movement which spread to other state institutions, such as the Queensland Institute of Medical Research and the State Library. However, it was almost certain that if a foundation were to be created for the Children's Hospital, each of the other Mater hospitals would want one too.[43] But four foundations on one campus could be unwieldy and incur substantial overhead administrative costs. In its search for funding from both the public and the private sectors, the Board contemplated some form of company concept or overarching Trust to support specialist activities, such as sleep studies, rather than creating separate trusts for each new area as it arose.[44]

Two methods could be used to create a fundraising foundation – establishment under the *Hospital Foundations Act 1982*, which required Cabinet approval, or establishment under companies legislation, which did not.[45] The Board wanted a broad structure to satisfy donors' preferences, the requirements of the individual Mater hospitals, and the Sisters' wish to appoint the foundation board to ensure that it would exercise Mercy values.[46] Late in 1987, draft articles and memoranda were prepared for a foundation known initially as The Mater Hospitals Trust. Incorporation under companies legislation provided several advantages, including limitation by guarantee. Major details, such as whether or not a donation of $25,000 paid over five years should be set as a qualification for Trust membership, had to be settled. 'Tiered' membership had been adopted by, for example, the State Library Foundation, which set various classes of members according to the size of donation, a useful strategy in appealing to the corporate sector.

The new company, officially titled Mater Hospitals Appeal Ltd, was incorporated on 6 March 1989. The Trust aimed high in appointing its first chairman, Sir Llew Edwards, AC, a former health minister, deputy premier and chairman of Expo 88.[47] The Mater Trust was launched with considerable fanfare by the Governor-General, Mr Bill Hayden, AC, on 14 April 1989. The New Life Centre at the Mater Mothers', the first step in a $10 million refurbishment plan, was a popular first objective, but there were numerous good causes pressing for priority. The Children's Hospital was to succeed the New Life Centre as the second target. Equipment was another pressing concern. Dr Jim Griffin, Director of Medical Services, reported with some frustration that the Mater public hospitals were millions of dollars behind in being able to procure new equipment, a situation which could mean reducing patient services, always an anathema to the Mater.[48]

With these pressures, the Trust's first few years were far from easy. Although fundraising in various forms had been a feature of Mater life since the first Mater was merely the inkling of an idea, the Trust structure was a new venture. Securing large donations from the corporate sector was difficult in a climate rife with competition from other worthy causes. The Trust did not achieve its first target, $3 million for the New Life Centre,[49] but it began to overcome original disappointments in the early 1990s, due in no small part to advocacy by Sir James Foots, former chairman of Mt Isa Mines. Substantial donations were received from the Westpac and National Australia banks, from the major resource development companies Mt Isa Mines Ltd and Queensland Alumina, and from the national retailer Coles Myer. The Variety Club, the charity wing of the entertainment industry, pledged a donation, and also offered to make a promotional video for the Trust.[50] Sister Angela Mary retired as the Sisters' Senior Director of Health Services late in 1993, and early in 1994 applied her energy and initiative as the new executive director of the Trust, where Mr Bernie Dawson had succeeded Sir Llew Edwards as chairman. Donor revenue improved significantly in the mid-1990s: in 1995 donations increased by 39 per cent and overhead costs were contained at 14 per cent. In 1996, the Trust distributed $1.1 million.[51]

All sorts of methods were used to raise money for the Trust, and to attract publicity. Mrs Betty McGrath OAM – by 2004, the longest-serving member of the Trust Board – and her husband, Brian, were indefatigable Trust fundraisers. Through the 1990s and into the twenty-first century, Betty McGrath ran many major events – the 'Rendezvous with Romance' Valentine's Day dinners, celebrity auctions, and novelty events such as the Great Race at the Southbank Parklands. The drawcard at one of the earliest auctions was a slouch hat donated by a rising local swimming champion, Hayley Lewis.[52] Success in achieving the Trust's objectives relied to a considerable extent on a high community profile. Publicity in all media was enthusiastically pursued. The young people's radio station FM 104 adopted the Mater Trust as one of its special interests in 1998. High-profile events such as the family walks, 5Ks for Kids, sponsored by prominent organisations such as Australia Post and the Bank of Queensland, were important in keeping the Mater name in the public eye, as well as raising considerable sums of money. The old stand-by, the art union, was revamped in 1994 and amalgamated with the Trust in 1997.

The Trust broadened its approach in the late 1990s. In 1997, for example, it joined with the Queensland Hotels Association to encourage hotels to hold fundraising events to assist the Mater, and secured support from several philanthropic associations, such as a large donation for the paediatric epilepsy centre from the Broncos Rugby League Club charities fund.[53] The Tzu Chi Buddhist Compassion Relief foundation, one of Sister Angela Mary's special interests, provided $180,000 to fund a research position in the paediatric development and rehabilitation clinic. Tzu Chi was introduced to Brisbane by Mrs Julia Wang who came to Brisbane from Taiwan in 1990. Obeying Master Cheng Yen's words – 'to be loved by others, you must love them first' – she became a volunteer at the Mater and met Sister Angela Mary. By 2002, Tzu Chi volunteers had donated $1.2 million to the Mater and had established the Mater Tzu Chi Research Scholarship.[54] The Brisbane Taiwanese community continued to be extremely generous supporters.

The Wu family from Taiwan became important benefactors of the cranio-facial unit, and in 2004 Tony and Lisa Teng donated $800,000 for research and were thanked at a special ceremony which included Sister Angela Mary's personal thanks in fluent Mandarin. The Mater's store of both financial and social capital was steadily increasing and being drawn from ever more diverse sources.

In 1997, the Mater Trust moved to its new offices on the ground floor of the original private hospital, by then renamed Aubigny Place.[55] Sister Angela Mary retired as executive director, and was succeeded by Nigel Harris, the Trust's director of fundraising. Sister Angela Mary remained on the board to chair a committee to generate community support for the establishment of a new Mater Medical Research Institute. By mid-1997, the Trust had raised $800,000 specifically for this purpose. In 1998, the Trust raised $3 million for all its projects, an increase of 12 per cent, but even this was not sufficient to support critical projects.[56] Terry Jackman and the businessmen on his capital campaign committee set themselves the ambitious target of raising significant capital sums to fund research initiatives and to defray the extra costs of building projects,

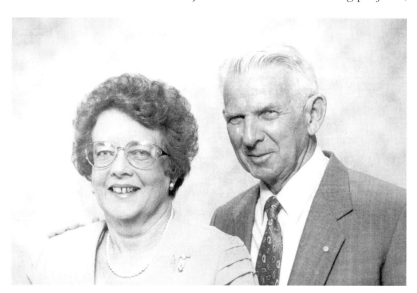

Mrs Betty McGrath, longstanding member of the Mater Trust Board and indefatigable fundraiser, photographed with her husband, Brian. MATER MEDICAL PHOTOGRAPHY

particularly the new Children's Hospital: a donation of $250,000 for the Children's Hospital from an anonymous donor in Hong Kong was gratefully received.[57]

By the end of the twentieth century, the Mater had become a large business, even more diverse than it had been in 1987 when the Governing Board was created as a major step in the Sisters' delegating power to lay management. The complexity of the Mater's business at the turn of the century required a modern corporate structure. The possibility of incorporating the Mater was an active topic for debate in the 1980s. J P Kelly, chairman of the Advisory Board until 1980, had not supported incorporation because, to him, it was inconceivable that a Catholic hospital would not be able to resolve contractual disputes or respond appropriately to a judgment against it.[58] The Board examined the advantages of incorporation as part of the 'future discernment' process in 1985.[59] The Mater, as part of the Corporation of the Trustees of the Order of the Sisters of Mercy in Queensland, had no legal authority to act on its own behalf, could not own property in its own name, but could assign its debts to the Sisters. The modern Mater needed to shoulder all its responsibilities.

Many different issues had to be weighed on both sides of the incorporation argument. Declining numbers of Sisters and the aging of the Congregation was a central issue in finding a way for Mercy values to continue at the Mater in the absence of the Sisters, perhaps by separating responsibility for the hospitals from the Sisters of Mercy, while continuing to enable the Sisters to own the Mater property and to control key appointments. Mother Patrick Potter, an abiding genius of the Sisters' business strategies, had ensured that the Sisters of Mercy had been an incorporated entity since 1927.[60] However, incorporation under Queensland's *Religious and Charitable Institutions Act 1861*, while providing a practical means of ensuring perpetual succession and a useful structure for negotiation with governments, was not a suitable model to address the needs of modern hospitals. Accountability for government funding, the management of huge commercial agreements and insurance against various liabilities was outside its scope.

As Congregational Leader, Sister Monica Stallard established task forces to examine all Mercy ministries, including the Mater.[61] The

Sisters were mindful that the Second Vatican Council had called upon all religious institutes to maintain their apostolic works while making adjustments in them according to changing times. For many years the Sisters had issued a strong 'call to partnership', encouraging Mater staff, volunteers, benefactors, government and the community to join them in pursuing their health care mission. Several signs seemed to point to incorporation: the responsibility to promote the role of the laity, the challenge of equitably distributing scarce resources, the ever-increasing costs of health care, and the ethical requirement to provide modern accountability mechanisms for the use of public resources.[62] Incorporation was seen as a way of enabling lay people to share more easily in the governance and mission of the hospitals, and of allowing the Mater to enter into its own contracts.

The Sisters also believed that a way had to be found to separate their various ministries from each other's legal liabilities.[63] In the 1990s, personal injury litigation and disputes over contracts had to be regarded as an unfortunate likelihood rather than an obscure possibility. In a legal system where litigants tried to identify the 'longest pocket' as a means of ensuring that large damages awarded by courts could be paid, the Congregation of the Sisters of Mercy, with its extensive holdings in schools, hospitals and other properties, was a very deep pocket indeed. It was evident, however, that even if the hospitals were incorporated, the Mater could never insure against the worst possible catastrophe. On the other hand, as Sister Kath Burke reminded the Board, if the Mater had a large judgment against it which it could not support, the Congregation could take the view that it should not jeopardise its other charitable institutions.

The Mater was formally incorporated as Mater Misericordiae Health Services Brisbane Limited on 1 July 2001. The incorporated structure created a civil law entity guaranteeing the secure continuation of the work of the hospitals into the twenty-first century, and allowed for delegations to maintain the partnership between the Sisters and the Board, a necessary framework to ensure the longevity of the mission. The Mater was one of the last Catholic hospitals in Australia to take this step. It is likely that the conservative approach to incorporation during the 1980s reflected concern that the eternally fragile relationship with the state government could be imperilled by corporate standards of accounting, which could end the advantage to government of the old arrangement whereby it did not pay rent for land and buildings or the Sisters' salaries.[64]

The 'working' name of the new entity, Mater Health Services, gave legal recognition to the metamorphosis from the original focus on hospital care to a broad range of services. The structure of the new company was ingenious, if complicated. The constitution provided for three separate tiers. The first, Class A, was the Congregational Leadership Team, which retained the power to appoint the Board of Directors and the chief executive officer, to approve the company's strategic plan, and to control the sale or lease of assets, as well as borrowings and expenditure outside defined limits. Class B was formed of advisors to the Congregation and Class C comprised the Board of Directors. The Board, as stewards of the Mater's resources, had authority to determine policies, practices and strategies – indeed all the management systems necessary to operate Mater Health Services – and was also charged with promulgating the Sisters' mission and health care objectives. The new Board set itself five key organisational goals: the integration of core values, enhanced clinical care and innovation, improved organisational performance, improved strategic positioning, and active programs of recruitment, education and development.[65]

Incorporation under the Australian *Corporations Law* also meant stringent accounting and formal reporting to regulatory bodies. The Board had the same responsibilities and obligations as boards of directors of commercial corporations, and faced the same legal sanctions if they were found wanting. Much of the early planning for incorporation had taken place during the chairmanship of the former Professor of Law at the University of Queensland and Supreme Court Justice, Kevin Ryan, who had been a member of the Board since 1976 and deputy chairman for five years before becoming chairman in 1989.[66] On his retirement from the Chair in 1996, Justice Ryan was succeeded by another University of Queensland professor, the civil engineer Colin Apelt. In 1954, Colin Apelt won a Rhodes Scholarship to Oxford University where he joined the Catholic Social Guild. His concern for social justice and the Church's duty to the poor was reflected in his paper, 'A reflection on poverty, power and the Church', discussed at an advisory board meeting in 1980. In the mid-1990s, Colin Apelt believed that maintaining the Mater's unique identity was a pivotal issue for the Board. Colin Apelt's deputy was the Honourable G E Fitzgerald QC, a former Justice of the Federal Court and chairman of the 1980s Royal Commission which exposed corruption in the Queensland police force and several areas of government.

In 2001, when the Mater entered its new era as a corporation, Colin Apelt retired from the chair to take up an appointment as a Class B member, and was succeeded by John McAuliffe. The new Board represented a wide range of business skills and health care knowledge. John McAuliffe was an authority on valuation, and the investment, development and management aspects of the modern built environment. He had been regional director of the Commonwealth Department of Administrative Services, where he honed his skills in property management. Brian Flannery came from the mining industry, a leading component of the Queensland economy, and had wide experience in developing and managing major projects. Sister Anne O'Farrell had a background in managing major educational institutions. Sister Patricia Kirchner, a member of the Congregational Leadership Team, had been at the Mater for thirty years and knew its every corner. Dr Laurel Moore was a general practitioner with particular interest in the health of Indigenous people and refugees, and the treatment of people with the human immunodeficiency virus and AIDS. Dr Elizabeth Davies, head of the School of Nursing at the Australian Catholic University's Brisbane campus, was a catalyst for change in nurse education and became foundation Professor of Nursing at the University of Queensland. Vince O'Rourke, former chief executive officer of Queensland Rail, had overseen the transition of Queensland Rail from a government department to a government-owned business entity. He was known for his skill at initiating and managing change in large organisations. Dr Elizabeth McDade, Director of International College at Queensland University of Technology had chaired the finance committee at the Catholic education office.

The new Mater corporation did not begin its life on solid financial ground. The underfunding problem was growing steadily and becoming unsustainable. The Mater had faced many perils in developing its health-care mission. In this respect, and in working towards achieving a dream, the early years of the twenty-first century had much in common with the first decade of the twentieth.

CHAPTER TWELVE

DEVELOPING A BOLD VISION

The staff and I share a vision for the Mater as . . . a strong and viable centre of international clinical excellence in service, teaching and research while providing holistic care to all without discrimination[1]

Dr John O'Donnell, 2003

Incorporation, which allowed the Mater to decide its own destiny, and innovations in clinical services, education and research, laid a firm basis to develop this bold vision. The new structure had been deliberately designed to ensure that both the spirit and the letter of the Mercy mission would be knitted into every aspect of the Mater's activities. The mission was distilled into five core values: mercy, the spirit of responding to one another; dignity, the spirit of humanity, respecting the worth of each person; care, the spirit of compassion; commitment, the spirit of integrity; and quality, the spirit of professionalism. These ideals were the purpose of the Mater's activities, but to advance towards any bold vision, many mundane issues needed to be tackled in the early twenty-first century. These included managing the Mater's new accountability and legal responsibilities, navigating relationships with governments, which had expanded to include the requirements of the Commonwealth *Corporations Law*, and planning a major capital

JOHN JAMES O'DONNELL, MB BS, DipRACOG, MHP, FRACMA, AFACHSE, was born in South Australia and educated at the Cleve Area School and Scotch College before graduating in medicine at the University of Adelaide in 1979. After residency terms at the Royal Adelaide Hospital and the Adelaide Children's Hospital, John O'Donnell was a registrar in neonatology and paediatrics in Calgary, Canada, before returning to general practice in Adelaide and two years as a visiting medical officer in the Department of Obstetrics and Gynaecology at the Flinders Medical Centre. After graduating dux of his year in the Master of Health Planning course at the University of New South Wales, he became deputy medical director at the Royal Adelaide Hospital from 1985–90. In the 1990s, he was, successively, Executive Director, Clinical Services and deputy general manager at the Royal Canberra and Woden Valley hospitals, commissioning chief executive of the Port Macquarie Hospital, chief executive officer of the St George private hospital and the Prince of Wales private hospital, and national director of clinical services and quality for Mayne Health Care, the owner of private hospitals around the nation. In 2001, John O'Donnell accepted appointment as the Mater's chief executive officer.

works program to modernise the Mater.[2] The Mater's financial position was, however, particularly pressing when Dr John O'Donnell arrived in September 2001 to begin work as the Mater's new chief executive officer.

Incorporation changed the relationship with the state government. Since 1978, state government funding for public hospital services had been provided under an 'Acknowledgment and Understanding' agreement between the Sisters of Mercy and the government. After twenty years, this agreement had become obsolete. The new twenty-year term of the agreement, signed in 2002, provided an element of security for the Mater: funding would be provided annually for the Mater, which would follow an agreed clinical services plan guided by policies and procedures developed by Queensland Health to manage its annual allocation from the state budget. The objectives of the new agreement included the government's undertaking to continue the 'quantity and quality' of the Mater's public health services by maintaining funding and the 'clinical viability of the delivery by the Mater of Mater health services'.[3] This was the rub: evidence was growing that state funding was not meeting the objectives of either viability or 'quantity and quality'.

In the early years of the new century, the state's effective debt to the Mater for under-funding public hospital services mounted steadily in all five of the components identified during the 1990s: the demotion of the Adult Hospital from the highest funding category; urgent capital works and equipment requirements; routine operating expenses, particularly the costs of medical and surgical supplies; insurance premiums; and provision for staff entitlements. This came to a total of $30.6 million over three years.[4] Even if all the Mater's private means were to be applied to making up the shortfall, it was becoming obvious that the day could come when debt would exceed private financial capacity. This scenario could mean that the Mater would need to consider withdrawing from public health services, a situation reminiscent of Sister Angela Mary's dilemma in the early 1970s when the Adult Hospital urgently needed replacement. Such a possibility remained unattractive to the Mater, which had continued to pride itself on its contribution to the health of Queenslanders. Any suggestion that the Mater might withdraw from adult public medicine, paediatrics, obstetrics and neonatology was also likely to alarm the government, which was continually besieged by accusations that its own hospitals were not addressing demand adequately.[5]

Although every effort was made to save each Mater dollar, often to the chagrin of clinicians who felt that their budgets were already threadbare, the cost of operating the Mater was approaching $1 million per day by 2003, a huge rise from the $2 million per week in 1993. After extensive consultation across Mater Hill, a new organisational structure was developed to centralise support services and to improve efficiency wherever possible. By 2004, the administration of the Adult, Children's and Mothers' hospitals had been combined under Dr Jenny King; the private hospitals at South Brisbane and

Redlands were combined under Don Murray as executive director; and support services – pathology, pharmacy, clinical risk management and general practice – were combined in Dr Julie Hudson's department. Mission services retained their primacy as part of the executive structure. The Education Centre developed its profile both internally in keeping staff up to date in international trends in management and clinical developments, and externally in holding national conferences on leadership in health education and on leadership to generate high performance.[6] The Corporate Services Division, with Chris Townend as executive director, was reorganised to recognise the essential service wings all large hospitals rely upon – finance, hotel, information management, engineering and environmental services, staff and supply.[7] Because the Mater was still paying commercial professional indemnity premiums for the public hospitals and their staff, and because the litigious climate showed little sign of abating and any claim would be a considerable impost, a new highly skilled clinical risk management team was established in 2002. Mater public relations expanded. Frank Pollard's marketing and communications division devised a

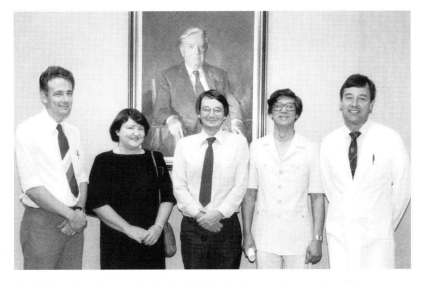

The William Dargie portrait of John P Kelly, chairman of successive Mater advisory boards for forty-two years, oversees the recipients of the first John P Kelly Research Foundation grants, who are photographed with his daughter, Margaret, second from left. The recipients are, from left, Dr Michael Irving, Dr David Tudehope, Professor Yee Hing Thong and Dr Dick Chalmers. MHHC

new, punchy phrase to better express the Mater spirit and promote its services: 'Exceptional People, Exceptional Care'.

Research was an essential element of the Mater vision. Indeed, research had been part of Mater activity ever since Sister Mary Chanel set up her microscope during the First World War. As the century progressed, Mater research spread among the various areas and departments in all the hospitals. Vital though it is, research is a voracious consumer of resources and a vigorous field for competitive activity. The Sisters had created the J P Kelly Research Foundation in 1982 to boost funding for Mater research and education. The Foundation attracted considerable financial support from various organisations and agencies.[8] Doctors on the J P Kelly research committee – in the early days, Dr John Bell, Dr Mervyn Neely and Dr John Burke – recommended grants for research in areas such as neonatal immunology, gastroenterology, the effects of neonatal death on families, the possibility of a vaccine to treat melanoma, and the potential of magnetic resonance spectroscopy for diagnosing tumour growth and evaluating the results of chemotherapy, a project conducted in collaboration with Griffith University.[9] By 1990, the J P Kelly Foundation had allocated more than $500,000. However, grants totalling $70,000 and $100,000 annually, the usual income on the Sisters' investment, would never be sufficient to assist all worthy research proposals.

The Sisters of Mercy had a much grander plan. At various times in the Mater's history, the vision of a special building devoted to medical research had sparkled amid more mundane concerns. As the 1990s progressed, the concept of stem cell and gene therapies to treat a variety of intractable conditions from spinal cord injury to cancer was reaching the public's consciousness. It had been a vigorous area of pure research for some years. Completing the mapping of the human genome in the early twenty-first century seemed to many lay people to be the end of a chapter, but to biomedical researchers it was merely an early breach in a new frontier. The era of biotechnology was well on its way to supplanting the knowledge economy for primacy in human society; 'stem cell' and 'gene therapy' became terms in common currency.

Although it often seemed that Australian medical research was based almost exclusively in the southern states in such august organisations as the Walter and Eliza Hall and the Garvan institutes, valuable medical research had also emanated from Queensland in areas ranging from the causes and effects of lead poisoning in children in the late nineteenth century, to mosquito-borne diseases in the twentieth century. The Queensland Institute of Medical Research, although under-funded, had developed a solid reputation, contributing the work of scientists such as Peter Bancroft and Josephine Mackerras to Australia's intellectual reputation.

In the 1990s, the Sisters of Mercy believed strongly that there was room for another medical research institute in Queensland. The work of many Mater doctors, among them Robyn Rodwell and Kerry Taylor in haematology, David Tudehope in neonatology and Michael O'Rourke, director of surgery at the Adult Hospital, in pursuing the possibility of harnessing the body's immune system to defeat melanoma, seemed to support the Sisters' view.[10] By the mid-1990s, plans were afoot for the Mater Medical Research Institute (MMRI). Bequests held by the Sisters would contribute a significant proportion of the $10 million start-up capital, the Tzu Chi Foundation promised to endow a perpetual scholarship,[11] and the Mater Trust was doing its utmost. Plans progressed at the Mater under the guidance of an expert steering committee which included Professor Laurie Powell from the Queensland Institute of Medical Research.[12] A worldwide search was launched for a leading scientist to direct the new institute, culminating in the appointment of Professor Derek Hart. While working as a Rhodes Scholar at Oxford in 1979, Derek Hart discovered dendritic cells, specialised white blood cells that play a critical role in initiating immune response; a precise understanding of their function was his next target.[13] Effective cancer immunotherapy through manipulation of stem cells became a central MMRI goal.

With the MMRI's first collection of frozen stem cells in his luggage, Derek Hart arrived in Brisbane to begin work on 1 July 1998. He had already attracted two scientists from Japan, complete with the necessary research funding, to begin work in six new laboratories constructed in the former operating theatres on the third floor of Aubigny Place, the original Private Hospital, with an animal house installed in the old fitter's workshop at the rear. With plans well underway to

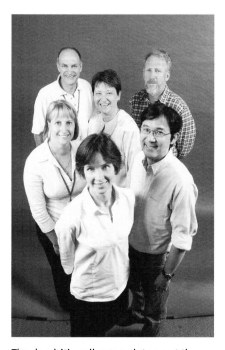

The dendritic-cell research team at the Mater Medical Research Institute (MMRI), from back, left to right, Professor Derek Hart, Dr David Munster, Dr Slavica Vuckovic, Dr Kirsten Radford, Dr Masato Kato and Dr Georgina Clark. MATER MEDICAL RESEARCH INSTITUTE

develop the Institute on a proper business footing, including purchasing patents on Professor Hart's previous work and setting up the mechanism to own the intellectual property on future discoveries, surprising news arrived from the other side of the river.[14] A $20 million cancer research centre was to be established at the Royal Brisbane Hospital, funded by an American benefactor, with a dollar-for-dollar contribution from the state government as part of its 'Smart State' initiative. This caused concern at the Mater. When the Sisters of Mercy had told the government it was giving $8 million plus buildings to start a research organisation, the state had claimed it had no available funds to help.[15]

But there was plenty of cancer research waiting to be done. The new Mater institute was officially opened by the Governor-General, Sir William Deane, in 1999. The Queensland-born Nobel Laureate in physiology and medicine, Professor Peter Doherty, accepted appointment as the Institute's scientific patron. Cancer was adopted as the Institute's first research theme, although plans were laid from the beginning to expand into other biomedical areas. Progress was startling. By 2001, there were several successes: a world-first process to count dendritic cells; a breakthrough in understanding the development of prostate cancer, with the real possibility that a vaccine could be developed to fight it; and the Mucin research team's internationally important discovery of the MUC13 gene, important in colo-rectal cancer.[16] The MMRI distinguished its approach from Brisbane's other research organisations by entering into several joint ventures with the various Mater hospitals. This concept of translational research facilitating the clinical application of new biological therapies was also seen as a key element in the Mater model, which would be important in attracting talented clinicians.[17]

The traditional Mater link to the wider community was not overlooked. From the beginning, the Institute held social functions to help the public understand the significance of its work. The point was not lost on a Brisbane businessman, Mr Bill Siganto, who donated $1 million in 2003 for prostate cancer research.[18] The next step in the search for a vaccine was a dendritic cell purification process which involved removing cells from a cancer patient, manipulating them to trigger an immune response to kill cancer cells, before returning the cells to the patient. Late in 2004, the Institute was ready to start its first clinical trials in dendritic cell immunotherapy for prostate cancer, with high hopes that immunotherapy could also be applied to multiple myeloma, melanoma and breast cancer. Work was also extending to include diabetes, and to a new approach to organ transplantation using the discovery that dendritic cells precipitate rejection of transplanted kidneys. A centre for innovative pathology was developed with the aim of applying cell biology advances to diagnosis. From its first days in 1999, the Institute fostered collaboration with universities to provide the opportunity for students to complete honours and master's degrees, and doctoral theses. In 2004, the MMRI's first 'home-grown' PhD was awarded to Dr Chris Ho; eleven other doctoral projects were progressing.[19]

In the twenty-first century, research institutes have to be highly effective business organisations, with strong accountable management, innovative commercial strategies and effective public relations. Under its chief of operations, David Wood, the MMRI worked hard to develop its financial resources. As well as important commercial collaborations with companies such as Pfizer, Becton Dickinson and Britannic Pharmaceuticals, and research grants from numerous organisations such as the Australian National Health and Medical

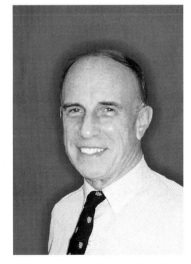

Professor Brian Hills, leader of the surfactant research team at the MMRI. MATER MEDICAL RESEARCH INSTITUTE

Research Council, the Queensland Cancer Fund, the United States National Institute of Health and the United States Army, it also developed its direct fundraising; Lord Spencer's signed eulogy for his sister, Diana, Princess of Wales, was auctioned at the Institute's annual dinner in 2004. By 2004, $10 million had been contributed by the state government from the Smart State Research Facilities Fund for imaging equipment and a further $3 million for other equipment; commercial partnerships contributed $2.6 million.[20]

The complexity of a research organisation of this kind needs careful shepherding. Living on the edge of knowledge and pushing forward is, like much in the Mater's history, a risky undertaking. It cannot work unless scientists feel valued and acknowledged, it cannot grow unless scientists appreciate the efforts of fundraisers and budget jugglers, it cannot progress unless new minds are inspired and taught, and it cannot feel satisfaction until its ideas become diagnosis and treatment realities. A 'warts and all review' was conducted in 2002 by Dr G F Mitchell, one of Australia's leading biological scientists, and Professor David Penington, well known for his work on AIDS. As is the case with all such examinations, the reviewers noted good points, identified areas which needed improvement and provided guidance for future development.[21] Professor Hart's strong scientific leadership, the teamwork and the research focus were all assets, according to the review, but there was a cautionary note: senior Mater staff needed the freedom to establish their own recognisable scientific reputations in order to attract grant support; and unless all researchers could establish themselves as creative, accomplished researchers, others might be dissuaded from joining the staff, limiting the potential for exciting new ventures; it was also necessary to create formal structures within the Mater hospitals to facilitate research activities across the complex so that research could be integrated with clinical practice.[22]

The reviewers also recommended incorporation to create an appropriate business model and to provide administrative independence from the Sisters of Mercy. The accountability of an incorporated organisation, would, they thought, enhance access to funding in a competitive climate where all Australian governments had identified biotechnology as a growth sector, and it would also remove some of the complexity from the management of intellectual property and the commercialisation of discoveries. Strategic partnerships would become increasingly necessary, the reviewers said, but industry in the pharmaceutical and biotechnology sectors preferred dealing directly with research providers as the owners of technology. All the risks of managing, securing, mobilising and exploiting patents would then be borne by the MMRI and not by either the Mater or the Sisters of Mercy. Incorporation would also provide an appropriate means of managing the inevitable scientific risk and, by differentiating the MMRI from the far broader mission of the hospitals, would facilitate the recruitment of top scientists. In its turn, it was hoped that the MMRI would become a better conduit bringing outstanding people into the hospital family. On the other hand, the reviewers warned that cautious souls would fear that incorporation could mean that the Institute could follow its own direction, without reference to either the Mercy mission or the values and interests of the hospitals. However, a 'tiered' structure, similar to the constitution of Mater Health Services Ltd, was suggested to protect the Sisters' and the Mater's large investments and to ensure that Mater values remained part of the MMRI.

These were big issues for the Institute council, chaired by Justice Martin Moynihan, with a team of eminent specialists: Andrew Greenwood, an intellectual property lawyer, the stockbroker Peter Evans, the mining company executive Brian Flannery, the nephrologist and long-term Mater board member Dr John Burke, the cytogeneticist and ethicist Sister Regis Mary Dunne, Professor John Mattick, Director of the Institute of Molecular Biosciences at the University of Queensland, Professor Peter Brooks, Executive Dean of Health Sciences at the University of Queensland, John McAuliffe, Mater Health Services chairman, the Institute's director, Professor Derek Hart, and Dr John O'Donnell, chief executive of Mater Health Services. Much would depend on strengthening links and nurturing trust between the Institute and the Mater administration, between researchers and clinicians, between Institute researchers and those in the Mater hospitals.

At the Adult Hospital in 2003, for example, Dr Kerry Taylor and Dr Robyn Rodwell were managing clinical trials of Glivec, which targets the molecular abnormality in chronic myeloid leukaemia cells, and by 2004 they were supervising bone marrow transplants as a day care service.[23] This was all part of the steady development of the clinical services at the Mater. Early in the new century, the Mater Mothers' initiated a direct link with St Joseph's hospital in Tampa, Florida, the base of the internationally renowned fetal surgeon, Dr Ruben Quintero.[24] This facilitated the development in 2003 of a treatment using intra-uterine laser surgery for twin-twin transfusion syndrome, a condition suffered only by identical twins where blood flows from one twin to the other through connected placental blood vessels, imperilling them both. The treatment was proclaimed in large posters with the telling epithet: 'These twins will have life-saving surgery. Then, they'll be born'.[25] In another respect, however, the development of maternal fetal medicine at the Mater was a reminder that difficult ethical questions would always be raised by scientific and technological advances: diagnosis of a serious fetal abnormality in the first trimester of a pregnancy could not, at the Mater, be regarded as a reason to terminate the pregnancy, unless the mother's life was threatened.

Outreach and partnerships continued to characterise many developments at the Mater. The pharmacy, for instance, looked outside the hospital and investigated a pharmacokinetic research centre partnership with Baxter pharmaceuticals.[26] At the Mater Children's, the cranio-facial 'Operation Smile' team planned an expedition to India early in 2005 to organise treatment for 150 children and develop training programs for local doctors and nurses.[27] Closer to home, the treatment of alcohol dependence in teenagers grew into the Queensland-wide Adolescent Drug and Alcohol Withdrawal Service (ADAWS) in 2003.[28] The website, Kids In Mind, was developed as Queensland's first interactive site for young people concerned about their mental health, a development of the Mater's Child and Youth Mental Health Service. In 2003, the mobile outreach service for health provided by integrated teams (MOSH PIT) continued help for homeless people in inner Brisbane, often visiting Musgrave Park, a traditional gathering place for Brisbane's Aboriginal community.

The Mercy values emphasised at the Mater during the 1990s found expression in addressing a new community need in the early twenty-first century. Hundreds of refugees came to Queensland from war zones and poverty-stricken regions on the other side of the world; many were sufficiently desperate to undertake the journey in defective ships run by people smugglers, and found themselves living in Brisbane on temporary visas which denied them full access to mainstream health services. In 2002, the Queensland Integrated Refugee Community Health Service, QIRCH (coordinated by the Community Liaison Section led by Kate Ramsay) was opened in a ceremony which included celebrants from the Hindu and Muslim faiths, as well as Christian denominations. Relationships already forged with general practitioners and community health services were particularly important, with many health professionals giving their time voluntarily to care for refugee patients.

New services and growing research opportunities were vital parts of the 'new look' Mater, which was also undergoing a physical renaissance. A new dimension to older government 'partnership' models was added when Queensland adopted from the southern states the idea of co-locating private hospitals with public hospitals, a feat the Mater had been managing for decades. The relationship between the Mater and the government was unique in Queensland, unlike New South Wales and Victoria where more privately owned hospitals were funded to provide public hospital services. Thus, in the Queensland health sector, the Mater was a pioneer of the 'Public Private Partnership' concept, developed more strongly by the Queensland government in the early 2000s. This policy development offered the Mater enticing opportunities to expand beyond South Brisbane. In 1996, the possibility of forging a partnership with the Rockhampton Mater to develop a private hospital on the Gladstone state hospital site was explored and discarded; in 1997, the idea of developing and managing a new public hospital at either Noosa, north of Brisbane, or Robina, to Brisbane's south, was researched, but there was too much uncertainty in the Queensland Health position; a proposal for the Caboolture hospital was briefly considered.[29]

The burgeoning growth area, Redland Bay, seemed a better fit with existing Mater services. Late in 1997, the Mater heard that it and the Wesley Hospital were on the shortlist for the Redland Shire development. In mid-1998, the Mater was the preferred tenderer and, in addition, was asked to consider managing obstetric services at the new Redlands public hospital.[30] By October 1998, with the ANZ bank continuing its traditional financial support, the Mater was ready to build its new fifty-bed private hospital to provide medical, surgical and obstetric services, at a cost of more than $20 million. Construction began during 1999 and the new low-rise hospital, the seventh child in the Mater family, tucked into its own corner of the Redlands public hospital site, was ready for its first patients in 2000, complete with light, airy wards, beautifully landscaped gardens, an elegant chapel and a cheerful coffee shop.[31]

Mater Redlands had also incorporated private radiology and pathology services. The Mater Private in Brisbane had developed similar services more than twenty years earlier, and, when the new Private Hospital was built in the early 1990s, suites for a range of specialists were constructed in an adjacent building. For the first few years, the medical suites seemed unable to attract sufficient numbers of doctors willing to buy their own consulting rooms. However, it wasn't long before space was at a premium and the decision to provide more suites and ancillary day surgery facilities had to be considered. The surgeon Dr Danny Lane had suggested providing specialists' rooms to Mother Damian decades earlier. The convenience of location close to the Private Hospital would, he thought, also encourage specialists in private practice to maintain visiting appointments to the Mater public hospitals.[32]

While doctors usually established their rooms near major hospitals, as in Macquarie Street in Sydney, directly opposite the Sydney Hospital, specialists' rooms in Wickham Terrace in Brisbane were some distance from the major hospitals. In addition, Dr Lane pointed out in 1957, the growing Australian suburban sprawl would mean that new public hospitals would be located outside the inner cities. Doctors' rooms located in the outer suburbs would be further from the centre of medical developments because the most up-to-date diagnostic infrastructure was likely to remain in the long-established public hospitals. The Royal Prince Alfred medical centre in Sydney was a pertinent example of this principle. Patients and specialists wasted less time travelling from place to place, and the hospital had specialists on hand at all times.

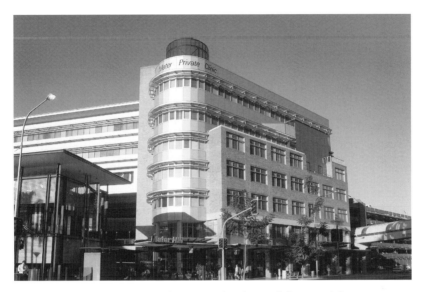

The Mater Private Clinic in Stanley Street showing, at left, part of the structure of the busway which provides rapid bus transport to and from the city. MATER PUBLIC RELATIONS AND MARKETING

Dr Lane's prescience was borne out by his remark that centralisation of expensive diagnostic and therapeutic services would be inevitable. Construction of the Mater Private Clinic, linked to both the Private Hospital and the main campus, went ahead in 1999. The Mater Private continued to develop its prominence in surgery, and by 2005 the tenth operating theatre had been opened. New teleconferencing technology allowed local surgeons to communicate with international specialists working in any teleconferencing venue in the world. Orthopaedics remained a prominent specialty. New trials of evidence-based clinical pathways and linkages to support services for orthopaedic patients enabled the Private Hospital to reduce patients' length of stay for total hip- and knee-replacement surgery.[33] This trend, if extended to all surgical procedures, would appeal to the private health funds, as well as benefiting patients through shorter hospital stays and enabling the Mater Private to admit more patients.

The Mater public hospitals benefited from the Queensland government's announcement in 1991 of a $1.5 billion capital investment plan for health over ten years, including funding for master planning for every metropolitan public hospital as part of a three-part program of asset review, functional assessment, and master planning. The Mater grasped this opportunity with relish, and, having decided not to move the Children's Hospital to Logan City in the 1990s, believed that an entirely new Children's Hospital should be built closer to the Adult and Mothers' hospitals.[34] Integration was to be expressed in the Mater's physical fabric, as well as in outpatient-inpatient services, and the research-clinical-teaching relationship. This became a time for thinking big, taking risks, living on the financial edge, negotiating with government – indeed all the features that had characterised each phase of the Mater's development: building the first two hospitals in the early years of the century, building the Children's Hospital during the Depression, building the Mothers' Hospital without money in the bank, playing hard-ball with government to build the new Adult Hospital.

The Sisters wanted to move the Children's Hospital from one side of the campus into an entirely new building on the opposite side, and to refurbish the Mothers' Hospital, which was really beginning to show the strain of forty hard-working years. Government was prepared to provide $50 million for the new Children's Hospital, but some $85 million for the rest of the construction program – the new private clinic, the Redlands Hospital, moving the Children's and Mothers' private hospitals – would have to be found by the Sisters and the Mater. Somewhat audaciously, the Mater hoped to persuade government to find many more millions to redevelop the Mothers' rather than merely renovate it. The $85 million from Mater funds included $15 million for property acquisition, provision of twenty-five private beds in the Children's Hospital, foyer retail outlets in Stanley Street and a bridge across Stanley Street to the Private Hospital.[35] This $15 million was to be found in existing reserves and borrowings repaid over a decade from the income generated by the new facilities. Expansion at the Private Hospital and the new medical centre proceeded only when it was almost certain that these facilities would generate sufficient income to service substantial borrowings.[36]

These seemed enormous sums, but there were substantial disadvantages in taking a cautious approach. If the Children's Hospital were to remain on its existing site, the inefficient separation from the

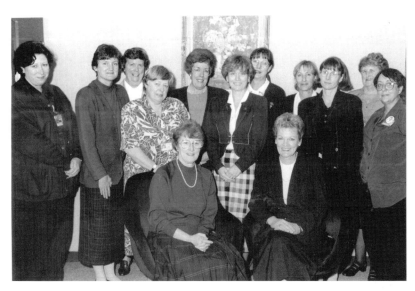

On her way to a new job – managing the move from the original Mater Children's Hospital to the new hospital – Mrs Rosalie Lewis (seated at left) is farewelled on her retirement as Director of Nursing, Mater Children's Hospital, by Pat Snowden, Director of Nursing, Mater Private Hospital (seated at right) and standing from left, Deborah Tanham, Linda Bogner, Sister Denise Downey, RSM, Karleen O'Reilly, Vivienne Devine, Margaret Fleck, Annette Wilcox, Margaret Smith, Fiona Brewin-Brown, Jeanne Kentish, Barbara Bryan. MHHC

Mothers' Hospital would remain, opportunities to integrate expensive services would be limited, and there would be a major decanting of paediatric services during any redevelopment of the Children's Hospital on its original site. In contrast, the advantages of co-locating the Adult, Children's and Mothers' hospitals would provide ease of patient access to all services, a physical link to the Queensland Radium Institute in Raymond Terrace, a central core of ambulatory care areas, and maximum sharing of operating theatre, intensive care and emergency facilities. This plan would also generate the greatest recurrent cost savings, through improved efficiencies, and be adaptable to future change.[37] This was an important point; changes in hospital care, such as mobilising patients very soon after surgery or childbirth, treating major medical conditions and many surgical procedures as day care services and keeping patients in hospital for as short a time as possible, had been so rapid and dramatic that older hospital designs were simply unsuitable, even in relatively recently constructed hospitals. If hospital planners and administrators, clinicians and researchers had learnt anything, they had learnt that the future was largely unpredictable.

There was more certainty in predictions of future growth in demand for Mater services. The population of Brisbane South was predicted to grow by 25.6 per cent by the Mater's centenary year, 2006. This would increase demands on the Adult Hospital by 25 per cent, on the Children's by 23 per cent, while demands on the Mothers' was likely to remain similar in quantity, but greatly increased in complexity.

Once decisions had been made, and all had recovered from an alarming moment in 1996, when it appeared that the new Children's Hospital had been deleted from the government's hospital redevelopment list, the new Mater Children's Hospital appeared remarkably quickly.[38] Although all new hospitals follow the modernist principle of form following function, the new Mater Children's, with its external façade designed to reflect the essence of Queensland – blue skies and brown land, sparkling seas and tranquil creeks – began to look entirely different from the new Royal Children's Hospital at Herston. From the beginning, it was to be family focused; all the extensive consultation with parents and the medical and nursing staff, both past and present, listed families as the priority. Parents, siblings and grandparents were to be given the greatest possible access, even to the sickest children. Overnight accommodation was provided for parents in every ward and single room, there were parent lounges with refreshments on tap, special relaxation areas for teenagers, indoor and outdoor play areas for younger children, oxygen and suction facilities on sunny balconies, ample space for visiting performers, and colour, bright colour, everywhere. Ceramic tiles designed by children were installed on many walls; windows and service counters were built at child height; the chapel was designed to be welcoming to children; and in 2003 a bright, light-hearted animal mural on a corridor wall led children from ward areas to play spaces.

Seriously ill children, particularly those who needed long periods of hospitalisation, were always a high priority. Efficiencies, such as fast and easy access from the emergency centre to the radiology department and operating theatres, and technologies, such as the latest in intensive care treatment technologies, did not mean that the environment for seriously ill children was all clinical sterility. Comfort was extremely important. The new Children's Hospital became the first Queensland children's hospital with a Starlight Room contributed by the Starlight Foundation, supported by the Australian tennis champion Pat Rafter. It was not long before the Starlight Room had touched 160,000 children.[39] Familiar features followed the patients to the new hospital – the Red Cross play scheme, Radio Lollipop, and education in a brand new school. Many old deficiencies were rectified. Separate areas where rosters were arranged so that young patients could be treated by familiar staff were provided for paediatric mental health patients and long-term cancer patients. Old traditions were not forgotten – a large mosaic was designed to emphasise healing and to unite the new hospital with the Mercy mission. The opening in 2001 was celebrated with a symbolic procession from the old hospital to the new. The new hospital rapidly became extremely busy: by 2004 it had cared for 15,000 inpatients, 120,000 outpatients and 25,000 children in the emergency department.

The Mater Mothers', with its overhead link to the new Children's Hospital, was looking very tired. It had exhausted its capacity to increase its services even though the New Life Centre extension, opened in 1991, had offered some relief. The Mater Mothers' had become Australia's busiest maternity hospital,[40] and was well on the way to recording an extraordinary statistic: in 2004, when the 250,000th Mater baby was born, one in six people living in Queensland had been born at the Mater Mothers'.[41] More and more at-risk pregnant women and pre-term babies were transferred to the Mothers' from other hospitals; in the early years of the new century, the Mater Mothers' was managing two out of three neonatal retrievals in Queensland.[42] Somehow, with the nurseries often more than 100 per cent occupied, the hospital's neonatal survival figures still equalled those of other centres of excellence. A great deal more than patching, mending and making do would be needed to keep up with demand, let alone maintain the Mothers' international reputation. However, the Mater had come a long way since the days when Queensland governments provided capital funding very reluctantly. During the 2004 Queensland state election campaign, the Queensland premier, Peter

Beattie, visited Mater Hill to announce that, if re-elected, the government would fund the new Mothers' public hospital.

The government was returned, and planning revved into top gear, and included plans to modernise the Adult Hospital, which was more than twenty years old. The planning team proceeded rapidly, led by the former Children's hospital physiotherapist and former director of mission and ethics, Dr John Gilmour, and Sister Michaeleen Mary, RSM, who had coordinated planning for the new Private and Children's Hospitals. Extensive consultation began to refine the layout and facilities. The new Mother's Hospital, linked directly to the Adult and Children's hospitals, would be an eight-storey building with concrete piers raising much of it above the ground, and would be reminiscent of a Queensland 'house on stilts' shaded by the huge Moreton Bay figs, a treasured feature in the Mater landscape.

Linkages, in modern health parlance, refer to cleverly integrated core services for several large hospitals, and to new methods of care maintained alongside older modes. At the Mater, linkages are also historical. As the Mater's first century draws to a close, continuing the Sisters of Mercy mission has been emphasised even more strongly: Mercy Week continues to be celebrated in September each year, senior executives participate in pilgrimages to Baggot Street, Dublin, where it all began, and the chief executive, Dr John O'Donnell, reminds all staff that:

> . . . continuing the Mission of the Sisters must be the foundation of all we do. Our Mission must be part of every process, policy and practice. This expectation relates not just to compassionate encounters with our patients, but extends into ensuring all staff know and understand the Mater Mission. We should all know the story of the Mercies in Brisbane; we should know Catherine McAuley, and we should know and experience a living culture within the Mater which expresses the values by which the Sisters live – without exception.[43]

Although business planning takes a hard-nosed approach to reduce the debt on public hospital services,[44] the Mater continues to maintain and develop services funded from its own resources or in partnership with universities and community organisation, because responding to need is a core Mercy value. These essential 'extras' include community support such as care for AIDS patients, immunisations and check-ups for homeless people and the Mater Child Youth and Mental Health Services which operate from suburban offices, outreach services such as Operation Smile and the refugee health service, innovative care such as maternal fetal medicine and the cord blood bank, as well as services such as the pastoral care team, which more obviously reinforce Mater values.

As the fundraisers gear up for yet another mammoth effort to pay for all the extras needed to put the final touches to the new Mater Mothers', the entrance to the new Mothers' building is planned for a shady space directly in front of the entrance to Aubigny, the first hospital on the Mater site. Indeed, the Mater's whole history can be read in the Mater Hill campus. The Baggot Street drive commemorates the original Mercy house in Dublin, and the first hospital across the river is commemorated in Aubigny Place, the name of the first hospital on Mater Hill. The first three hospitals, testaments to the 'waste not, want not' aphorism, are alive with new functions – administration, research and education in the original Private Hospital, clinics and meeting spaces in the first Adult Hospital, community services in the first Children's Hospital. At the beginning of the Mater's second century, many more babies will be born in the first Mater Mothers', soon to be replaced by the new Mothers' Hospital rising nearby.

In endings, there are many new beginnings.

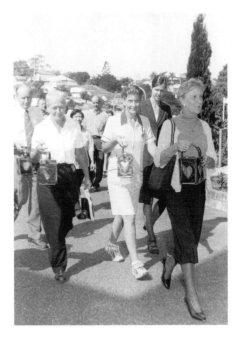

A procession of Mater people, each with a golden lantern, led the way from the old Mater Children's Hospital to the new, in time for its opening in May 2001. MHHC

ENDING THE BEGINNING

Late in 2005 in the final weeks of the Brisbane Mater's 100th year, while a chef checks that all the vegetables on the hundreds of plates about to leave her kitchen are fresh and enticing . . .

- the CEO drafts a letter to the Health Minister
- a helicopter clatters in with a very ill tiny baby from far south-western Queensland
- a plumber from engineering services sets out to vanquish an irritating knock in a water pipe
- a young registered nurse at the Adult Hospital devises a care plan for a disabled elderly patient who wants to go home
- the executive director at the Mater Foundation refines his approach to a major corporation
- a security officer raises the boom gate for a Board member's car
- a medical student feverishly searches her mind for the answer to a question about chemotherapy
- the children in the hospital school practise Christmas songs
- a farmer feels almost amused that his long-awaited bone marrow transplant has arrived in a small plastic bag
- several surgeons scrub for surgery on a little boy from the Philippines with a malformed face
- an administrative assistant searches for that last address for an invitee to an important function

- a woman at Mater Redlands blinks into consciousness without her troublesome gall bladder
- an ambulance brings a woman with chest pain to the Mater Adult Hospital in South Brisbane
- the Holy Cross laundry truck trundles to the service entry
- a speech pathologist watches a three-year-old's face as he hears for the very first time
- a teenager discusses her love for hamburgers with the nutritionist at the diabetic clinic
- financial officers scrutinise the latest budget forecast
- a volunteer 'cuddlema' rhythmically pats a restless baby at the Mother's Hospital
- a doctor at the specialist centre tries to keep pace with the patients arriving in the waiting room
- a planner struggles to fit yet another service into the community services building
- a radiologist is reading a worrying scan
- the Mater Redevelopment Project reviews submissions for space against the plans for the new Mothers' Hospital
- a Rugby international is wheeled to the theatre at the Private Hospital for his knee reconstruction
- a young scientist at the MMRI rubs her glasses and prepares to start again
- an Imam contacts the Refugee Health Service about a new Afghani family . . .

. . . the Sisters at lunchtime Mass in the chapel pray for them all.

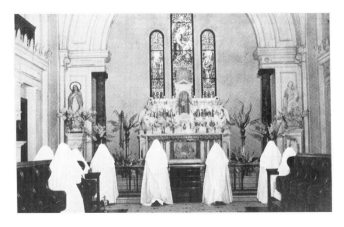

ACKNOWLEDGMENTS

Every aspect of researching and writing the history of Brisbane's Mater hospitals has been an exhilarating experience. I am extremely grateful that Mater Health Services Ltd, the modern corporate entity encompassing the seven Mater hospitals, established this project with foresight and more than a little courage. There was plenty of time: the project was commissioned in October 2002 with the stipulation that a final draft be ready for submission to University of Queensland Press in January 2005. This generous allocation of time for large projects is essential to ensure that research can be thorough, interpretation carefully considered, and drafts revised adequately.

The Chairman of Mater Health Services, Mr John McAuliffe, and the chief executive officer, Dr John O'Donnell, never flagged in their support or in their enthusiasm for the project. Dr O'Donnell's perceptive criticisms of the draft, based on his broad experience of medicine and hospital administration, and the doors and drawers he opened for me were invaluable. Mrs Christa Henry, Dr O'Donnell's secretary, was splendid in her cheerful and prompt support, organising mountains of photocopying and arranging numerous meetings and interviews.

The project Steering Committee was established with excellent representation of the skills and experience necessary to supervise a project of this kind. I thank Dr Grace Croft, the project manager who chaired the Steering Committee, Sister Angela Mary Doyle, former Sister Administrator, Sister Madonna Josey, former Director of Nursing at the Mater Adult Hospital, Mr Pat Maguire, former Chief Executive Officer, Mr Bill Concannon of Mary Ryan Books, Dr Neil Carrington, the Mater's first director of education, and Mr Nigel Harris, Executive Director of the Mater Foundation. It was a pleasure to report to them and discuss the various issues in research and interpretation which inevitably arise; all scrutinised the drafts with perception and shared willingly their vast knowledge of the Mater. They were professional to the very end, offering constructive criticism and ideas, but never interfering or insisting that something be included or deleted. Sister Angela Mary and Mr Pat Maguire devoted many extra hours to answering numerous questions and contributing their memories and reflections. I appreciate their support and friendship greatly.

The oral history project conducted by Dr Grace Croft and Ms Rosalie Lewis with many Sisters of Mercy provided essential information and insight. I am very grateful to them, and to the participants, Sisters M. Collette Anderson, Norah Boland, Kath Burke, Pauline Burke, Ursula Byrne, Carmen Coffey, Catherine Courtney, Josephine Crawford, Gwen Doan, Regis Mary Dunne, Marie Fitzgerald, Etienne Flynn, Deirdre Gardiner, Germaine Greathead, Loyce Gordon, Anne Hetherington, Flora Heany, Catherine Heffernan, Brigid Hirschfeld, Claire Irving, Mary C Johnson, Win Johnson, Madonna Josey, Margaret Kanowski, Margaret Mary King, Patricia Kirchener, Mary Denise Lanigan, Mary Lawson, Sandra Loth, Sandra Lupi, Camillus Mary Lynch, Anne McDonnell, Fay McMeniman, Patrice Nally, Mary Francesco O'Brien, Anne O'Farrell, M Cephas Philben, Patricia Plint, Eileen Pollard, Clo Quinlan, Patricia Reordan, Marie Therese Rosenberg, Margarita Shannon, Susan Smith, Peg Slack, Monica Stallard, Helen Stanley, Caroline Steiner, Jill Stringer, Jacinta Weidmann and Ruth Wyatt.

Any history relies greatly on archival sources. Sister Josephine Crawford, manager of the Mater Archives since 1987, willingly contributed her extensive knowledge of the Mater and its people, as well as opening all the records in her charge. The morning teas she provided for a sometimes weary researcher were, as was all she did, received with great appreciation, as was the support of Sister Regis

Mary Dunne and Sister Loyce Gordon when Sister Josephine was away.

Researching in the Sisters of Mercy Congregation Archives at Bardon was a pleasure: Sister Germaine Greathead, Sister Helen Mary Perrott and Sister Kay Lane allowed free rein to the important records in their charge, answered endless questions and searched valiantly for necessary details. The conversations and laughter I shared with other members of the Congregation and the staff at Bardon enlivened many days.

New staff frequently comment that the Mater is a friendly, welcoming place: I share this view. Wherever and whenever I roamed through wards and departments, I was inevitably greeted with a smile. So many people answered questions, opened their records, shared their photographs and responded to emails and telephone calls, often more than once, that it is impossible to name them all. However, I would like to thank individually: Sister Michaeleen Mary Ahern, Vicki Adams, Professor John Bell, Dr John Burke, Dr Steve Costello, Sister Catharine Courtney, Professor Derek Hart, Ms Vicki Franklin, Dr John Gilmour, Dr John Hinds, Dr Jenny King, Mr Norbert Konecki, Sister Marcia Maranta, Ms Sharon Mickan, Mr Frank Pollard, Ms Kate Ramsay, Mrs Pat Snowden, Dr John Thearle, Mr Chris Townend, Dr David Tudehope and Mr Mark Young.

Professional scrutiny is extremely important when any history is written under contract. Dr Ross Johnston, a 'guru' of Queensland history recently retired from the University of Queensland, read drafts and identified issues requiring resolution and questions needing answers. Jane Greenwood's careful attention to matters of expression and writing style immensely improved the drafts. They both have my profound appreciation. Felicity McKenzie, my University of Queensland Press editor, performed her task with grace, perception and insight. Her help was valuable.

Dr Grace Croft, the project manager, has a very special place in this project. After decades in nursing and nursing research, she gave up a huge amount of time in her 'retirement' to support this project. She was immensely supportive until the last moment, meticulously scrutinising every detail. I doubt she will ever really know how grateful I am.

An historian usually feels relieved when a large project of this kind is finished and the proofs returned. This time I feel sad: being trusted with writing the history of Brisbane's Mater hospitals has been a profound privilege and a great pleasure.

Helen Gregory
Brisbane, May 2005

NOTE ON SOURCES

Any history of a complex human institution provides a rich lode for the historian. There are many ways a century in the life of a hospital could be interpreted and written: it could be a history of medical practice in the hospital setting; it could be a history of patients and their ailments; or it could be a broad-brush approach which sets the history of the hospital in the context of the times it has passed through. This history of the Mater hospitals takes the third of these possible approaches, with a focus on the special nature of the Mater as it evolved into seven separate, but integrated, hospitals.

There is, therefore, an exploration of the Brisbane Congregation of the Sisters of Mercy from its establishment in the 1860s, through the Sisters' decision to build the hospitals, the pressures which influenced later developments, and the Sisters' gradual withdrawal from hospital management. In Queensland, with its traditional state dominance of public hospital services, the existence of three Mater public hospitals for, respectively, adults, children and mothers and babies has consistently challenged state policy. Interaction between the Mater and the state is, therefore, an important theme. Since the Second World War, the role of the Commonwealth government in health policy and funding has grown considerably, which, in the Mater's case, has set up some interesting tensions with state policy. Funding is a critical issue both in the Mater's relationship with the state and in accommodating patients' and doctors' needs for the latest in technologies. Co-location of public and private hospitals on single sites has become prominent in government health systems in recent decades: the Mater has been managing a co-located system since 1911, a factor which requires consideration of the management of the four Mater private hospitals and their ancillary facilities. The Mater was established to service Brisbane's southern suburbs: the development of this part of the city weaves its way through various eras in the Mater's history.

Sources for this type of social history of the development of a hospital system were, inevitably, rich for some periods and somewhat sparse for others. Each chapter contains comprehensive references to the sources. The core sources were the minutes of successive Mater Boards, records of the building of the hospitals, and medical developments and biographical records of staff, both Religious and lay, held in the Mater History and Heritage Centre. The Sisters of Mercy Congregational Archives at the Congregational centre at Bardon provide valuable material on the Congregational perspective on the Mater, which was only part of a broad mission that included numerous schools and diverse social works. Records of Cabinet discussions at various periods in the Mater's history and government departmental records at the Queensland State Archives were valuable aids to explanation. The oral history program with many Sisters of Mercy, conducted by Dr Grace Croft and Mrs Rosalie Lewis, provided important insights from the Sisters' points of view. Hospital histories and the history of state health services generally is not a highly developed genre in Australia. The first histories of the Mater, Harry Summers' *They crossed the river. The founding of the Mater Misericordiae hospital by the Sisters of Mercy* (Brisbane, University of Queensland Press, 1979) and Robert Longhurst's *A history of nursing at the Mater Misericordiae hospitals, Brisbane* (Brisbane, Mater Misericordiae Hospital, 1992), were important starting points. Anthea Hyslop's *Sovereign remedies. A history of Ballarat base hospital 1850s to 1980s* (Sydney, Allen & Unwin, 1989) and Bryan Egan's *Ways of a hospital. St Vincent's Melbourne 1890s to 1990s* (Sydney, Allen & Unwin, 1993) are two of the more modern Australian hospital histories which were particularly helpful; others are documented in the endnotes, as are relevant histories of Australian health policy and medical developments. This history of the Mater hospitals is only a start; much more can be done to flesh out the histories of individual Mater hospitals and departments within them. The ending of this century of the Mater's life should be seen as just one stage.

ENDNOTES

ABBREVIATIONS

MHHC   Mater History and Heritage Centre, Mater Health Services, South Brisbane

RSM   Religious Sister of Mercy

QSA   Queensland State Archives

SOMCA   Sisters of Mercy Congregational Archives, Bardon, Brisbane

PART 1
GETTING ESTABLISHED

1. BEGINNING A 'BIG WORK'

1   D W Martin, *The foundation of the Catholic Church in Queensland*, Toowoomba, Church Archivists Society, 1988, pp. 1–12. Polding's mission to the Aborigines, staffed by Passionist fathers, did not succeed.

2   For background on this period, see W Ross Johnston, *Brisbane. The first thirty years*, Brisbane, Boolarong, 1933; P Statham, ed., *The foundation of the Australian capital cities*, Cambridge, Cambridge University Press, 1989; G Greenwood and J R Laverty, *Brisbane 1859–1959*, Brisbane, Ziegler, 1959; W Ross Johnston, *The call of the land. A history of Queensland to the present day*, Brisbane, UQP, 1983.

3   See J D Lang, *Cooksland in north-eastern Australia: the future cottonfield of*

Great Britain: its characteristics and capabilities for European colonization, with a disquisition of the origin, manner and customs of the aborigines, London, Longmans, 1847, for an account of Lang's vision for the region; J Mackenzie Smith, *Moreton Bay Scots 1841–59*, Toowoomba, Church Archivists' Press, 2000.

4   *Daily Guardian*, 25 September 1963, p. 2.

5   The *Benevolent Asylums Wards Act 1861* and the *Hospitals Act 1862*. See P R Patrick, *A history of health and medicine in Queensland 1824–1960*, Brisbane, UQP, 1987, p. 45.

6   *Moreton Bay Courier*, 6 May 1848.

7   C K Killerby, *Ursula Frayne. A biography*, Perth, University of Notre Dame, 1996, pp. 172, 239.

8   M B Degnan, *Mercy unto thousands*, Dublin, Browne and Nolan, 1958, pp. 20, 25–7.

9   For background on Ireland in this period, see A Jackson, *Ireland 1798–1998*, Oxford, Blackwell, 1999; R Dudley Edwards, *Daniel O'Connell and his world*, London, Thames and Hudson, 1975; R B McDowell, *Public opinion and government policy in Ireland, 1801–1846*, Studies in Irish History, vol. 5, London, Faber and Faber, 1952; N Davis, *The Isles. A history*, London, Macmillan, 1999.

10   Degnan, *Mercy unto thousands*, p. 54.

11   Degnan, *Mercy unto thousands*, p. 92.

12   Degnan, *Mercy unto thousands*, p. 117.

13   Degnan, *Mercy unto thousands*, p. 54; R Longhurst, *In the footsteps of the Mercies. A history of nursing at the Mater Misericordiae public hospitals, Brisbane*, Brisbane, Mater Misericordiae Hospitals, 1992, pp. 15–17; B Abel Smith, *The hospitals 1800–1948*, London, Heinemann, 1964.

14   M X O'Donoghue, *Mother Vincent Whitty. Woman and educator in a masculine society*, Melbourne, MUP, 1972, p. 10.

15   William Howard Russell in the *Times,* quoted in E Bolster, *The Sisters of Mercy in the Crimean War*, Cork, Mercier, 1964, p. 11.

16   Quoted in Bolster, *The Sisters of Mercy in the Crimean War*, p. 29.

17   Mother Vincent to Reverend Mother, 14 July 1860, 15 November 1860, Sisters of Mercy, *Mercy women making history from the pen of Mother Vincent Whitty*, Brisbane, Congregation of the Sisters of Mercy, 2001, p. 1.

18   E M O'Donoghue, 'Ellen Whitty', *Australian dictionary of biography*, vol. 6, Melbourne, MUP, 1976, pp. 394–5.

19   Mother Vincent to Rev. Mother, 22 November 1860, in *Mercy women making history*, p. 22.

20   Mother Vincent to Sr M. Joseph in Hull, 24 March 1841, in *Mercy women making history*, p. 19.

21   Mother Vincent to Rev. Mother, 13 May 1861, in *Mercy women making history*, p. 25.

22   For example, *Moreton Bay Courier*, 20 May 1848; C A C Leggett, 'The social significance of the Brisbane hospital' in *Brisbane retrospect. Eight aspects of Brisbane history*, Brisbane, Library Board of Queensland, 1978; J H Tyrer, *History of the Brisbane Hospital and its affiliates. A pilgrim's progress*, Brisbane, Boolarong, 1993, pp. 51–3.

23   Mother Vincent to Rev. Mother, 18 September 1863, in *Mercy women making history*, p. 66.

24   Mother Vincent to Rev. Mother, 19 July 1863, in *Mercy women making history*, pp. 62, 81.

25   Mother Vincent to Rev. Mother, 17 June 1863, in *Mercy women making history*, p. 54.

26   Mother Vincent to Rev. Mother, 18 July 1863, in *Mercy women making history*, p. 66.

27   E Campion, *Australian Catholics*, Melbourne, Penguin, 1985, p. 44.

28   M X O'Donoghue, *Mother Vincent Whitty*, pp. 85, 86, 94.

29   J M Mahoney, *Dieu et Devoir*, Brisbane, Boolarong, 1985, p. 14; M X O'Donoghue, *Mother Vincent Whitty*, p. 34.

30   Mother Vincent to Rev. Mother, 19 October 1863, in *Mercy women making history*, p. 72.

31   Florence O'Reilly to Mother Vincent, 21 February 1871, Florence O'Reilly information, box 87, Florence O'Reilly, Sisters of Mercy Congregational Archives [SOMCA].

32   Florence O'Reilly to Mother Vincent, 28 January 1872, Florence O'Reilly information, box 87, Florence O'Reilly, SOMCA.

33   B Crouchley, 'George Wilkie Gray', *Australian dictionary of biography*, vol. 9, Melbourne, MUP, 1983, pp. 84–5. Gray persuaded the government to extend scholarship benefits to Catholic schoolchildren so they could enjoy the same subsidy for secondary education as state school children.

34   Mother Vincent to Bishop Quinn, 10 October 1880, in *Mercy women making history*, p. 106.

35   O'Donoghue, *Mercy unto thousands*, p. 99; *Mercy women making history*, p. 89; box 87, Florence O'Reilly, SOMCA.

36   N J Byrne, *Robert Dunne, 1830–1917. Archbishop of Brisbane*, Brisbane,

UQP, 1991, p. 43, pp. 66–7, 224; O'Donoghue, *Mercy unto thousands*, p. 103.

37 P R Patrick, 'Ernest Sandford Jackson', *Australian dictionary of biography*, vol. 10, Melbourne, MUP, 1983.

38 For an account of Brisbane in the depression era, see R Lawson, *Brisbane in the 1890s: A study of an Australian urban society*, Brisbane, UQP, 1973.

39 Father Andrew Quinn, brother of Bishop James Quinn of Brisbane and Bishop Matthew Quinn of Bathurst, appealed to the Superior at Athy to train sisters for their Australian dioceses. Mother Patrick Potter, ADB file, box 4: Mother Patrick Potter, SOMCA.

40 Mary Jackes to Sr. M. Chanel, 26 December 1927, Mother Patrick Potter ADB file, SOMCA.

41 Mother Patrick's correspondence files, box 4: Mother Patrick Potter, SOMCA.

42 Mother Patrick's funeral file, box 4: Mother Patrick Potter, SOMCA; K M O'Brien, 'Norah Mary Potter', *Australian dictionary of biography*, vol. 11, Melbourne, MUP, 1988, pp. 265–6; Undated unsigned letter, the 'late Bishop's secretary' said Miss O'Reilly is thinking of giving land at Samford for an ecclesiastical college and seminary and that the St Killian's site was for a college and seminary which Samford is designed to maintain. Florence O'Reilly information file, box 87, SOMCA; A J Thynne to Rev. Mother, 28 September 1887, Miss Florence H O'Reilly 1871–1967: Accounts and correspondence, box 87, SOMCA.

43 The Blessing of our new Mater Children's Hospitals, 16 May 2001 (commemorative booklet); R Kidd, 'Aboriginal history of the Princess Alexandra Hospital site', paper prepared for the Diamantina Health Care Museum of the Princess Alexandra Hospital, 1997, p. 2.

44 Woolloongabba is derived from 'woola' meaning talk, 'woolloon' meaning fight-talk and 'gabba' meaning place of.

45 William Clark, cited in R Kidd, 'Aboriginal history of the Princess Alexandra Hospital site'.

46 C Maggs, *The origins of general nursing*, London, Croom Helm 1983, p. 63.

47 E Nolan, *One hundred years. A history of the School of Nursing and of developments at Mater Misericordiae Hospital 1891–1991*, Dublin, Sisters of Mercy, 1991, p. 16.

48 *The Queenslander,* 8 December 1900, p. 1169, quoted in R Longhurst, *In the footsteps of the Mercies*, p. 25.

49 Mother M. de Chantal, 'The Mater Private Hospital story', unpublished manuscript, Mater History and Heritage Centre [MHHC]; *History of the movement for the establishment of the Mater Misericordiae Hospital from 1 January 1906–31 October 1911*, MHHC; The Mater Misericordiae Hospital, *Illustrated Publication*, Brisbane, Innes Millbank, 1934, p. 3; H J Summers, *They crossed the river*, Brisbane, UQP, 1979, pp. 4–14; R Longhurst, *In the footsteps of the Mercies*, p. 26.

50 D Watson, *Nineteenth century Queensland architects: a biographical dictionary*, Brisbane, Queensland Museum, 1994; Aubigny file, MHHC. In Davis's time, the house was called 'Rosalie Villa'. Patrick Perkins, born in Tipperary, had joined the rush to Victoria's goldfields in 1855 and became a successful storekeeper and brewer in the town of Castlemaine. After opening a brewery in Toowoomba in 1869, Perkins arrived in Brisbane in the mid-1870s and opened a brewery in Mary Street which became famous for its Castlemaine XXXX brew. Patrick Perkins was elected to the Queensland Parliament for the Darling Downs seat of Aubigny in 1877, but lost his electorate in the midst of a scandal in which he was accused of buying votes with beer. He came to the fore again as Member for Cambooya, before becoming a Member of the Legislative Council until his death in 1901.

51 Mother Patrick to Dottie, 27 February 1906, letters from Mother Patrick Potter to G W Gray, box 139: Mother Patrick Potter, SOMCA.

52 N J Byrne, *Robert Dunne*, pp. 5, 224.

53 *Brisbane Courier*, 4 January 1906.

54 *Brisbane Courier*, 4, 5 January 1906.

55 H Gregory and C Brazil, *Bearers of the tradition. Nurses of the Royal Brisbane Hospital, 1888–1893*, p. 3. The year of the award of Minnie Brosnan's certificate was taken from the official records of the Royal Brisbane Hospital.

56 Mother Mary de Chantal, RSM, 'The Mater Hospital story', vol. 1 of a 2 volume unpublished manuscript, MHHC.

57 Mater Private Hospital, Patients Record Book, 4 January 1906–29 October 1922, MHHC; Ross Patrick, *A history of health and medicine in Queensland 1824–1960*, Brisbane, UQP, 1987, p. 254. The dengue outbreak was so serious that the Commissioner for Public Health, Dr Burnett Ham, estimated that almost three-quarters of the Brisbane population had been affected.

58 L Williams, *No easy path. The life and times of Lilian Violet Cooper*, Brisbane, Amphion, 1991, p. 41; R Patrick, *A history of health and*

medicine in Queensland, p. 355; J Tyrer, *History of the Brisbane Hospital*, pp.193–4.

59   Patient numbers calculated from Mater Private Hospital, Patients Record Book, 4 January 1906–29 October 1922, MHHC; *Brisbane Telegraph*, 7 March 1908.

60   R Patrick, *A history of health and medicine in Queensland*, p. 368.

2. ADVANCING TO 'GREATER TRIUMPHS'

1   Mother Patrick to Gray, 20 October 1907, letters from Mother Patrick to G W Gray, box 4, Mother Patrick, SOMCA.

2   Mother Patrick Potter, appeal letter [1907], Mater Private Hospital scrapbook, MHHC.

3   *Brisbane Telegraph*, 7 March 1908; *Brisbane Courier*, 7, 9 March 1908; *Warwick Argus* (undated cutting), Mater Private Hospital scrapbook, MHHC; *The Telegraph*, 30 May 1908; Mother M. de Chantal, 'The Mater Hospital story', 2 vol. unpublished manuscript, MHHC; undated newspaper cutting, Mater Private Hospital scrapbook, MHHC.

4   D Watson and J Mackay, *Nineteenth century architects: a biographical dictionary*, Brisbane, Queensland Museum, 1994.

5   H J Summers, *They crossed the river. The founding of the Mater Misericordiae Hospital, South Brisbane by the Sisters of Mercy*, Brisbane, UQP, 1979, p. 35.

6   'The Mater Story 1908', MHHC; *The Queenslander*, 27 August 1910; undated cuttings, Mater Private Hospital Cutting Book, MHHC.

7   Mother M. de Chantal, 'The Mater Hospital story', vol. 1; *Brisbane Courier*, 27 July 1910.

8   *Brisbane Courier*, 15 August 1910; undated press book account of the first annual meeting of the Mater Public Hospital, Mater Private Hospital Cutting Book, MHHC; 'The Mater Story 1908', MHHC.

9   For background on Sir William MacGregor, see R B Joyce, *Sir William MacGregor*, Melbourne, MUP, 1971. In his speech at the Mater Private Hospital opening, MacGregor referred to a friendship with Archbishop Dunne of twenty years standing, formed during MacGregor's frequent trips to Queensland during his years in New Guinea, N J Byrne, *Robert Dunne 1830–1917. Archbishop of Brisbane*, Brisbane, UQP, 1991, pp. 223–4.

10   Undated cutting, Mater Private Hospital Cutting Book, 'The Mater Story 1908', MHHC.

11 Dunne to Maria Dunne, 6 May 1911, cited in Byrne, *Robert Dunne*, p. 225.

12 Mother Patrick to Mother Bridget Conlan, 13 October 1908, box 139, Mater Private Hospital, early days, SOMCA.

13 Mater Public Hospital, Annual Report for the year ending 31 December 1912. This report also included results for 1911, which had not been a complete twelve-month period.

14 Calculated from Mater Public Hospital Annual Reports, 1912–1915, and Ledger, Receipts and Expenditure, 1908–1928, MHHC.

15 J H Tyer, *History of the Brisbane Hospital and its affiliates. A pilgrim's progress*, Brisbane, 1993, pp. 175–9.

16 Mater Public Hospital, Annual Report for year ending 31 December 1912.

17 Patient statistics compiled from Annual Reports, 1911–1915.

18 Mother Patrick to the Home Secretary, 11 November 1912, Correspond-ence, Records and Reports re Hospitals and Hospital Boards, Brisbane, 1 January 1885–31 December 1926, PRV8699, Queensland State Archives (QSA).

19 Crown Solicitor's memos, 22 August 1912, 7 January 1913, PVR8699, QSA; J G Appel's note, dated 10 December 1912, on Mother Patrick's letter, £2 subsidy for every £1.

20 *Darling Downs Gazette*, 21 March 1913; cutting included in file PRV8699, QSA.

21 N J Byrne, *Robert Dunne*, p. 197.

22 Mother Patrick to J G Apple, Home Secretary, 13 June 1913, box 146, Mater Public Hospital, SOMCA.

23 Mother Patrick to Home Secretary, 28 August 1913, PRV8699.

24 Mater Public Hospital, Annual Report, 1913; account of Governor's speech at the first annual meeting, undated cutting, Mater Private Hospital Cutting Book, 'The Mater Story 1908', MHHC.

25 J H Tyer, *History of the Brisbane Hospital*, pp. 175–9; *Brisbane Courier*, 18 November 1912.

26 Mater Public Hospital, Annual Report, 1914.

27 Mater Misericordiae Public Hospital, honorary medical staff, Register 1914–18, MHHC.

28 T J B Kelly to Mother Patrick, 13 February 1913, box 139, Mater Private Hospital, early days, SOMCA; T J B Kelly to Mother Patrick, 3 October 1912, box 139, Mater Private Hospital, early days, SOMCA.

29 M F Windor, ed., 'The Australian memoirs of Dr H J Windor 1914–76 in his own words', unpublished manuscript, MHHC, p. 62.

30 *Telegraph*, 25 May 1908.

31 For an account of legislation and other measures in this period, see P R Patrick, *A history of health and medicine in Queensland* 1824–1960, Brisbane, UQP, 1987.

32 N J Byrne, *Robert Dunne*, p. xvii; Mater Public Hospital, Annual Report, 1913.

33 Mater Public Hospital, Annual Report, 1913. The original registration regulations provided that nurses with three years practical experience before 1 January 1912 could be registered without having passed examinations.

34 Sister Mary Dominica Phelan, Memoirs, Sisters of Mercy collection, Mater Convent. For more on the early days of the nursing school at the Mater, see R Longhurst, *In the footsteps of the Mercies. A history of nursing at the Mater Misericordiae Hospitals*, Brisbane, Mater Misericordiae Public Hospitals, 1992, p. 30.

35 R Longhurst, *In the footsteps of the Mercies*, p. 38; H Gregory, *A tradition of care: A history of nursing at the Royal Brisbane Hospital*, Brisbane, Boolarong, 1988, sets out the system at the Brisbane General Hospital.

36 P O'Farrell, *The Catholic church and community. An Australian history*, Sydney, University of New South Wales Press, 1985, pp. 329–30.

37 By the end of 1915, 40 wounded soldiers, some of them Gallipoli survivors, had been treated. Mater Public Hospital, Annual Report, 1915; Mater Public Hospital, Annual Reports, 1915, 1916, 1917.

38 Mater Public Hospital, Annual Reports, 1915, 1916.

39 Sister Mary Borgia Byrne to Home Secretary, 30 June 1915, Home Secretary to Sister M. Borgia, 8 December 1915, PRV8699, QSA.

40 Mother Patrick to Home Secretary, 27 August 1919, PRV8699, QSA; notes on Mother Patrick to Home Secretary, 27 August 1919, PRV8699, QSA.

41 Bourne to Sister Administrator, 1 February 1919, and Sister Administrator to Bourne, 4 February 1919, box 146, Mater Public Hospital, SOMCA; J B McLean, Medical Superintendent, Brisbane General Hospital, speech to Brisbane and South Coast Hospitals Board, typescript, John Oxley Library; Mater Public Hospital, Annual Report, 1919.

42 Home Secretary to Mother Patrick, 27 August 1920, box 145, Mater Building Fund, art union, appeals, SOMCA.

43 Mater Public Hospital, Annual Report, 1920.

44 Sister Mary Chanel, 'Hospital nursing in Australia', in *Hospital Progress*.

Official Magazine of the Catholic Hospital Association of the United States and Canada, vol. v, no. 1, January 1942, pp. 1–5; *Brisbane Courier*, 12 June 1924; Mater Public Hospital, Annual Reports, 1928, 1930; Tyrer, *A pilgrim's progress*, p. 219. The Governor opened the Mater cancer centre on 20 December 1928.

45 Mater Public Hospital, Annual Report, 1926.

46 H Gregory, *Vivant Professores. Distinguished members of the University of Queensland, 1910–1940*, Brisbane, Fryer Library Occasional Publications Series, 1987, p. 31. Dr Duhig was a tireless campaigner for the establishment of a medical school in Queensland and became its first Professor of Pathology.

47 'A tribute to Sister Mary Chanel England', Sister Mercia Mary Higgins file, MHHC.

48 Sister Mercia Mary Higgins, 'The Mater Laboratory (in the good old days)', Sister Mercia Mary Higgins file, MHHC.

49 Mater Public Hospital, Annual Report, 1927.

50 'A tribute to Sister Mary Chanel', Sister Mercia Mary Higgins file, MHHC.

51 H J Summers, *They crossed the river*, p. 72.

52 T P Boland, *James Duhig*, Brisbane, UQP, 1986, pp. 72–5, 182, 192; E Campion, *Australia Catholics*, Melbourne, Penguin, 1988.

53 Mater Building Fund file, Art Unions, 1914–41, box 145, SOMCA; T C Beirne to Mother Patrick, 3 February 1920, box 145, SOMCA.

54 Mater Public Hospital, Annual Report, 1927.

55 Longhurst, *In the footsteps of the Mercies*, p. 44.

56 R S Dods wrote to Mother Patrick on the 14 October 1916 assuring her that he had not mentioned the proposed chapel to anyone, even his architectural partner, R F Hall; R S Dods to Mother Patrick, 15 March 1917. Mater Private Hospital, early days, box 139, SOMCA.

57 R S Dods to F R Hall, 30 July 1917, box 139, SOMCA.

58 Mother Patrick engaged in a vigorous correspondence during 1925 and 1926 with Mr H Creddington, of Italian Art Reproductions, Melbourne, who imported the artworks from Italy. Box 139, SOMCA; The Mother de Chantal James Story, MHHC.

59 Mater Public Hospital, Annual Report, 1924.

60 W C Horstmann to Mother Patrick, 13 April 1922, 7 June 1929; Sisters of Mercy balance sheet 1925, box 13, Property, SOMCA.

61 Sister Mary Chanel, 'Hospital nursing in Australia', *Hospital Progress. Official magazine of the Catholic Hospital Association of the United States and Canada*, 1924, p. 2.

62   Mater Public Hospital, Annual Report, 1924.

63   P Hall, *Royal Children's Hospital Brisbane, 1878–1978. A century of care*, Brisbane, Royal Childrens Hospital 1978, pp. 49–50.

64   Mater Public Hospital, Annual Report, 1924; Thynne and Macartney to Rev. Mother Patrick, 26 June 1918, re Gray transferring Shalimar to the Sisters, box 13, Property, SOMCA.

65   *Daily Mail*, 12 June 1924.

66   Mater Children's Hospital, Annual Report, 1932; Mater Public Hospitals, Annual Report, 1935.

67   Mother Patrick funeral file, box 4, Mother Patrick Potter, SOMCA.

3. CHALLENGING MANAGEMENT

1   Sister Mary Ursula Lavery to Honorary Staff, Mater Children's Hospital, 14 April 1931. Mater Children's Hospital collection, MHHC.

2   Mother Alban Salmon file, box 5, Sisters of Mercy Brisbane, SOMCA; M X O'Donoghue, *Beyond our dreams. A century of the works of Mercy in Queensland*, Brisbane, Jacaranda, 1961, pp. 258, 260–1.

3   O'Donoghue, *Beyond our dreams*, p. 284.

4   Mater Public Hospitals, Annual Reports, 1931, 1932.

5   Fr English, St Leo's College to Mother Alban, 30 May 1927, box 13, Property, SOMCA; see for example, S Hegerty, Secretary Mater Misericordiae Hospitals to Rev. Mother re expenditure and rentals, 15 May 1941, Cameron Brothers to Mother Alban, 20 July 1933; S Hegerty, Secretary Mater Misericordiae Hospitals to Rev. Mother re expenditure and rentals, 15 May 1941, box 13, SOMCA.

6   Sr Patricia Reordan, eulogy for Sr M St Rita, Sisters of Mercy obituaries file, MHHC.

7   Minutes of Mater Ball committee, 16 July 1936, box 145, SOMCA.

8   Mother Alban to Scanlan, 11 September 1939, box 145, SOMCA; Morris Industries Exports Ltd to Sister Administrator, 16 February 1937, box 146, SOMCA.

9   Mother Alban to H A Hegerty, 2 July 1934, File: Public Hospitals Assistance Fund 1934–1946, box 145, SOMCA.

10   Mother Alban to H A Hegerty, 2 July 1934; M F Windsor, ed. 'The Australian memoirs of Dr H J Windsor 1914–76 in his own words', unpublished manuscript, MHHC, p. 123.

11   The Act established the principle of hospital districts throughout

Queensland, each of which would be controlled by a district hospital board. However, the district to be controlled by the Brisbane and South Coast Hospitals Board was the only district initially proclaimed.

12 Robertson had considered it a 'great honour' to be a member of the Mater's honorary staff. Mater Public Hospital, Annual Report, 1927; *Courier-Mail*, 12 June 1924; Minutes of meeting, 21 August 1934, Minutes of the Medical Board, Mater Misericordiae Public Hospital, 12 September 1930, 5 November 1936, MHHC.

13 D Gordon, 'Social, political and economic background to the genesis of the Faculty of Medicine', in R L Doherty, ed., *A medical school for Queensland*, Spring Hill, Boolarong, 1986, p. 11.

14 Mother Alban to Dr Ellis Murphy, secretary of the Mater Medical Board, 24 November 1935, box 145, SOMCA; Mother Alban to H A Hegerty, 25 September 1934, box 145, SOMCA.

15 Document setting out working of the scheme from 1 September 1935 to 28 February 1936, box 145, SOMCA.

16 P R Patrick, *A history of health and medicine in Queensland* 1824–1960, Brisbane, UQP, 1987, pp. 115, 357.

17 Mother Alban to H A Hegerty, 8 January 1936; Hegerty to Mother Alban, 15 January 1936, box 145, SOMCA; Minutes of Mater Medical Board, 6 March 1936.

18 Minutes of Mater Medical Board, 6 March 1936.

19 Minutes of Mater Medical Board, 1 September 1933, MHHC; Medical Board rules, 1935, box 150, Mater Public Hospitals Advisory Board, SOMCA.

20 Minutes of Mater Medical Board, 1 September 1933.

21 Minutes of Mater Medical Board, 6 November 1933, 6 July 1934.

22 Queensland Parliament, Legislative Assembly, *Debates*, vol. CCLXX, 1936, p. 1813.

23 P R Patrick, *A history of health and medicine in Queensland*, pp. 22, 82.

24 Mother Alban to Medical Board, 29 July 1936; Minutes of Medical Board, 25 August 1936, MHHC.

25 Minutes of Meeting of the Administration of the Mater Misericordiae Hospitals and the Public Hospitals' Advisory Board, 11 August 1936, box 150, Mater Public Hospitals Advisory Board, SOMCA.

26 Queensland Parliament, Legislative Assembly, *Debates*, vol. CCLXX, 1936, p. 1815.

27 Mother Alban to H A Hegerty, secretary of the Advisory Board, 24 May 1937, box 150, SOMCA.

28 Mother Alban's response to decisions of the Medical Board, 25 May 1937, box 150, SOMCA.

29 Mother Alban to honorary medical staff, 17 June 1937.

30 English to Dr Ralph Weaver, secretary of the Medical Board, English to Dr Weaver, 12 July 1937 and 29 July 1937 in response to Weaver's letter 20 July, 1937, box 150, SOMCA.

31 F Fisher, *Raphael Cilento: A biography*, Brisbane, University of Queensland Press, 1994, p. 22.

32 Minutes of combined Advisory Board, 25 March, 7 April, 12 April, 5 May; Mother Alban to Advisory Board, 11 May 1938, 5 May 1938.

33 Mother Alban to Apostolic Delegate, 4 April 1938.

34 Monsignor John Panico, Apostolic Delegate to Mother Alban, 5 April 1938.

35 Sister Gertrude Mary's handwritten account of her life, file: Sisters of Mercy A–G, MHHC.

36 D C Jackson, 'Recollections and reflections concerning the development at the Mater Children's Hospital clinical school', in R L Doherty, *A medical school for Queensland*, p. 217.

37 Minutes of meeting between Mother Alban and representatives of the Medical Board, 23 August 1936, MHHC.

38 Mother Alban to Sisters, Palm Sunday, 1938, SOMCA.

39 Sisters of Mercy file A–G, MHHC; Paddy Lundy to Sister Germaine Greathead, 15 August 2003, *Mercies Link*, September 2003.

40 Sister Gertrude Mary's handwritten account of her life, file: Sisters of Mercy A–G, MHHC; eulogy for Sister Gertrude Mary, 29 October 1992. File: Obituaries, Sisters of Mercy, MHHC; Mater Private Hospital Memorabilia, MHHC.

41 B L W Clarke to Sister Superior, Mater, 26 March 1935.

42 Mother de Chantal, 'The Mater Private Story', vol. 1, p. 18, MHHC.

43 *Courier-Mail*, 15 November 1941.

44 Mother Superior to Registrar, University of Queensland, 18 February 1936.

45 Minutes of Meeting of the Administration of the Mater Misericordiae Hospitals and the Public Hospitals' Advisory Board, 11 August 1936.

46 R Longhurst, *In the footsteps of the Mercies: A history of nursing at the Mater Misericordiae public hospitals*, Brisbane, Mater Misericordiae Hospitals, 1992.

47 Sister Mercia Mary Higgins, The Mater Misericordiae Hospitals, typescript, MHHC.

48 H O'Brien, N Buckingham, L Dyer, 'The early medical technologist of the Mater Hospital', in L Williams, *Hygeia's daughters*, Brisbane, L Williams, 1997, p. 45.

49 Mother Alban's obituary, unsourced cutting, MHHC.

PART 2
GROWING UP

4. MAKING A LARGE BRICK STATEMENT

1   Archbishop Duhig to Mother Alban, 9 October 1946, box 147, Mater Mothers' Trust, Nurses Quarters, Public Hospital, SOMCA.

2   The 1943 amendments created a power to declare certain hospitals as medical schools.

3   Minutes of Advisory Board, 12 July 1937, box 150, SOMCA; Mother Alban to Hanlon, 29 October 1935, box 147, SOMCA.

4   J P Kelly, speech in booklet 'Notes of speeches given to the hierarchy and clergy on the occasion of the Solemn Blessing of the Mater Mothers' Hospital as a tribute of appreciation from the Sisters of Mercy, 30 November 1960, MHHC.

5   *The Hospital Benefits Act (Cwlth) 1945.*

6   T A Foley, Minister Health and Home Affairs to Mother Alban, 27 February 1946, box 146, Mater Public Hospital, SOMCA; J P Kelly, 'Notes on speeches'.

7   Eakin's speech at the official dinner to celebrate the laying of the foundation stone, 16 May 1948, Mater Mother's collection, MHHC. Mother M de Chantal, 'The Mater Misericordiae Public Hospital', MHHC.

8   R Patrick, *The Royal Women's Hospital, Brisbane*, Boolarong Press, Brisbane, 1988, p. 31.

9   Stephenson and Turner to Mother Alban, 1, 13 May 1946, box 147, SOMCA.

10 R Patrick, *Royal Women's Hospital*, p. 32.

11 Hall and Phillips to Mother Alban, 2 July 1946, box 147, SOMCA.

12 Archbishop Duhig to Mother Alban, 9 October 1946, box 147, SOMCA.

13 M J Eakin, speech in booklet 'Notes of speeches given to the hierarchy and clergy on the occasion of the Solemn Blessing of the Mater Mothers' Hospital', MHHC.

14 Biographical material on Dr Eakin from Annual Report 1969–1970; box 147, Mater Mothers' Trust, SOMCA.

15 Hanlon's speech at the official dinner to celebrate the laying of the foundation stone, 16 May 1948, Mater Mothers' collection, MHHC. Mother M de Chantal, 'The Mater Misericordiae Public Hospital', MHHC.

16 *Catholic Leader*, 25 August 1966

17 M J Eakin, 'The Mater Mothers' Hospital Appeal', in Mater Misericordiae Hospitals, *Golden Jubilee, 1910–1960*, Opening of Mothers' Hospital, 1 December 1960, p. 55.

18 Unidentified newspaper cutting, 18 August 1966, box 147, SOMCA.

19 CBC to Rev. Mother, 12 November 1952, box 12, Banks, SOMCA.

20 A tall, active man, and father of six children, McCann enjoyed bushwalking and also wrote radio plays. Undated newspaper cutting from 1961, file: Mater Appeal Meetings 1946–1971, box 145, SOMCA.

21 *Courier-Mail*, 1 February 1955, p. 5.

22 Interview with John McCann, *Courier-Mail*, 10 September 1982, Art Union; Cecilia McNally file, Cabinet 3, MHHC; Queensland Parliament, Legislative Assembly, *Debates*, vol. 208, 1953–54, p. 1796.

23 *Telegraph*, 11 March 1967; 2 June 1966.

24 H G Noble, Minister for Health and Home Affairs to Mother Superior, 30 August 1957, box 147, SOMCA.

25 Mater Public Hospital, Annual Report, 1958–59.

26 Mother Alban to Manager, CBC, 27 November 1958, box 12, Banks, SOMCA.

27 Mother Mary Benigna Burke, Secretary General to Apostolic Delegate, 20 September 1958, box 147, SOMCA.

28 Biographical information on J P Kelly from F Hills, *The rise and fall of the Aquinas Library*, Brisbane, published by the author 1992; H Summers, *They crossed the river. The founding of the Mater Misericordiae Hospital, South Brisbane by the Sisters of Mercy*, Brisbane, UQP, 1979; *Catholic Leader*, 4 September 1977, 15 January 1978, 24 December 1978, 24 June 1984.

29 Mater Misericordiae Hospital, *Golden Jubilee, 1910–1960*, Opening of Mater Mothers' Hospital, MHHC.

30 R Patrick, *Brisbane Women's Hospital*, p. 35.

31 *Golden Jubilee, 1910–1960*, Opening of Mothers' Hospital, p. 33.

32 Oral history interview, Sister Josephine Crawford.

33 Sister Mary Virgina, Matron, Mater Public Hospital, Annual Report, 1960–61.

34 Oral history interviews, Sister Josephine Crawford, Sister Jill Stringer.

35 Oral history interview, Sister Jill Stringer.

36 Oral history interviews, Sister Peg Slack and Sister Josphine Crawford.

37 Mater Mothers' Hospital, Honorary Medical Officers' staff meeting, 11 May 1961, box 147, SOMCA; Mater Public Hospital, Annual Report, 1966–67.

38 *Courier-Mail*, 8 May 1968, 26 December 1964.

39 *Courier-Mail*, 19 May 1964, 1 June 1967.

40 Mater Mothers' Hospital, Honorary Medical Officers' Association, 14 May 1964, box 147, SOMCA; Annual Report, 1964–65, p. 27.

41 Mater Mothers' Hospital, Honorary Medical Officers staff meeting, 13 April 1961; J J O'Brien to Dr C F Marks, 30 August 1961; minutes of committee on antenatal care in the Brisbane area, 31 July 1961, box 147, SOMCA.

5. NAVIGATING TURBULENCE

1 Sister Angela Mary to Tooth, 12 May 1971, Dept of Health correspondence, 1944–45, box 152, Catholic health care, SOMCA.

2 See G Bolton, 1942–1988. *The middle way*, Melbourne, Oxford University Press 1996, for background on this period.

3 Sandra M Schneiders, 'Religious life' (*Perfectae Caritatis*) in A Hastings, *Modern Catholicism*, London, SPCK 1991, p. 157. The decree was based on a 1960 draft called 'The States that aim at perfection'.

4 Schneiders, 'Religious life', p. 159.

5 Sister Angela Mary, discussion with Helen Gregory, 29 April 2004.

6 Mater Public Hospitals, Annual Report, 1958–1959.

7 Dr Brian Purssey, first Director of Medical Services, Annual Report, 1960–61. The administration asked the Medical Advisory Board for its help in ensuring that patients did not stay any longer than necessary, e.g. Minutes of Medical Advisory Board, 17 March 1947, MHHC; Annual Report, 1958–59.

8 Mater Public Hospital, Annual Report, 1960–61.

9 Medical Advisory Board minutes, 1 August, 3 October 1949, MHHC.

10 Minutes, Advisory Board, 22 June 1946 to 1 November 1948, MHHC.

11 Oral history interview, Sister Marie Therese Rosenberg.

12 K Wilkinson, J Craig, J Bourke, anaesthetic registrars to O'Callaghan, 27 April 1962, file: Mater Children's Hospital 1926–1986, box 146, SOMCA.

13   Medical Advisory Board minutes, 1 November 1965, MHHC.

14   Minutes of Children's Hospital Committee, 23 September 1964, file: Mater Children's Hospital 1926–1986, box 146, SOMCA.

15   Professor Rendle-Short arrived in Brisbane in May 1961. For more information, see John Pearn, *Focus and innovation. A history of paediatric education in Queensland*, Brisbane, Amphion, 1986.

16   Medical Advisory Board minutes, 22 April 1949.

17   Education Department to O'Callaghan, 10 September 1962, File: Mater Children's Hospital 1926–1986, box 146, SOMCA.

18   T J Rendle-Short, 'Mater Children's Hospital', a report for St Mary St Gabriel circa 1961, box 146, SOMCA.

19   Mater Public Hospitals, Annual Report, 1961–62.

20   Mater Public Hospital, Annual Report, 1961–62.

21   Mater Public Hospital, Annual Reports, 1966–67, 1967–68.

22   Mater Public Hospital, Annual Report, 1960–61.

23   Ibid.

24   Mater Public Hospital, Annual Report, 1960–61.

25   Mater Public Hospital, Annual Report, 1964–65.

26   Preliminary Appraisal for the Sisters of Mercy, W D Scott and Co. Pty Ltd, March 1969, p. 10, Sister Angela Mary box, MHHC.

27   D R McLeod of W D Scott to Mother General, 17 March 1969, box 144: Mater Public Relations, SOMCA.

28   'Preliminary Appraisal for the Sisters of Mercy', W D Scott and Co. Pty Ltd, March 1969, SOMCA.

29   Section 24.

30   Kelly to Mother Damian, 25 October 1961, box 146, SOMCA.

31   Mater Misericordiae Public Hospitals, study of community attitudes and analysis of financial resources, confidential report, Compton Associates, 1969, p. 1, box 145, SOMCA.

32   Minutes of a meeting of people interested in the development of the Mater Hospitals, 2 October 1970, box 151, SOMCA.

33   *Courier-Mail*, 29 July 1966.

34   Mater Public Hospital, Annual Report, 1964–65.

35   Mater Public Hospital, Annual Report, 1963–64.

36   *Sunday Mail*, 21 June 1970.

37   W M Johnstone, Report to the Sisters of Mercy, 28 October 1970, box 145, Mater Hospital Project Board, Fundraising 1970, SOMCA.

38   Minutes of Appeal Board, 28 May 1969, file: Mater Appeal Meetings

1946–1971, box 145, SOMCA; T J Heike, paper presented at Mater Appeal Committee meeting, 26 November 1969, box 145, SOMCA; Compton to Kelly, 25 September 1969, op. cit.

39 Appeal committee minutes, 28 October 1970; *Catholic Leader*, 6 June 1971.

40 *Catholic Leader*, 19 April 1970; Appeal Board, 28 May 1970, file: Mater Appeal Meetings 1946–1971, box 145, SOMCA.

41 *Courier-Mail*, 24 May 1971; Sister Angela Mary to Mother Damian, 28 January 1971, file: Reports to General Council 1970–1974, box 151, SOMCA.

42 Sister Angela Mary to Tooth, 4 March 1971, file: Dept of Health correspondence 1944–75, box 152, Catholic Health Care, SOMCA.

43 Sister Angela Mary to Tooth, 12 May 1971, ibid.

44 Mater Public Hospitals, Annual Report, 1970–71; Mater Children's Hospital, 'Booklet commemorating the opening of the new hospital', MHHC.

45 Sister Angela Mary, Story of the Mater Children's Hospitals; *Brisbane Telegraph*, 20 May 1971; *Catholic Leader*, 14 June 1971 and 25 June 1971; Leonard to Sister Angela Mary, 30 July 1971, box 145, Appeal Board meetings, SOMCA; Casey, the auditor, to Mother General, 23 August 1971, box 145.

46 Submission 14254, 'Mater Public Hospitals', Cabinet meeting, 13 July 1971, Z6866, QSA.

47 Sister Angela Mary to Health Minister, 1 June 1971, attached to Submission 14254.

48 Sister Angela Mary, report to General Council, 31 July 1971, box 151, SOMCA.

49 Sister Angela Mary's notes, Sister Angela Mary collection, MHHC.

50 Mater Public Hospital, Annual Report, 1970–71.

51 Submission 14254, 'Mater Public Hospitals', Cabinet meeting, 13 July 1971, Z6866, QSA.

52 S Sax, *A strife of interests. Politics and policies in Australian health services*, Sydney, Allen & Unwin, 1984; J A Gillespie, *The price of health. Australian governments and medical politics 1910–1960*, Melbourne, Cambridge University Press, 1991, p. xii.

53 Sax, *A strife of interests*, pp. 78–91.

54 Submission 14254, 'Mater Public Hospitals', Cabinet meeting, 13 July 1971, Z6866, QSA.

55 Summary of meeting, 13 August 1971.

56 Decision 16588, 20 December 1971, Z6869, QSA.

57 *Courier-Mail,* 28 October 1974.

58 *Courier-Mail*, 28 October 1974; information from Sister Angela Mary, 15 February 2005.

59 H Summers, *They crossed the river: the founding of the Mater Misericordiae Hospital Brisbane by the sisters of Mercy*, St Lucia, University of Queensland Press, 1979, p. 201.

60 Submission 15203, Cabinet meeting, 30 May 1972, Z6870, QSA.

61 Meeting with Health Dept, 6 December 1973, attended by Dr Ross Patrick, Director General, Mr Dick Strutton, Dr O Powell, Dr Peter Livingstone and J J O'Brien, E D O'Callaghan, Sister Angela Mary, Pat Maguire. File: Negotiations with government, Sister Angela Mary collection, MHHC.

62 Recommendations of Mater Public Hospital Advisory Board planning committee to General Council, 22 April 1974, box 151, SOMCA.

63 Sister Angela Mary, record of meeting with Dept of Health, 6 December 1973, Sister Angela Mary collection, MHHC.

6. BREAKING THROUGH

1 Press release 29 October 1975, Sister Angela Mary collection, MHHC.

2 Draft of letter, 1974, Sister Angela Mary to Strutton, Sister Angela Mary negotiations with government file, MHHC.

3 Sister Angela Mary's handwritten note on her letter drafted in 1974.

4 Mater Advisory Board minutes, 3 February 1975, MHHC.

5 Queensland Parliament, Legislative Assembly, *Debates*, vol. 266, 1974, p. 1104; Medical Advisory Board minutes, 1 July, 6 September 1974.

6 Draft submission presented to Board, Mater Advisory Board minutes, 3 February 1975, MHHC.

7 Sister Angela Mary, recommendations to board, 3 February 1975, MHHC.

8 Submission 14445, Purchase of land for hospital purposes, Inala, Decision 16245, 13 September 1971, Z6868, QSA.

9 Mother Marcella McCormick was particularly keen to explore this opportunity. Sister Claire Irving, oral history; S Sax, *A strife of interests. Politics and Policies in Australian health services*, Sydney, Allen and Unwin, 1984, pp. 97–104.

10 Medical Advisory Board minutes, 3 February 1975, MHHC.

11 Sister Angela Mary's handwritten notes of events in 1975–76, Sister Angela Mary file, MHHC.

12 J P Kelly, Memorandum of a meeting with Mr Strutton, 19 March 1976, Sister Angela Mary collection, MHHC.

13 Medical Advisory Board minutes, 4 October, 1 November 1976; notes of a discussion between J P Kelly and Dick Strutton, 3 March 1976, Sister Angela Mary file, MHHC.

14 Sister Madonna Josey, oral history.

15 Medical Advisory Board minutes, 6 February, 22 May 1978, MHHC.

16 Sites and symbols of spiritual interest on the Mater complex, pamphlet, MHHC.

17 Sister Patricia Plint, Sister Madonna Josey, oral history interviews.

18 Sister Catharine Courtney, oral history interview.

19 J C Kable, Report on organisation of Mater public hospitals for the Sisters of Mercy, February 1973, Sister Angela Mary collection, MHHC.

20 Sr Angela Mary's report to General Council, All Hallows', 30 November 1972, box 151, SOMCA; Kable, p. 8.

21 Sister Madonna Josey, discussion with Helen Gregory, 4 May 2004.

22 Information provided by Sister Angela Mary Doyle.

23 *The Misericordian,* December 1945, p. 1.

24 *The Misericordian*, December 1949–50, p. 6.

25 *The Misericordian,* December 1947, p. 18.

26 T R Hall and Phillips to Director, Building Control Division, 12 February 1946, box 146, SOMCA.

27 Sister Eileen Pollard, oral history.

28 Sister Angela Mary, Report and recommendations from the sub-committee appointed May 1970.

29 Ibid.

30 Sister Claire Irving, oral history; Mater Public Hospital, Annual Report, 1969–70.

31 *Queensland Government Gazette*, No. 7, 15 January 1970.

32 Sister Madonna Josey, discussion with Helen Gregory, 4 May 2004.

33 Information from Sister Madonna Josey and Miss Jill Marshall, 25 January 2005.

34 Sister Eileen Pollard, Director of Nursing, Annual Report, 1969–70.

35 Biographical material on P A Earnshaw from *The medical journal of Australia*, 28 June 1980, p. 678; J Pearn, ed., *Focus and innovation. A history of paediatric education in Queensland* including an account of the

Department of Child Health within the University of Queensland, Department of Child Health, University of Queensland, 1986. Biographical material on Geoffrey Toakley from doctors' obituary file, MHHC.

36 Investigating committee, HMO staff, papers and report, MHHC; J A Gillespie, *The price of health. Australian governments and medical politics 1910–1960*, Sydney, CUP, 1991, pp. 28–30.

37 M Dickenson and C Mason, *Hospitals and politics. The Australian Hospital Association 1946–86*, Canberra, 1986, pp. 9–11.

38 Mater Public Hospital, Annual Report, 1968–69.

39 Preliminary appraisal for the Sisters of Mercy, W D Scott and Co. Pty Ltd, March 1969, p. 10, Sister Angela Mary box, MHHC.

40 Sister Administrator's Report to General Council, 2 February 1971, box 151, SOMCA.

41 Scott report, MHHC.

42 For example, submissions from Dr W J Arnold, Dr V Youngman, Dr J F McCaffrey and Dr K O'Reilly; Dr J C A Dique, 11 October 1967, and Dr I Ferguson's report of discussions with staff, 24 April 1967; Dr R P Yaxley, 29 June 1967, HMO staff, papers and report, MHHC.

43 Eye department submission, 16 November 1967.

44 Dr G Carroll, 29 September 1967.

45 P J Landy to M J Gallagher, 10 October 1967, Investigating Committee, HMO staff, papers and report, MHHC.

46 Minutes of general meeting of the Honorary Medical Staff, 26 May 1966, MHHC; Dr H J Windsor, 24 August 1967, HMO Investigating Committee, MHHC.

47 Medical Advisory Board minutes, 6 September 1974, MHHC.

48 Mater Public Hospital, Annual Report, 1969–70.

49 Mater Public Hospital, Annual Report, 1968–69.

50 Confidential report, Compton Associates, 1969, p. 1, box 145, SOMCA.

51 Meeting at the Mater Hospital, 18 March 1973, between Mother Damian, Sister Angela Mary, J P Kelly, and other senior Sisters of Mercy with J C Kable, MHHC.

52 Sister Angela Mary, discussion with Helen Gregory, 29 April 2004.

53 Sister Mary Camillus Lynch, oral history interview.

7. FACING DIFFICULT QUESTIONS

1   Mater Adult Hospital, opening booklet, 1981.

2   P M Dunn, 'Newborn care in the UK since 1928', in Bernard Valman, ed., *The Royal College of Paediatrics and child health at the millennium*, London, 2000, p. 41. The term 'neonatal medicine' was first used in 1960 and the first special-care nurseries were introduced into British maternity hospitals during the 1960s.

3   Dr M J Thearle, discussion with Helen Gregory; J Pearn, ed., *Focus and Innovation. A history of paediatric education in Queensland* including an account of the Department of Child Health within the University of Queensland, Child Health, University of Queensland, 1986.

4   *Australian*, 8 September 1972.

5   Minutes of Mater Board, 16 October 1972, MHHC.

6   Dr A Dugdale, paper on the future of the Mater Hospitals, 1 May 1974, file: Building projects public hospital, box 147, SOMCA; Sister Peg Slack was awarded a Wyeth Travelling Scholarship.

7   Biographical information on D I Tudehope from *Courier-Mail*, 17 January 1981; D I Tudehope, 'Memoirs', typescript, Mater Mothers' Hospital.

8   D I Tudehope, 'Memoirs'.

9   Oral history interview, Sister Jill Stringer; D I Tudehope, 'Memoirs'; *Sunday Sun*, 10 June 1979.

10 Information from Rosalie Lewis, 24 August 2004.

11 *Catholic Leader*, 29 February 1976.

12 *Courier-Mail*, 23 February 1979, *Daily Sun*, 18 March 1971.

13 Mater Mothers' Hospital, Clinical Report, 1979, MHHC; *Courier-Mail*, 3 November 1982.

14 *Courier-Mail*, 3 November 1982.

15 *Sunday Sun*, 5 June 1982; *Courier-Mail*, 26 May 1981; *Catholic Leader*, 11 October 1983.

16 *Courier*-Mail, 19 June 1981; *Telegraph*, 24 November 1982.

17 Mater Mothers' Hospital, Clinical Report, 1979.

18 *Telegraph*, 10 June 1980; *Daily Sun*, 10 September 1982.

19 *Courier-Mail*, 16 November 1984.

20 Oral history, Sister Kath Burke; information from Sister Angela Mary; AIDS folder, MHHC.

21 *Telegraph*, 4 March 1985; *Courier-Mail*, 21 November, 1981, Esler to O'Callaghan, 20 October 1962, box 154, SOMCA.

22 *Courier-Mail*, 13 January 1983; *Sunday Mail*, 16 August 1981; *Courier-Mail,* 3 February 1983; *Sunday Sun*, 12 June 1983; E J Esler, report, 9 July 1982, box 141, SOMCA; Sister Angela Mary, 18 November 1982 to Sister Jill Stringer, enclosing a position paper on Mater Private Hospital, box 141, SOMCA.

23 E J Esler to O'Callaghan, 20 October 1982, box 145; Esler to O'Callaghan, 8 March 1982; Esler to Sister Angela Mary, 13 April 1983, box 154, SOMCA.

24 Minutes, Hospital Council, 10 November 1982, box 151, SOMCA; Mater Public Hospitals, Annual Report, 1984.

25 Mater Mothers' Hospital, Clinical Report, 1979.

26 Advisory Board minutes, 9 September 1985; information supplied by Rosalie Lewis, 28 August 2004.

27 Advisory Board minutes, 10 March 1986; 26 May 1986.

28 Sister Alison Anderson and Sister Claire Doherty were the first coordinators of the course.

29 *Catholic Leader*, 16 October 1983.

30 Sister Angela Mary to Sister Kath Burke, box 154, SOMCA; *Sunday Mail*, 12 September 1983.

31 Minutes of Hospital Council meeting, 7 November 1985. The Sisters of Mercy donated $10,000 to sponsor this meeting.

32 Dr O'Callaghan's report, Mater Public Hospitals, Annual Report 1974–75; information on Sister Mary Dorothea from Sister Madonna Josey's eulogy, Sisters' obituaries file, MHHC; L Shields, 'Celebrating nursing achievement: Sister Mary Dorothea Sheehan RSM, 1916–1999'. *Neonatal, paediatric and child health nursing*, 1999, vol. 2, no. 4, pp. 5–7; *Catholic Leader*, 15 September 1986.

33 Minutes of Mater Misericordiae Public Hospitals' Board, 16 October 1972, file: Reports to General Council 1970–1974, box 151, Mater Public Hospitals to General Council, SOMCA.

34 Dr A Dugdale to Sister Angela Mary, 1 May 1974, file: Building projects public hospital, 1962–71, box 147, SOMCA.

35 *Courier-Mail*, 3 February 1983; Mater Public Hospitals, Annual Report, 1985.

36 box 146: Mater Public Hospital, file: Mater Children's 1926–1986.

37 box 154, 1983 correspondence.

38 Information from Sister Angela Mary Doyle.

39 *Sunday Sun*, 23 January 1983.

40 Sister Angela Mary to Dr Livingstone, 17 February 1983, file: Government policy, box 154, SOMCA; Mater Advisory Board minutes, 3 August 1983.

41 Heyworth to Sister Angela Mary, 2 December 1983, Heyworth to Sister Kath Burke, 13 April 1984,

42 Advisory Board minutes, 11 April 1984.

43 Mater Public Hospitals, Annual Report; 1984; Advisory Board minutes, 13 March 1985.

44 Mater Public Hospitals, Annual Report, 1979–80. The 1989-90 figures were the same; it seems the reduction in patient days had stalled.

45 Mater Hospital Committee, 8 June 1982, box 151, SOMCA.

46 Sister Angela Mary to Sister Kath Burke, 3 December 1985.

47 Mater Public Hospitals, Annual Reports, 1984, 1985, 1986.

48 Hospital Council minutes, 21 August 1985.

49 Mater Health Services Governing Board; inaugural meeting 18 March 1987, box 153: SOMCA; Reg Leonard House, Ronald McDonald House blue file, MHHC; *Telegraph*, 2 October 1978.

50 Information from Rosalie Lewis, 24 August 2004; Mater Public Hospitals, Annual Report, 1989–90, Mater Children's Hospital section.

51 Mater Public Hospitals, Annual Report, 1980.

52 Advisory Board Minutes, 7 November 1985; Mater Mothers' Hospital, Clinical Report, 1979.

53 Mater Mothers' Hospital, Clinical Report, 1979.

54 Minutes of Hospital Council, 12 June 1985, box 151, SOMCA; QRI (T P Tolhurst) to Sister Angela Mary, 16 October 1985: QRI will approve calling tenders for Hemicentre at the Mater with 2 linear accelerators.

55 Minutes of Hospital Council, 21 August 1985.

56 Mater Public Hospitals, Annual Report, 1980.

57 Meeting with Paul Gross, 9 September 1981, Sister Angela Mary box, Cabinet 6/7, MHHC.

58 Mater Public Hospitals, Annual Report, 1984.

59 Mater Public Hospitals, Annual Report, 1989–90.

60 Sister Angela Mary, 'Medical/technological developments and their ethical implications', Sister Angela Mary box, Cabinet 6/7, MHHC.

61 For example, Archbishop Quinn of San Francisco, cited in Paul F Gross, 'Health technology and health care ethics in the 1980s: The future of the Catholic hospital in Australia', 9 November 1979, box 152: file Qld Catholic Health Care Assoc 1982–5, SOMCA.

62   Archbishop Rush, Foreword to the Mater Adult Hospital opening booklet, 1981.

63   Information on Sister Regis Mary supplied by Sister Regis Mary, January 2005; Sister Regis Mary Dunne file, MHHC.

64   Mater Public Hospitals, Annual Report, 1981; Dr Esler, 1982, box 154, SOMCA.

65   Philosophy of health service under the care of the Sisters of Mercy, file: Mater Futures task force, October 1984, box 155, Mater Futures, SOMCA.

66   1977 philosophy of health service under the care of the Sisters of Mercy, box 155, Mater Futures, SOMCA.

67   Ibid.

68   Advisory Board minutes, 23 March 1981.

69   Advisory Board, 9 November 1983.

70   K J Ryan, draft policy of the Mater hospitals, 1983, box 154, SOMCA.

71   Psychiatrist to E D O'Callahgan, 15 September 1982; E D O'Callaghan's response, 22 September 1982, box 145, SOMCA; minutes of medico-moral committee, 29 October 1984, box 145, SOMCA; Sister Deirdre Gardiner, E D O'Callaghan, 15 February 1984, box 154, SOMCA.

72   Minutes of Hospital Council, 20 February 1985, box 151, SOMCA; minutes of Advisory Board, 5 October 1983.

73   David Tudehope; oral history, Sister Deirdre Gardiner.

74   Report to Hospital Council, 8 May 1985.

75   Advisory Board minutes, 10 September 1980.

PART 3
MATURING

8. ADAPTING, RENEWING, GROWING

1   Dr O'Callaghan's presentation to doctors beginning work at the Mater, cited by Professor J S Biggs, D O'Callaghan, obituary file, MHHC.

2   *Mater News*, No. 12, June 1983. Sister Stephanie was awarded an OBE for her services. She had served as a Flight Lieutenant in the Air Force during World War II, before entering the Sisters of Mercy.

3   Sister Catharine Courtney, oral history interview.

4   By this time, the Sisters' responsibilities extended widely across Queensland and New Guinea.

5   Sister Kath Burke, oral history interview.

6   Anne McLay, 'Mercy sponsorship of an institution', H M Burns, RSM, 'The leadership role of major superiors in the health care ministry', box 155, SOMCA.

7   Sr Anne Tormey, RSM, 'Setting the context. Theological and sociological trends affecting trusteeship/administration of religious institutions', box 155, SOMCA.

8   Sr Kathryn Grant, RSM, Detroit, 'The environment'; Sister Angela Mary, 'How can private hospitals of the future relate to Christian ethics', box 154, SOMCA.

9   Sister Angela Mary, 'Laity in Catholic health care facilities', address to ACHCA, Melbourne, 30 April 1985. Sister Angela Mary collection, MHHC.

10   E J Connors & J W Glaser, 'Health care: ministry or industry? A critical question', box 155, SOMCA. The Vatican II Decree on Apostolate of lay people reiterated this view: '. . . the church . . . showed itself as one body around Christ united by the bond of charity . . . it claims charitable works as its own mission and right. That is why mercy to the poor and the sick, and charitable works, for the alleviation of all kinds of human needs, are held in special honour by the church.'

11   Mater Public Hospitals, Annual Report, 1983.

12   Advisory Board minutes, 18 February 1985; Sister Catharine's postgraduate degree in educational administration had placed emphasis on these topics. Sister Catharine Courtney, oral history interview.

13   Advisory Board minutes, 21 May 1985.

14   Dr A McSweeny, motion at Advisory Board meeting, 26 October 1984.

15   ISMA Plenary Council, 7 November 1985, box 151.

16   Sister Angela Mary presentation, October 1984, box 155, SOMCA. The Brisbane Sisters of Mercy had already started to share their expertise. Sister Michaeleen Mary had been lent to the Calvary Hospital in Cairns to prepare it for Diocesan management, and to the Rockhampton Mater.

17   D Gottemoeller, RSM, 'Evaluation of corporate effectiveness: SMHC five-year evaluations'; Sister Dorothy Campion, National President ISMA to Sister Kath Burke, 21 August 1985, box 155, SOMCA.

18   Report to ISMA by US team, 15 October 1985, box 155, SOMCA.

19   Sister Angela Mary, Report to Hospital Council, 20 February 1985, box 151, SOMCA.

20   Paul F Gross 'Health technology and health care ethics in the 1980s: The

future of the Catholic hospital in Australia', oration at 40th anniversary of Sacred Heart Hospital, Coburg, 9 November 1979, box 152, SOMCA.

21   C J Apelt, 'A reflection on poverty, power and the Church'. Discussion of this took place at Mater Advisory Board meeting on 12 November 1980.

22   Advisory Board minutes, 10 June 1982.

23   Minutes, Hospital Council, 10 March 1982.

24   Sister Angela Mary, discussion with Helen Gregory, 19 December 2004.

25   Sister Angela Mary, Report to Hospital Council on the status of Mater Hospital employees vis-à-vis State Health Department employees, 8 July 1985.

26   Sister Angela Mary, Proposals for reorganisation of Mater Hospitals, Brisbane, June 1986, box 157, SOMCA.

27   Mater Health Services Governing Board, induction manual, 1987; *Mater News*, No. 27, July 1987.

28   Sister Kath Burke to Sister Angela Mary, 4 November 1986, filed with 1980s Board minutes, MHHC.

29   Stan Walsh had left the Mater for eighteen months to manage the laboratories at the Princess Alexandra Hospital, and returned to the Mater as Executive Director, Administrative Services in 1980.

30   Sister Angela Mary, 'Laity in Catholic health care facilities', address to ACHCA, 30 April 1985, box 152, SOMCA, and published with the conference proceedings.

31   Sister Angela Mary, Annual Report, 1983; information supplied by Sister Angela Mary, 19 December 2004.

32   Mater Health Services Governing Board manual, 1987.

33   Sister Angela Mary, Sister Administrator's report, Mater Public Hospitals, Annual Report, 1984; Mater Public Hospitals, Annual Report, 1989–90.

34   Minutes of Advisory Board, 15 February 1984; Sister Angela Mary, Annual Report, 1983.

35   Pat Maguire, address to Mater Futures workshop, 25 October 1984, box 155, SOMCA.

36   D Limerick, 'Planning for structural changes in organisations', Mater Futures workshop, 25 October 1984, box 155, SOMCA.

37   R Longhurst, *In the footsteps of the Mercies. A history of nursing at the Mater Misericordiae public hospitals, Brisbane*, Mater Misericordiae Hospitals, 1992, pp. 77–8.

38   *Catholic Leader*, 13 March 1988.

39 The medical staff establishment, for instance, grew from 107.5 to 125.5, the ancillary medical staff from 32 to 33, the pathology staff from 48 to 61, the social workers from 9.2 to 9.7, the radiology staff from 38 to 42, student nurses from 280.6 to 292, enrolled and assistant nurses from 152.8 to 163.4, senior and registered nurses from 247.6 to 338.4; artisans and engineers remained at 48; housekeeping had declined from 140.6 to 129.8, mainly due to a reduction in cleaning staff. Visiting medical officers' sessions had increased from 206 each week to 222.

40 Statistics file: Mater hospitals – public, box 155, SOMCA.

41 Sister Angela Mary report to Mater Hospital Council, 18 November 1986, box 151, SOMCA.

42 Justice Department to Maguire, 26 April 1985, box 151, SOMCA.

43 Hospital Council, minutes, 9 May 1985, Sir Llew Edwards to Sister Angela Mary, 30 April 1985; box 151, SOMCA

44 Minutes of Governing Board, 21 October 1987.

45 Sister Catharine Courtney, oral history interview; Sister Margaret Ryan, Bursar-General to P J Maguire, 27 March 1978; Health Dept to ED, Administrative Services, MM Public Hospitals, replying to letter dated 7 April 1982, file: Capital works report, MAH, 10 August 1983, box 151, SOMCA.

46 Sister Angela Mary, Report on Status of Mater Hospital employees vis-à-vis State Health Department employees, 18 July 1985; minutes of Hospital Council Meeting, 21 August 1985, box 151, SOMCA.

47 Sister Eileen Pollard, oral history interview.

48 R Longhurst, *In the footsteps of the Mercies*, p. 111; *Catholic Leader*, 12 March 1978.

49 Sister Eileen Pollard, oral history interview.

50 Nursing Division Report, in Annual Report, 1989.

51 Rex Ducat's report, 1 September 1983, box 154, SOMCA; oral history, Sister Eileen Pollard; *Mater News*, No. 24, March 1986.

52 R B Scotton and J S Deeble, 'Compulsory health insurance for Australia', in J R G Butler and D P Doessel, *Health economics. Australian readings*, Sydney, Australian Professional Publications, 1989, p. 203; Board minutes, 15 February 1984, MHHC.

53 Annual Report, 1989–90, p.19.

54 Annual Report, 1989–90.

55 S Wilde, *Practising surgery. A history of surgical training in Australia*,

1927–1974, PhD, University of Melbourne, 2003, pp. 37–8.

56   Mater Advisory Board minutes, 7 April 1975, 6 December 1976, 7 March 1977. Mater Public Hospitals, Annual Reports, 1982, 1985. There were nine registrars in the medicine training program in 1985.

57   Medical Director's report, Annual Report, 1974–75.

9. KEEPING THE FAMILY TOGETHER

1   Sister Catharine Courtney, speech at opening of Mater Private Hospital extensions, 19 July 1980, file: Extension MPH 1978–80, SOMCA.

2   P Maguire, 21 March 1977, Report of special committee formed to investigate the future of the MPH, SOMCA, box 147, file: Building projects public hospital, 1962–71.

3   Paul F Gross, 1979, box 152, SOMCA.

4   S J Duckett, 'Structural interests and Australian health policy', in J R G Butler and D P Doessel, *Health economics. Australian readings*, Sydney, Australian Professional Publications, 1989, pp. 73–4, describes the doctors' lobby as the prime example of the professional monopolist structural interest in Australian health policy.

5   Paul F Gross, 'Health technology and health care ethics in the 1980s: The future of the Catholic hospital in Australia', 9 November 1979.

6   *Sunday Mail*, 2 September 1977.

7   Sister Mary St Gabriel to Sister Catharine Courtney, 21 March 1977.

8   W D Scott report.

9   Pat Maguire, 22 November 1979 (Asst Hosp Admin), Report to Superior-General on managerial aspects of the MPH and recommendations for its future, box 141 – Mater Private Hospital 1978–1983, SOMCA.

10   Ibid.

11   Sister Josephine Crawford, oral history interview.

12   Sister Josephine Crawford, oral history interview.

13   Sister Josephine's report to Hospital Council, 2 April 1982.

14   Sr Mary C Johnson to Fr T J Connolly, 27 February 1982; Sister Mary C Johnson re committee reviewing pharmacy at the Mater Private Hospital, 9 August 1982. The Mater retains this private pharmacy licence.

15   Mater Hospital Council, 10 August 1982.

16   Mater Private Hospital finance committee, 24 June 1982.

17   File: MPH Project Group 1981–84, meeting 9 November 1981; Sister Bernard Mary's report, 20 February 1985.

18 Sister Bernard Mary to Sister Kath Burke, 11 June 1982; Drs R Morgan and J Bolger to Congregation, 2 August 1982.

19 Increased income of $72,000 was estimated.

20 Sister Josephine Crawford, oral history; the Health Dept approved using part of 3rd floor for obstetric patients Sister Bernard Mary to Sister Kath Burke, 1 April 1981; Dr E J Esler to Sister Kath Burke, RSM, 5 October 1982; minutes of meeting at MPH at 1 pm on 4 October 1982.

21 The July–December 1980 loss was $128,764.

22 Mater Private Hospital finance committee, 24 June 1982.

23 MPH Report, 1 November 1985, box 151, SOMCA; Pat Maguire report, October 1984, box 155, SOMCA; File: MPH, 1983, box 141, SOMCA. Bed occupancy for first three months of 1983–84 was much higher than the previous year, with a daily average of 98.6 in March and 75.29 in January, and 99.57 in February.

24 Peddle Thorp to Sister Bernard Mary, 24 March 1982; Sister Bernard Mary's report, 9 March 1983; Peddle Thorp to Sister Bernard Mary, 24 March 1982.

25 Budget 1981–82; Budget paper for 1983–84 showing the fees comparison in October 1983:

	MPH	St Andrew's	Holy Spirit	Wesley
Wards	$118	$120–130	$130–140	$130
Private rooms	$135–155	$150–155	$160–180	$155–168
Suites (4)	$167			
Twin rooms with ensuite	$140	$130–145		

26 Sister Bernard Mary to Sister Kath Burke, 6 January 1984.

27 M Dickenson and C Mason, *Hospitals and politics. The Australian Hospital Association 1946–86*, Canberra, Australian Hospital Association, 1986; pp. 21, 35–36, 128; S Sax, *A strife of interests. Politics and policies in Australian health services*, Sydney, Allen and Unwin, 1984, p. 133.

28 *Sunday Mail*, 20 November 1983.

29 Meeting, 9 September 1983.

30 *Catholic Leader*, 1 April 1984.

31 J S Deeble, 'Health care under universal insurance: the first three years of Medicare', in Butler and Doessel, pp. 189, 202, 203. The Commonwealth compensated the states substantially for patients who moved from private hospital care to public hospitals.

32 Australian Catholic Health Care Association Newsletter, No. 4, December 1983.

33 Sister Bernard Mary's report, 20 February 1985.

34 Submission for redevelopment of Mater Private Hospital, 24 April 1984.

35 Finance and project committee, 4 July 1984.

36 Dr Patrick O'Dwyer to Sister Kath Burke, 20 November 1984.

37 E D O'Callaghan to Sister Kath Burke, 19 August 1985.

38 Dr M Redmond to Sister Angela Mary, 25 July 1985.

39 Dr M Redmond to O'Callaghan, 24 June 1985. Advanced neurosurgery was expensive. The Mater Private Hospital needed a cavitron which cost $100,000.

40 Sister Bernard Mary to Sister Kath Burke, 18 September 1985, box 154, SOMCA; Mater Private Hospital Report to General Council, 1 November 1985, box 151, SOMCA.

41 Alexander Browne Cambridge and Partners, to H L Chapman, hospital architect, 20 December 1984:

42 Dr L Brunello to Sister Bernard Mary, 18 February 1985, Dr H Barry, co-ordinator, Medical services, Mater Private Hospital to Sister Bernard Mary, 22 February 1985, Dr A McSweeney to Sister Bernard Mary, 19 February 1985 in Agenda papers, Hospital Council meeting, 14 March 1985.

43 Sister Bernard Mary's report, 9 April 1985.

44 Sister Bernard Mary, report to hospital council on Mater Private Hospital, 20 February 1985, box 157; minutes of meeting of medical specialists to discuss future of Mater Private Hospital, 13 June 1985; Mater Private Hospital, reports to Hospital Council, 1985, box 151.

45 Campbell and Associates interim report on the recommended redevelopment strategy for the MPH, February 1986.

46 R Pavlyshyn, 'Options for redevelopment', 1986, Mater Private Redevelopment Committee file, box 157, SOMCA.

47 Sister Bernard Mary's report, 14 March 1985.

48 Oral history interview, Sister Kath Burke.

49 Oral history interview, Sister Madonna Josey; meeting of Sisters at the convent, 23 April 1986; Mater Private Hospital redevelopment committee meeting, 28 August 1986, informed of decision at Hospital Council meeting 21 July 1986 that a scheme which includes convent is not acceptable.

50 J B Cope, FRACP, to Sister Angela Mary, 15 September 1986.

51 Hospital Council meeting, 22 December 1986; information from Pat Maguire, 11 February 2005.

52   Mater Private Hospital report to Hospital Council, 8 May 1985.

53   Sister Michaeleen Mary's report on Mater Private Hospital, 2 September 1988.

54   Doctors J Edwards and A Fitzgerald to Sister Mary Michele Quinlan, 11 December 1986.

55   Medical Benefits Fund to Sister Bernard Mary, September 1986.

56   Finance and project committee, 7 August 1987.

57   Early in 1991, both Mater private hospitals resigned from the Association due to concern about its direction and management. 'The Management Committee has adopted an entrepreneurial approach looking at great methods of cost saving, reaping benefits for the bigger hospitals and completely losing sight of the smaller hospitals.' The main benefit of belonging to the association had been help with negotiating with health funds about benefits and with the unions about awards. Minutes of Board, 20 February 1991.

58   Medical Benefits Fund of Australia, fees and rebates booklet, 1 March 1987.

59   Finance and project committee, 22 June 1987.

60   Special committee meeting, 21 March 1987; Mater Private Hospital project committee, 25 March 1987.

61   Mater Private redevelopment committee, 1, 7 April 1987.

62   Oral history interview, Sister Kath Burke.

63   Sister Kath Burke to Kevin Cronin, 16 February 1988.

64   Pat Maguire, Report to Gov Board on financial feasibility of new Mater Private Hospital, 6 September 1988.

65   'Dee' to Sister Madonna Josey, 5 October 1988.

66   Graham Wright Associates, management consultants, to Pat Maguire, 8 November 1988.

67   Minutes of Board, 29 August 1990, 20 March 1991.

68   Annual Report, 1989–90.

69   *Sunday Sun*, 17 September 1989.

70   *The Sun*, 26 July 1990; *Courier-Mail*, 25 January 1991, 22 February 1991.

71   *Courier-Mail*, 16 September 1991, 17 August 1994.

72   *Sunday Mail*, 16 November 1984.

73   *Courier-Mail*, 16 March 1988.

74   Mater Private Hospital, opening booklet, 1993.

75   *Catholic Leader*, 10 March 1993.

76   Minutes of Board, 20 September 1989, 23 August 1989.

77 Paediatric Society of Queensland to Mater Board, 30 April 1990, enclosing the Society's submission on green paper on organisational arrangements for Queensland public sector health services.

78 *AMA Bulletin*, May 1982, vol. 21, no. 5.

79 Report on the feasibility study into the relocation of the Mater Children's Hospital, Phase 1, 1992, box 143, SOMCA.

80 14 May 1992. Special board meeting to discuss tertiary paediatric services in the Brisbane South Region.

81 Report on the feasibility study into the relocation of the Mater Children's Hospital, Phase 1, 1992, box 143, SOMCA.

82 Information from Sister Angela Mary Doyle.

83 Sister Angela Mary Doyle's notes on the 1992 proposal, MHHC.

84 Dr John Burke, submission to Board, June 1992.

85 Minutes of Mater Board, 17 June 1992.

86 Minutes of Mater Board, 8 September 1992.

87 Minutes of Mater Board, 18 November 1992, 17 February 1993.

88 Information from Sister Angela Mary, 20 February 2005.

10. INTEGRATING CARE

1 Professor K W Ryan, Chairman's report, Mater Public Hospitals, Annual Report, 1992.

2 Radiation therapy services were extended to the Royal Brisbane Hospital in 1940.

3 Cancer clinic file, MHHC.

4 Mater Health Services, Annual Report, 1995.

5 Mater Health Services, Annual Report, 1991. The Board considered renovating old Ward 3 to accommodate day care QRI patients. Minutes of Board, 20 June 1990.

6 Mater Health Services, Annual Report, 1996. Even melanoma of the eye was treated by day radiology.

7 D Wood, 'Queensland Radium Institute recollections', Cancer clinic file, MHHC.

8 The Leukaemia Foundation opened accommodation for out-of-town patients.

9 Minutes of Board, 19 April 1995.

10 Mater Health Services, Annual Reports, 1995, 1997.

11 *Catholic Leader*, 24 November 1999.

12 Mater Private Hospital file: visit/opening Diabetic Centre, Mary McAleese, 9 September 1998, box 157, SOMCA.

13 Mater News, vol. 17, issue 1, April/May 1997.

14 Minutes of Board, 25 September 1996.

15 Mater Health Services, Annual Report, 1993.

16 Mater Health Services, Annual Report, 1991.

17 Information from Dr John Hinds, 2004; Mater Health Services, Annual Report, 1999.

18 Information from Michael Enright, 2004; Mater Health Services, Annual Reports, 1997–2000.

19 Mater Health Services, Annual Report.

20 Bob Marshall, oral history interview, 12 November 2004.

21 Mater Health Services, Annual Reports, 1991, 1992.

22 Minutes of Board, 16 March, 19 April 1995; Mater Health Services, Annual Report, 1995; minutes of Board, 19 April, 1995; *Weekend Australian*, 14 May 1977; *Courier-Mail*, 25 March 1989.

23 Mater Health Services, Annual Report, 1996.

24 Minutes of Board, 17 November 2003; Mater Health Services, Annual Reports, 1994, 1996.

25 Minutes of Board, 21 November 1995.

26 *Catholic Leader*, 2 December 1992.

27 Minutes of Board, 15 July 1992.

28 Mater News, vol. 17, issue 1, April/May 1997.

29 Sister Angela Mary Doyle, 'The story of the Mater Children's Hospital', Sister Angela Mary collection, MHHC; *Brisbane News*, 9–15 June 2004.

30 Mater Health Services, Annual Report, 1992.

31 Mater Health Services, Annual Report, 1994; 'Volunteer profile – Dr Leigh Atkinson, *Smile*, September 2004.

32 Queensland Profile, May 1984, Cranio-facial clinic file, MHHC.

33 Ibid.

34 Mater Public Hospital file: Children's Hospital, 1926–86, box 146, SOMCA.

35 Minutes of Board, 23 February 1997, 29 November 1996.

36 Sister Angela Mary, 'The story of the Mater Children's Hospital', Sister Angela Mary Doyle collection, MHHC.

37 Mater Health Services, Annual Reports, 1998, 1999.

38 Mater Children's Hospital, Nursing Division Report, 1989, minutes of Board, 17 April 1993.

39 Sister Angela Mary Doyle, 'The story of the Mater Children's Hospital

cranio-facial unit', Sister Angela Mary collection, MHHC.

40 *South West News*, 29 October 1997; *Courier-Mail*, 19 March 1986, 2 September 1991.

41 *Smile*, September 2004.

42 Booklet commemorating the opening of the New Life Centre, 14 April 1991.

43 Minutes of Board, 21 February, 21 March 1990.

44 Minutes of Board, 16 May 1990, 20 June 1990.

45 Minutes of Board 18 September 1991.

46 Minutes of Board, 20 September 1995; information supplied by Dr Grace Croft.

47 Mater Health Services, Annual Report, 1994; minutes of Board, 15 September 1993.

48 Minutes of Board, 28 September 1994.

49 *Courier-Mail*, 23 February 1995; *Southern News*, 23 February 1995.

50 Mater Health Services, Annual Report, 1997; minutes of Board, 20 October 1993.

51 Mater Health Services, Annual Report, 1995.

52 Minutes of Board, 18 May 1994.

53 Mater Health Services, Annual Report, 1993.

54 G Croft, Mater Misericordiae Hospitals Nursing Research Centre discussion paper, October 1999.

55 Mater Health Services, Annual Report, 1999.

56 She was a surveyor with the Australian Council on Hospital Standards and an Associate Fellow of the Australia College of Health Service Executives.

57 Mater Health Services, Annual Report, 1992.

58 Mater Health Services, Annual Report, 1998.

59 *SpiritED*, No. 45, November 2004.

60 Mater Health Services, Annual Report, 1999.

61 Doctors' file, MHHC.

62 Information from Pat Maguire, 11 February 2005.

63 *South East Advertiser*, 31 August 1988.

64 *Courier-Mail*, 26 October 1988.

65 Minutes of Board, 21 October 1987; AIDS file, MHHC.

66 Mater Health Services, Annual Report, 1991.

67 Mater Health Services, Annual Reports, 1990–91; Mater Children's Hospital files, MHHC.

68 Mater Health Services, Annual Reports, 1996–2001.

69 Hospital Council minutes, 9 May 1985, box 151, SOMCA; Sir Llew Edwards to Sister Angela Mary, 30 April 1985.

70 Discussion between Sister Madonna Josey and Helen Gregory, 4 May 2004.

11. MANAGING PARTNERSHIPS

1   G R Palmer and S D Short, *Health care and public policy. An Australian analysis*, Sydney, Macmillan, 1989, pp. 32, 239. The extent of public–private and state–Commonwealth interactions in Australia makes it unique, even among federations.

2   S J Duckett, *The Australian health care system*, Melbourne, OUP, 2nd edn, 1994, pp. 31, 36.

3   S Leeder, 'Achieving equity in the Australian healthcare system', *Medical Journal of Australia*, 2003, 179 (9), pp. 475–8.

4   S Sax, *A strife of interests. Politics and policies in Australian health services*, Sydney, Allen and Unwin, 1984, p. 209; Duckett, p. 13.

5   M Dickenson and C Mason, *Hospitals and politics. The Australian Hospital Association 1946–86*, Canberra, Australian Hospital Association, 1986, p. 127.

6   Ever since a Commonwealth Senate review, chaired by Senator Michael Macklin in 1991, foreshadowed health policy integration.

7   Minutes of Board, 15 February 1984.

8   Mater Health Services, Annual Report, 1995. Mary Rita Lane, Dr Danny Lane's daughter, coordinated the process.

9   Sister Monica Stallard, Congregational Leader, speech on accreditation, 18 December 1993, box 8, SOMCA.

10 S Duckett, pp. 44–5.

11 Mater Health Services, Annual Report, 1993.

12 Mater Health Services, Annual Report, 1995; minutes of Board, 20 September 1995.

13 Mater Health Services, Annual Report, 1999; Blake Dawson Waldron, 'Strategic advice concerning funding arrangements with the State of Queensland', for Mater Misericordiae Health Services Brisbane, 2004, p. 6.

14 Mater Health Services, 'A new healthier partnership', submission to the

Queensland Government, Case 1 – Quality: Category A or B?, November 2004, p. 2.

15 Pat Maguire's Chief Executive Officer's report, Mater Health Services, Annual Report, 1993; 'A new healthier partnership', submission to the Queensland Government, Case 1 – Quality: Category A or B?, November 2004, p. 2, and Case 4 – Indemnity and insurance, p. 1.

16 Sax, *A strife of interests*, pp. 185, 193.

17 M Charlesworth and S Gifford, *The place of ethics in health care resource allocation. Where to now?*, Ethics of Resource Allocation in Health Discussion Paper 1, Canberra, Australian Health Ethics Committee Secretariat, 1992.

18 Minutes of Board, 19 February 1992, 18 March 1992, 17 June 1992.

19 Minutes of Board, 24 April 1996.

20 Mater Health Services, 'A new healthier partnership', Case 4 – Indemnity and insurance, p. 3.

21 Minutes of Board, 21 May 1985.

22 Information from Sister Angela Mary, 30 November 2004.

23 'A new healthier partnership', Case 5 – Employee provisions, p. 1.

24 Estimated from the 2004 figure in 'A new healthier partnership', Appendix 1: The value of the Mater Public Hospitals, p. 8.

25 S Wilde, Report on unfunded/under-funded services provided by Mater Misericordiae Health Services Brisbane, 2004; D Cohen and L Prusak, *In good company. How social capital makes organizations work*, Boston, 2001, p. 4; R Putnam, ed., *Democracies in flux: The evolution of social capital in contemporary society*, New York, 2002.

26 Mater Health Services, Annual Reports, 1991–95; file: Mater Ladies Auxiliary Fundraising, MHHC; file: Mater Appeal Meetings 1946–1971, 1947–48, box 145, SOMCA.

27 Mater Health Services, Annual Report, 1991–99; *Mater News*, vol. 17, issue 1, April/May 1997.

28 In 1995, important new ophthalmology equipment was funded by two bequests totalling $360,000. Minutes of Board, 20 September 1995.

29 *Bayside Bulletin*, 20 July 2004.

30 *Courier-Mail*, 29 January 1983; *Daily Sun*, 6 August 1984; *Daily Sun*, 18 February 1987; Cecilia McNally file, MHHC.

31 *Courier-Mail*, 14 August 1997; *Sunday Mail*, 5 October 1997.

32 Public Affairs Management to Sister Angela Mary, 27 November 1986, file: Inaugural meeting, 18 March 1987, box 153: Mater Health Services Governing Board.

33 Public Affairs Management to Sister Angela Mary, 27 November 1986, file: Inaugural meeting, 18 March 1987, Mater Health Services Governing Board, box 153, SOMCA; minutes of Board, 19 April 1995.

34 Mater Public Hospital, Annual Report, 1989–90, p. 6, Mater Health Services, Annual Report, 1993.

35 Minutes of Board, 16 May 1990. Mission statement accepted by Strategic Planning committee, 5 April 1990.

36 Sister Angela Mary's message, Mater Public Hospitals, Annual Reports, 1991, 1992.

37 Ryan's chairman's report, 1995, Mater Public Hospitals, Annual Report.

38 Mater Public Hospitals, Annual Report, 1995–96. In 1996, Mater staff attended the 'Mercy Alive' conference in Canberra celebrating 150 years of the Sisters' work in Australia.

39 Minutes of Board, 21 June 1995.

40 Medical staff file, MHHC.

41 Secretary, Mater Staff Association to Sister Angela Mary, 28 November 1986, Mater Health Services Governing Board, file: Inaugural meeting, 18 March 1987, box 153, SOMCA.

42 Minutes of Board, 21 June 1995. Peter Forster from the Consultancy Bureau assisted the Trust to tailor its business plan to specific objectives, including ways of developing a reasonable level of working capital.

43 Minutes of Board, 26 May 1986.

44 Minutes of Board, 15 June 1994, 28 September 1994.

45 Minutes of Board, 6 October 1986.

46 Minutes of Board, 21 October 1987.

47 Minutes of Board, 18 November 1987; Mater Health Services, Annual Report, 1990.

48 *The Sun*, 22 February 1989, *Courier-Mail*, 27 February 1989; minutes of Board, 20 September 1989; Mater Health Services, Annual Report, 1990.

49 Minutes of Board, 21 March 1990, recorded that the Trust Board was gravely concerned at its deficit.

50 Minutes of Board, 20 September 1989, 1 August 1990, 19 September 1990, 21 November 1990.

51 Mater Health Services, Annual Reports, 1994, 1995.

52 *The Sun*, 14 February 1991.

53 *Highlights*, MPH staff newsletter, June 1997.

54 Li Wei-huang, 'When east meets west', in *Tzu Chi. Buddhism in Action*, Spring 2002, pp. 70–4, 72.

55 Mater Children's Hospital Art Unions 1983–1990; Mater Health Services, Annual Report, 1997. In 2005, the Mater Foundation moved to a street-front office in Stanley Street.

56 *Mater News*, vol. 17, issue 1, April/May 1997; Mater Health Services, Annual Report, 1998.

57 Sister Angela Mary, story of the Mater Children's Hospital; minutes of Board, 19 August 1992, 17 February 1993, 17 August 1995.

58 Justice M Gobbo, 'New legal structures for religious health care bodies', paper delivered at conference, 21 September 1979, box 25, SOMCA; James Gobbo, 'Religious orders and advisory bodies' circa 1983–4; minutes of Board, 11 April 1985; information from Sister Angela Mary, December 2004.

59 Minutes of Board, 11 April 1984, 18 February 1985.

60 Thynne and Macartney to Mother Patrick, 4 October 1926, box 4, Mother Patrick Potter, SOMCA. Incorporation under the Religious, Educational and Charitable Institutions Act was an important means of husbanding the Sisters' resources in an expansionist era.

61 Minutes of Board, 20 February 1991; Sister Monica Stallard, oral history interview.

62 Theology of incorporation, 28 October 1965, cited in pamphlet 'Why incorporate?', circulated to Mater staff, 2001.

63 Minutes of Board, 18 November 1987. The Sisters continued to be advised by Sir James Gobbo.

64 Pamphlet 'Why incorporate?', 2001, Mater Health Services, Annual Report, 2001; minutes of Board, 11 April 1985.

65 Sister Kath Burke, foreword to Mater Health Services, Annual Report, 2001.

66 Kevin Ryan had been a member of the Law Reform Commission, President of the Council of Consumer Affairs, Garrick Professor of Law at the University of Queensland and an Australian trade commissioner.

12. DEVELOPING A BOLD VISION

1 Dr O'Donnell to Sister Pauline Burke, 15 April 2003.

2 Mater Health Services, Annual Report, 2000.

3 Mater Hospital Funding Agreement, 16 December 2002.

4 Data used in the submission 'A new healthier partnership' was calculated by the economics consultancy Access Economics; Executive summary, 'A new healthier partnership', p. 2.

5   See, for example, AMA, Queensland Branch, press releases, 5 June, 4 August, 19 August 2004.

6   *SpirtED*, no. 45, November 2004.

7   Chief Executive Officer's Report, Mater Health Services, Annual Report, 2001–02.

8   Dr Tony McSweeny, 'Medical research in hospitals', paper presented to Board, 10 June 1981.

9   Minutes of Board, 17 March 1982; minutes of Hospital Council, 8 September 1982, 7 November 1985, box 151, SOMCA; Sister Angela Mary to Dr Ken Donald, Chair Cancer Fund, 8 October 1986, box 151, SOMCA; J P Kelly Foundation reports, MHHC; Mater Health Services, Annual Reports, 1982–86.

10 *Courier-Mail*, 24 November 1995.

11 Mater Health Services, Annual Report, 1997.

12 Minutes of Board, 28 May 1997.

13 Minutes of Board, 30 July 1997.

14 Minutes of Board, 36 August 1998. The University of Otago agreed to sell the patents for NZ$300,000 (A$262,000) and a share of the royalties.

15 Minutes of Board, 24 June 1998.

16 The role of PSA in blocking the body's immune system and ability to fight prostate cancer. The Mucin team was then able to set up the first model for human gastric ulcer.

17 MMRI, *The earth is flat*, Report, 2004.

18 *Courier-Mail*, 1 August 2003.

19 *Discovery*, November 2004.

20 Ibid.

21 G F Mitchell, D G Pennington, 'A review of the Mater Medical Research Institute (MMRI) and Research Activities and support across the Mater Hospitals Complex', for the Mater Misericordiae Health Services Brisbane Ltd by Foursight Associates, May 2002.

22 Ibid.

23 Mater Health Services, Annual Reports, 1995, 1997.

24 Mater Health Services, Annual Report, 1996.

25 Mater Health Services, Annual Report, 2003.

26 Minutes of Board, 26 June 1996.

27 *Smile*, September 2004.

28 Mater Health Services, Annual Reports, 1996, 1999.

29 Minutes of Board, 28 February 1996; minutes of Board, 27 August 1997,

special Board meeting, 26 August 1997. The Noosa/Robina concept would cost $37 million in capital and $16 million in annual operating costs.

30 Minutes of Board, 17 December 1997, 24 June 1998, 29 July 1998.

31 Minutes of Board, 28 October 1998, 16 December 1998.

32 Dr D Lane to Mother Damian, 28 November 1957, enclosing 'The one roof plan', *The Australian Medical Digest*, November 1957, file: Mater Redevelopment, box 157, SOMCA. The one-roof plan was followed at the Mayo Clinic.

33 Sano Consulting, 'Impact of evidenced-based pathways and an integrated delivery system on health outcomes and hospital funding', report for the Mater Private Hospital, November 2003.

34 Minutes of Board, 18 May 1995, 20 September 1995.

35 box 151, 9 May 1985, Hospital Council MAH – looking at Annerley Road property. General Council supports buying the property. Price down to $2.36 million. May do a future commercial development on this property which is opposite the Mater. Will sell 'Webster' land (opposite Boggo Road jail) if Annerley Road is purchased.

36 Monica Stallard to Sisters, 2 May 1996; Sister Elizabeth Hepburn, IBVM, facilitated the two sessions.

37 This was the plan recommended by the master planning consultants. Mater Health Services, Annual Report, 1996.

38 Minutes of Board, 25 September 1996.

39 Sister Angela Mary, 'The story of the Mater Children's Hospital', Sister Angela Mary collection, MHHC.

40 In 1990, with 6,428 births. Annual Report, 1989–90, p. 3; *Courier-Mail*, 6 April 1989.

41 Mater Health Services, Annual Report, 2003.

42 Mater Health Services, Annual Report, 2003.

43 Dr John O'Donnell, message to all staff, 8 March 2005.

44 C Towned, chief financial officer, P Rogers, group financial officer, to heads of departments, 9 March 2005.

INDEX

Page numbers in *italic* indicate an illustration.